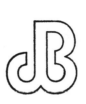

# HANDBOOK OF COMMUNITY MENTAL HEALTH PRACTICE

*The San Mateo Experience*

*H. Richard Lamb*
*Don Heath*
*Joseph J. Downing*
Editors

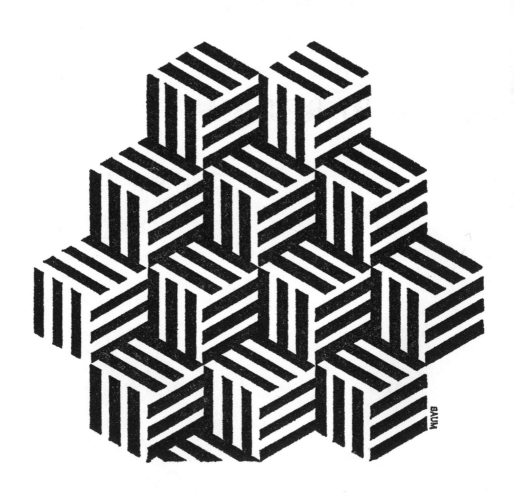

# Handbook of Community Mental Health Practice

Jossey-Bass Inc., Publishers
615 Montgomery Street • San Francisco • 1969

HANDBOOK OF COMMUNITY MENTAL HEALTH PRACTICE
*The San Mateo Experience*
          Edited by H. Richard Lamb, Don Heath, Joseph J. Downing

*Jossey-Bass Inc., Publishers*
*615 Montgomery Street*
*San Francisco, California 94111*

**Library of Congress Catalog Card Number 72-92886**

**Standard Book Number SBN 87589-040-7**

Manufactured in the United States of America
          *Composed and printed by York Composition Company, Inc.*
          *Bound by Chas. H. Bohn & Co., Inc., New York*
          *Jacket design by Willi Baum, San Francisco*

FIRST EDITION

*6911*

# THE JOSSEY-BASS BEHAVIORAL SCIENCE SERIES

*General Editors*

WILLIAM E. HENRY, *University of Chicago*
NEVITT SANFORD, *Stanford University and
Wright Institute, Berkeley*

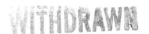

# Foreword

The San Mateo program was the first in the United States to link together the essential and the supplementary elements of a community mental health program. This book describes that ten-year experience. It is not only worth reading in itself, but is also a useful handbook that supplies the "how-to-do-it" that should improve the quality of similar programs.

The Joint Information Service of the American Psychiatric Association and the National Association for Mental Health studied community mental health programs in various parts of the country and recently published "The Community Mental Health Center: An Interim Appraisal." The authors of that study noted many problems which limit the growth and efficiency of community mental health programs. The San Mateo group has faced these many problems, and in this book shows how they have been successful in solving many of them.

They call particular attention to key problems in community mental health programs: inadequate conceptualization of mission; lack of comprehensiveness; failure to provide complete services for a catchment area; absence of services to children and old people; various interpretations of continuity of care; the change in therapists when one goes to the outpatient department; role-blurring between professionals; a tendency for a minimal role to be filled by psychiatrists who principally service the medication patients require; the failure to utilize general practitioners; the difficulty in identifying short-term and long-term patients at admission; the almost complete absence of day hospitals and partial hospitalization; deficient emergency care without personnel around the clock; poor understanding of consultation; the expressed need for training in community health; the absence of relationships in state hospitals; and the absence of evaluation for effectiveness as a measure of the worthwhileness of the program. Obviously, much remains to be done to bring community mental health programs up to a quality standard of performance.

Good administration and charismatic leadership are often responsible for the success of an outstanding program. It seems to be so in San Mateo. Is administration an art? Must leaders be born with qualities that require only maturation over time? I think not. There is now a body of knowledge on administration that can be taught. Strategy and technique can be mastered and are powerful tools for the administrator.

The authors provide delightful and intensely human evidence that the learning process can be as enjoyable as it is frustrating at times. Downing says, "the clinically adept can be an organizational ignoramus . . . the administrator requires an incredible range of highly sensitive responses," and he must get out of his office to set the style for the staff and serve as a role model in community relations. He correctly cautions against oversimplification and notes that "convictions are the forerunners of principles."

In response to community pressures, more services to children were provided; more support for juveniles in trouble; more resources for the treatment of adults in order to make it possible to retain the seriously ill in the community. There are risks involved in maintaining patients on open wards and in partial hospitalization status. These must be assumed and understood by staff and by the community.

My own experience in Boston with a home visiting program was replicated by the authors, who found that over 50 per cent of the patients in San Mateo County recommended for inpatient care could be cared for in the community on extramural status.

Building a service that is truly responsive to needs of the community requires talking to many people and involving them in the planning process. There also must be clarification of the nature of mental health services, for the public indulges the unrealistic expectation that community mental health can and should solve the major social problems in the service region.

I was pleased the authors began their description of the elements of a community mental health program with a chapter on integrating the community services with the state hospital. This places the emphasis and the priority where they belong—on new services for the mentally ill. Too many mental health programs have not included the state hospital. The seriously ill, the poor, the disadvantaged, and the aged have been served by the public mental hospital. The revolution in administrative management, first insulin therapy, then EST and new drugs, has contributed to the decline in census and the shortened need for inpatient care that made management of the sick patient in the community psychiatric facility possible.

San Mateo assigned public health nurses to participate in the planning for release of state hospital patients and to supervise the maintenance of their health after release. An imaginative county inpatient service, a social club, day hospital, vocational services, and transitional living arrangements were established. This achieved a net drop of 31 per cent in state hospital admissions from San Mateo County at a time the population in the county increased by 25 per cent and admissions from other Bay Area counties to state hospitals increased by 24 per cent.

But if state hospital admissions fall, admissions for service to other agencies providing mental health services will inevitably increase. The high rate of utilization of local psychiatric services made some critics of the program uneasy.

Community mental health needs more explicit guidelines on how to evaluate the effectiveness of its programs. The chapter on program evaluation is a chronological account of San Mateo's experience in examining its goals to see if they were on target and effecting changes to insure that they were. For instance, it was found in San Mateo that when there was a wait of three weeks to a month between the family's initial call and the first child guidance clinic appointment, there was a 40 per cent dropout rate for this group of families. When the wait for a response was less than two weeks, the dropout rate fell to 15 per cent. One of the attempts initiated to improve functioning of the program actually increased the dropout rate. Another study determined the time that was spent with a patient, the time on the telephone, in travel, in staff meetings, in activities, in supervision, and in training.

Portia Bell Hume, in the Epilogue to this book, says, "the San Mateo County mental health services are the embodiment of a public mental health program with the potentiality for serving, both directly and indirectly, the whole population of a particular community. It is a program which seeks to integrate psychiatric with nonpsychiatric services to people and to maximize both the comprehensiveness and the continuity of these elements by means of interagency and interprofessional sanctions and relationships that are both ethically considered and technically refined. . . . the feature that gave added depth to the San Mateo program is its recognition of the mental health functions performed by the nonpsychiatric agencies and professions in behalf of the individuals who either are at risk of, or have already experienced, mental breakdown: (1) the psychosocially deprived, (2) the persons experiencing a life crisis, (3) cases requiring referral for psychiatric evaluation, and (4) the mentally disabled who need either habilitation or rehabilitation. . . ."

In the development of community mental health programs, responsive to the needs of complex and ever-increasing communities, every day is a day for evaluation and reevaluation, for adaptation and readaptation. As is amply demonstrated in this volume, enduring stability comes by flexibility and by renovating the structural elements of a program in response to changing needs, rather than relying upon fixed structures which may be unresponsive to new functions.

A rich reward awaits the reader of this book, in chapters on the therapeutic community, inpatient services, day hospitals, halfway houses, vocational services, children's services, mental retardation,

preventive services, and program evaluation. If community mental
health programs are to grow and to serve their intended function,
such program analyses and evaluations as are presented here are vital.

WALTER E. BARTON

*Washington, D.C.*
*September, 1969*

# Preface

First and foremost this book was written for those fortunate people who are able to learn from the hard-won experience of others rather than exclusively through the expensive process of trial and error. We hope it is a practical book. Though there have been a number of excellent books written in recent years on the broad principles of community mental health, our wide and varied contacts with professional visitors to the San Mateo County program have made us aware that there has not been sufficient emphasis on how to put these principles into operation at the day-to-day working level. We have attempted to do this here by drawing from the San Mateo experience. However, our goal has been to focus on issues and problems which are not limited to the specifics of San Mateo or California but which we perceive as issues that would arise in any part of our nation where efforts are under way to set up comprehensive community mental health services. Our twenty years of experience in San Mateo County have helped to clarify many important concerns for us and have generated a rich body of knowledge of practical solutions as well as an equally valuable sensitivity to the pitfalls and blind alleys that await the mental health program developer.

We hope our book will prove useful to mental health professionals and subprofessionals of all disciplines and callings who will be staffing the new community mental health centers springing up across our nation. Included are those professionals at high (state and local) administrative levels entrusted with the tasks of overall program planning and maintenance of standards of practice, as well as those who are setting up, conducting, and administering the actual specific services. In these endeavors a host of issues inevitably arise—treatment philosophy, continuity of care, how to set priorities of service, how to go about providing consultation to community agencies, how do "traditional" treatment methods fit into community mental health, what are the advantages and disadvantages of regionalization of services.

It was our intent to make this book useful in academic training centers as well as in operating community programs. We wanted to supplement available books by producing a handbook of practical experience. We hoped this would supply an input currently too fragmentary in academic settings: an operational or functional input to help the trainee prepare for a dismaying collection of competing reality issues that will confront him in the pragmatic environment of community practice. We have consciously tried to capture some of the exciting atmosphere of adventure and the pioneering challenge to which we have seen ourselves responding in San Mateo. Perhaps this will help both student and teacher to recognize some of the intangible rewards that are held out by community mental health.

But we hope our book will be valuable to other important segments of our professional and nonprofessional population, as well. Members of local mental health associations wanting to become more involved in mental health issues in their communities and other concerned members of the lay public are people we hope to reach with this book. It was our intent to help them see that promoting mental health is no easy task and that a myriad of hard-to-balance, hard-to-resolve issues must be faced by many dedicated citizens; at the same time, we want to share our conviction that solutions to these problems can be found.

Some of the ideas expressed in the section on aftercare in Chapter 5 and in Chapter 8 first appeared in *Hospital and Community Psychiatry*. Some of the ideas expressed in the section on public health nursing in Chapter 7 first appeared in the *American Journal of Nursing*.

We acknowledge the immense contribution that Margaret Fitzsimons, administrative coordinator for the program chief, has made not only to this book but to the development of our program. Many of the ideas in this book, both administrative and "professional," came from her during her twenty years of service to San Mateo County's mental health program. We also acknowledge the contribution of Marjorie Clarke and her clerical staff, who managed to find time to work on this book in addition to their regular duties. Finally, for their editorial assistance, we express our appreciation to Arlene Reiff, staff psychiatric social worker, and to Pamela Miller, who at the time was an intern from the mental health information specialist program at Syracuse University.

We dedicate this book to Ernest M. Gruenberg, who drew the preliminary sketches for a true community mental health program; to H. D. Chope, who turned the sketches into blueprints and contracted to build the program; and to Margaret F. Fitzsimons, who made the thing work.

H. RICHARD LAMB
DON HEATH
JOSEPH J. DOWNING

*San Mateo, California*
*September, 1969*

# Contents

# Contributors

All of the contributors are, except as noted, on the staff of the County of San Mateo Mental Health Services Division.

Theodore I. Anderson, M.D., former Chief of Consultation Services, now with the Department of Mental Hygiene, Boston

Dorothy M. Asbury, A.C.S.W., Social Work Supervisor, Psychiatric Social Services

Walter E. Barton, M.D., Medical Director, American Psychiatric Association

Bernice Birchess, A.C.S.W., Social Work Supervisor, Adult Psychiatric Outpatient Clinic

Pauline A. Bowen, R.N., M.S., Supervising Nurse, Psychiatric Rehabilitation Services

Harold D. Chope, M.D., Director, Department of Public Health and Welfare

Joseph J. Downing, M.D., former Program Chief, now in private practice

Howard Gurevitz, M.D., Program Chief

Clarice H. Haylett, M.D., Psychiatrist, Consultation Services

Don Heath, Demonstration Officer

George Hexter, M.D., Chief, Developmental Evaluation Unit

Gary Heymann, Ph.D., Chief Clinical Psychologist, Psychological Services

Portia Bell Hume, M.D., Director, Center for Training in Community Psychiatry and Mental Health Administration, Berkeley, Department of Mental Hygiene, State of California

Isadore Kamin, M.D., Chief Psychiatrist, Adult Psychiatric Outpatient Clinic

H. Richard Lamb, M.D., Chief, Psychiatric Rehabilitation Services

Richard J. Levy, M.D., Chief of Psychiatry, San Mateo County General Hospital

Gerald Lutovich, M.D., Home Visiting Psychiatrist

Cecile Mackota, Supervisor, Psychiatric Vocational Services

Leah B. McDonough, Ph.D., Chief, Courts and Corrections Unit

Mildred L. Mouw, R.N., M.A., Mental Health Consultant (Public Health Nursing)

John F. Odenheimer, A.C.S.W., Social Work Supervisor, Psychiatric Rehabilitation Services

Charles Richmond, A.C.S.W., Executive Director, El Camino House, a private voluntary agency

Norman R. Rogers, M.D., Assistant Superintendent, Agnews State Hospital

David J. Schwartz, M.D., Psychiatrist, Consultant to Juvenile Probation Department

Paul I. Wachter, M.D., Director of Training and Chief of Professional Education

Harry A. Wilmer, M.D., Ph.D., Clinical Professor of Psychiatry, University of California and Langley-Porter Neuropsychiatric Institute, Department of Mental Hygiene, Director of Youth Drug Study Unit

Lina S. Wygant, R.N., Supervisor of Nursing In-service Training, Psychiatric Inpatient Service

Lois Wynn, A.C.S.W., Social Work Supervisor, Child Guidance Clinic

# HANDBOOK OF
# COMMUNITY
# MENTAL HEALTH
# PRACTICE

*The San Mateo
Experience*

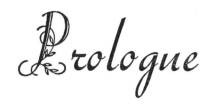

# Prologue

# Program Antecedents and Public Health

*Harold D. Chope*

Community mental health and public health have much in common. Nevertheless, each has sometimes found it difficult to embrace and support the other. In San Mateo County, the common denominator between them has been a concern, not universally shared elsewhere, for preventive procedures to reduce the toll of chronic illness and severe impairments that prove to be of major cost and concern to the community. Consequently, the community mental health program is very obviously a public health service in San Mateo County. It has clearly adopted public health principles in attempting to meet the mental health needs of the community.

This book, which might be characterized as an in-depth study of an emerging community mental health service, describes many of the concepts that have evolved in the work of prevention—which, in public health, includes active treatment and rehabilitation services—in the field of mental illness. The exposition covers a ten-year span, from 1958 to 1968.

For a decade prior to 1958, the San Mateo County Department of Public Health and Welfare had taken a growing interest in creating new patterns of service to meet the needs of victims of chronic illness. It had learned from its own experiences and those of others that these disabilities are frequently characterized by symptom complexes that are physical, social, and emotional in origin. Having observed the multi-determined nature of these costly disabilities, the department placed heavy emphasis upon interdisciplinary approaches. This emphasis, in turn, demanded the invention of integrative mechanisms designed to bring about closer collaboration between our public health, public welfare, county hospital, and rehabilitation services.

As it has emerged in San Mateo, community mental health has creatively implemented many of these same principles. It, too, has taken a broad view of disability, tending to assume that many conditions to which it directed its attention were produced by the interplay of diverse variables. Among these were some that were intrapsychic, some interpersonal, and some psychosocial in nature. Our most innovative workers have been willing to utilize the formulation of the social breakdown syndrome (Gruenberg, 1967), rather than to insist upon the narrower and more conventional diagnostic precision that is seldom replicable by two or more therapists.

Consequently, this program has willingly imposed upon itself certain tasks which required clear and rigorous thinking to redefine and extend clinical responsibilities to include attention to many community problems and groups that, until quite recently, often have been ruled out as objects of psychiatric concern. These tasks have included vigorous consultative and collaborative work with all other divisions of the multiphasic department, as well as with a wide range of local agencies whose services to people frequently contribute potently to the prevalence, incidence, and control of mental illness in the community. Given such an orientation, it is not surprising that the goals of San Mateo's mental health service emphasized prevention rather than remedy and rehabilitation.

In the course of developing our mental health program, we have found that many well-established public health techniques—such as demonstration methods, health education, and community organization, to name a few—and certain administrative issues, including continuity of care and service integration, have been further shaped, improved, and clarified. In other words, our experience suggests that public health and community mental health have much to contribute to one another.

San Mateo County is today a progressive county of an estimated 560,000 population, lying immediately to the south of San Francisco, with a flourishing commercial-industrial establishment, based upon electronics, air transportation—both passenger and freight—publishing, insurance, warehousiing, and building trades. Because of the type of industry, a high percentage of the adult population consists of college graduates. It is a youthful population, only 6.9 per cent being over sixty-five and 33.5 per cent under eighteen. The county is relatively wealthy, having a gross average annual family income of $11,728 and an annual payroll in 1967 of $1,005,596,174, as compared with $16,000,000 in 1937.

Since 1933 all health and welfare services have been combined in one department with a physician as director. In the last twenty years, the budget of the San Mateo County Department of Public Health and Welfare has increased from $2,908,373 in 1947–48 to $35,743,464 in 1968–69. In addition to the Division of Public Health, the Division of Social Welfare, the Division of Hospitals, and the Tuberculosis Sanatorium existing in 1948, three new divisions have been added: a two hundred-bed rehabilitation center (1954), a Division of Administration (1957), and Mental Health Services Division (1958). During the twenty years, a new 120-bed Tuberculosis Sanatorium, now used principally for extremely sick geriatric cases (fifteen beds being reserved for tuberculosis), was constructed (1951); a fifty-bed addition and all new basic services for the county hospital was completed (1956); a health and welfare building was erected (1953), was then enlarged twice (1963, 1967), and is still inadequate for the staff; a modern addition was attached to the old "poor farm," making a modern inpatient rehabilitation center of two hundred beds; a new district health center was constructed in the north end of the county

(1959) and then enlarged (1966), and a regional mental health center was located in the northern part of the county (1965).

The early history of mental health in San Mateo follows a pattern not uncommon in many communities; that is, the citizen is often ahead of the professional in delineating problems. In 1946, a group of citizens formed a mental health association. Perhaps influenced by the pioneering work of the Commonwealth Fund in 1924, they decided that the place to start would be with youth and the organization of a child guidance clinic. The officers of the association appealed to the Board of Supervisors for funding, and a small appropriation ($12,-000) was made. Emphasis was placed on early detection without professional guidance. One of the citizens who had had some training and experience in psychology and another who was trained in social work were the staff.

The second definitive step came in 1950. The Director of Health and Welfare considered alcoholism to be an emotional disease, and he asked the psychiatrists of the county to meet and discuss the problem. Five of the seven psychiatrists then in practice in the county responded to the invitation and spent many nights discussing the problem. The final recommendation formulated for the Board of Supervisors was that each psychiatrist would be glad to donate four hours per week to the clinic, providing: that the county employ a well-trained psychiatric social worker as a "core" person to operate the clinic, and that the clinic be known as an "adult psychiatric clinic," not as an alcoholic clinic. Though a significant step forward, it foreshadowed what we have found to be a persistent problem—the reluctance of mental health professionals to give priority to the treatment of alcoholism.

The next incident was initiated by the department. In 1952, the voters approved a bond issue to enlarge the county hospital and provide all new basic services, including a thirty-bed psychiatric ward. The four locked, windowless cubicles, known as holding cells and constituting the only public psychiatric inpatient facilities in the county, were a humanistic monstrosity. On the assumption that modern medicine could improve upon this dismal situation, the psychiatric ward was included in the plans.

Our views on mental health in general and hospital treatment in particular were greatly influenced by the work of Thomas Main and Maxwell Jones, brought particularly to our attention by Harry Wilmer, who opened a therapeutic community unit at the Oak Knoll Naval Hospital across the bay in Oakland. Fortuitously, Wilmer stopped in the department one afternoon, and we proudly showed him the plans for our new ward with twelve isolation rooms, a continuous bath, chamberlain screens on all windows, and an elegant array of security features. He took one look and gasped. He then explained the techniques he had learned in England and described his experiences at Oak Knoll. The idea of treating emotionally disturbed patients with dignity and providing comforts and the discarding of all barriers or restraints, whether physical or architectural, seemed most appealing. Although it was too late in the construction to make any definitive changes, it was perfectly possible to alter the policies and the treatment methods. On December 1, 1956, the ward was opened over the objections of exactly 50 per cent of the psychiatrists in the community. (The psychiatric section of the medical society, polled as to the desirability of an open-door ward, cast a tie vote.)

Administrative efforts were guided by the basic elements of good administration, best remembered by the mnemonic *POSDCORB,* as designated by Gulick (1937). These letters stand for the following administrative processes: Planning, Organizing, Staffing, Directing, Coordinating, Reporting, and Budgeting.

The mere listing of the elements of administration does not encompass the total process. Planning and budgeting generally have been collaborative ventures between the mental health program chief and the director of the department. Organization and direction of the Mental Health Services Division have fallen almost entirely upon the shoulders of the program chief. The coordination problems, however, have been shared responsibilities, since other segments and specialists in the department frequently have been involved; among those units whose efforts have been coordinated with those of the mental health program are the public health nurses (Health Division), social workers (Social Service–Welfare Division), and medical care specialist (Hospital Division). Coordination within the mental health services has been the responsibility of the program chief. Both he and the director have been deeply involved in reporting to the community, to professional associates through published papers and the extensive visitor program, and to state and federal officials around program and budgets. Staff members from all of the mental health disciplines and all services have also been involved in these services in varying degrees.

It used to be, and perhaps is still, a lively and provocative question within schools of public health whether administration can be taught. After several years as an instructor of public health administration and forty-five years of practical experience, I remain convinced that rules can be imparted and that trainees can benefit from the experiences of others but that administration basically requires a certain distinct temperament and personality. It demands ability to respond to different stimuli and rewards than those to which the skillful diagnostician and therapist responds. At the same time, therapeutic and diagnostic talents and training offer some valuable models that can be translated into highly significant administrative applications.

San Mateo's mental health program, as is also true of the Department of Public Health and Welfare as a whole, has been a medically-administered program. This has produced benefits, as well as liabilities. Because of a staunch public health tradition, however, we have avoided one common major liability. Despite our medical heritage, we have not been unresponsive to the multifarious needs of a total population.

One must not lose sight, however, of the fact that new social inventions require surpassing patience and disciplined attention to their implications. We must steel ourselves to withstand inducements to impulsive and unreasonable behavior. Despite a clamor for change and a hunger for improvement, we must make certain that we know that our next steps have clinically and professionally sound bases before we irrevocably disengage ourselves from traditional practices, no matter how evident it seems to us that they have become archaic.

Public health, a kind of maverick within the medical establishment, provides a reasonably sound and responsible tradition for invoking viable change without too radically disturbing the most cherished and rewarding aspects of our heritage. From the standpoint of San Mateo's administrative climate, one might submit that this tradition has been a kind of dominant underlying theme. Professionals have received a cordial sanction to be dissatisfied and to invoke and test new ideas. They have, at the same time, been reassured by an aware-ness that change is not valued for its own sake, that the traditions in which they had been schooled were valid and relevant sources of ref-erence.

PART I

*Before getting into the specifics of each segment of a comprehensive community mental health program, we feel it useful to have a brief overview of the underlying philosophy of that program. Thus, what follows are, in our opinion, the essential elements of the philosophy of community mental health as it has evolved in San Mateo.*

*Community mental health in San Mateo has borrowed heavily from public health and has adopted public health principles in attempting to meet the mental health needs of the community. Thus, there is much emphasis on prevention, on considering the needs of a total population, on the epidemiology of mental illness in our community, on actively becoming involved with the community and other community agencies, on health education and demonstration tech-*

# PHILOSOPHY, ADMINIS-
# TRATION, AND LIAISON

*niques. There is a recognition of the importance of social and cultural factors in addition to the intrapsychic as crucial determinants of human behavior.*

*We believe that community mental health should utilize its limited manpower in a way that will best meet the needs of a total population and not focus on a selected "motivated" few. This means providing service to all categories of patients, including those who are often regarded by mental health professionals as unattractive to treat, and extensively using mental health consultation to facilitate the work of caregivers in the community who are not mental health professionals.*

*The indirect or preventive services are accorded a high priority. These services do not involve clinical transactions with identified patients, but rather include the activities of mental health professionals as they work with presumably healthy individuals or organizations to expand their potential for the prevention of mental illness or the promotion of mental health. It is recognized that clergymen, physicians, nurses, social workers, policemen and probation officers, school personnel, and many other community service professionals are more strategically situated for sensitive intervention at times of life crisis than mental health clinicians. Included in the indirect services are mental health consultation, community organization, and mental health education.*

*A high priority is placed on the treatment and rehabilitation of the severely and chronically mentally ill. Thus, liaison with the state hospital is stressed as well as the conviction that the local public program and the state hospital serving the community must inevitably share responsibility for every severely impaired person needing treatment which cannot be obtained in the private and voluntary sectors. Providing treatment for patients coming out of state hospitals is not "somebody else's responsibility."*

*Our tendency is increasingly in the direction of reserving one-to-one outpatient psychotherapy for crisis-oriented brief treatment and to use group and activity therapies for those patients who need longer-term outpatient treatment. We do not restrict our concept of treatment to a resolution of unconscious conflict in psychotherapy. Vocational services, milieu therapy, a relationship with a teacher or a probation officer, are all seen along with group and individual psychotherapy as part of treatment. Continuity of care is stressed, both in terms of liaison between the local program and the state hospital and among the different services within the local program. The reorganization of our services on a regionalized basis, as described in Chapters 17, 18, and 19, has continuity of care as one of its major rationales.*

*The concept of the therapeutic community is of central importance. Thus, we are committed to the idea that socioenvironmental and interpersonal influences play an important, though not exclusive, part in the treatment program. Our treatment programs are oriented to restore patients to more healthy, normal social roles by so altering the hospital or institutional structure that these roles are expected of patients while they are still in the institution—for example, by assum-*

*ing patients can help in the treatment of other patients and can share in decision-making with the staff.*

*Program evaluation and research are, as far as possible, built in to the fabric of the ongoing clinical services.*

*Hospitalization remains a key part of community mental health. But hospitalization, except for a small number of patients who need a longer period of "sanctuary" in the state hospital, should be brief and crisis-oriented and not a setting for long-term residential treatment to "cure" severe mental illness.*

*Chapter 1 describes some of the lessons we have learned about administration in the development of our program. Chapter 2 then turns to the vital relationship between a community program and the state hospital.*

# Building the Program

*Joseph J. Downing*

In little more than a decade, community mental health has produced a distinctive institutional format, the mental health center, and has developed and partially explored some essential concepts and principles. Given a broad spectrum of services and the active collaboration of a wide range of other caregivers, community mental health has shown that it can respond to the mental illness and health challenges of a given total population.

The early goals of community mental health, those we aspired to in 1958 or 1963, now seem possible to attain. Yet, paradoxically, what appeared to be the urgently needed goal of yesterday turns out to be merely a stepping stone to different needs of the future. It is a not unfamiliar situation for workers in mental health to find that their problems have no final solutions—or to find that they themselves have become the old guard. The great present danger, it seems to me, is that today's champions will assume that the earlier goals, aspired to when Congress passed the Community Mental Health Centers Act, continue to express the legitimate needs of the present and immediate future. Needed now, no less than a decade ago, is the flexibility, the willingness to reconsider the need to reshape old assumptions and traditions to suit the requirements of a rapidly altering social reality.

We want to present our errors as well as our successes. In brief, three stages or aspects of this community mental health program have evolved: first, providing direct care by coordinating existing services and establishing new ones; second, through consultation introducing psychological concepts into related community activities, such as schools, jails, and churches; third, evolving novel patterns through joint participation in our fantastically exploding social system. We work in poverty programs and family life education curriculums, aid developing family planning programs, and initiate mental health evening courses for teachers. We have done fairly well in the first, clinical aspect; quite well in the second, consultative aspect; and made a slight beginning in the third. Our staff time use reflects this proportion: 80 per cent for clinical services, 15 per cent for consultation, and less than 5 per cent for community organization.

In 1958, I took the then new position of program chief of the San Mateo Mental Health Services Division. Our guide to a model program was the new program elements set down in the Milbank Memorial Fund Conference reports (Milbank Memorial Fund, 1956, 1957). The three major clinical goals established then are relevant today: first, we wanted to develop a truly unified service—so that the individual patient could be served by closely cooperating clinical elements joined under single record, budgetary, and administrative direction. Second, major clinical program emphasis was on identifying and serving the chronic and severely mentally ill person in the community rather than in the state hospital. (In 1958, we believed community services could supplant state hospitals, but could not prove it.) And third, active program research and development was to be integrated into the fabric of the ongoing clinical services. In 1969, these goals are national policy and accepted as old hat. In those days, they were visionary, to be tested against existing service patterns before they could be accepted and implemented. But even today they remain, in some mental health centers, pious hopes rather than actual accomplishments.

Three clinical services were in existence in 1958: (1) the child and (2) the adult outpatient clinics, and (3) the unique open-door therapeutic community inpatient unit at the County Hospital. The consultation service was newly established as well. The pioneering work of Harry Wilmer and Maxwell Jones had been successfully applied by Calvin Young to the psychiatric emergency and the acute psychotic patient. The consultation service was being formed at about the time I arrived, so its service patterns had not yet evolved.

Aiming at non-hospital community services, within a matter of months we launched a rehabilitation service by the simple expedient of organizing an ex-patient club. In the following year this service was expanded by the addition of a rehabilitation clinic for alcoholics and their families, followed by a day hospital, a vocational counseling service, a sheltered workshop, and, most recently, an affiliated halfway house. We have been most fortunate in having few inpatient beds (thirty-seven beds for a half-million population); we have been forced to develop non-hospital services.

Having previously stumbled interminably in chronic frustration between the various autonomous public agencies of a tradition-encrusted eastern county, I was quick to appreciate the advantages offered by the multiphasic San Mateo County Department of Public Health and Welfare. It supplied more than could have been expected as an environment in which to create an effective, integrated system of local mental health services. Program innovation—once a dream—became a possibility; coordinating services became inevitable rather than a painful, frustrating chore. In many jurisdictions the patient finds little continuity or coordination of services as he is directed from hospital to clinic, from welfare to medical care to psychiatric clinic to rehabilitation program. As one mentally retarded unwed mother of six children said about the nine public servants who regularly visited her family, "It sure is hard to give all those people what they want!"

I had anticipated that my major administrative problems would include obtaining needed funds, attracting qualified staff, and developing the essential network of relationships which would be so necessary, if mental health was to take advantage of the opportunities presented by the multiphasic department—those of working toward integrated and systematic linkage with local welfare, public health, and public hospital services. In general, none of these proved as difficult as one major unanticipated problem: the resistance among some professionals to the kinds of changes necessary to produce the unified patient-centered services I had in mind. I mention this matter openly, because it is of pressing importance to every medical service innovator. For instance, our early efforts in program development and evaluation led to a major upheaval in which virtually the entire staff of the adult clinic resigned in protest. This experience demonstrated to me that changes in clinical patterns can be effective only when the administrator has obtained the active participation and concurrence of the professionals involved (Blum and Downing, 1964).

The community must be informed, and agree to the goals of the professional in any area—mental health, social welfare, police and corrections, or the schools. Early on, the community mental health administrator must actively gain this general agreement to his plans, or risk failure. In my talks to San Mateo County organizations, I made it unmistakably clear that our inpatient service was calculated to head off long-term custodial care in a state hospital by keeping the mentally ill person at home. Our community never blinked at taking local responsibility for its own citizens, never categorized them as a "state responsibility." Nor has the community flinched at the real social risks involved in serving such seriously disturbed people in open-door wards and part-day settings. This, too, was a constant theme in speeches I delivered during the first five years. There are risks; they are tangible; they are worth taking. Today, though incidents have occasionally occurred, it no longer seems necessary to warn of such risks; San Mateo has learned what we have constantly preached to our professional visitors: the occasional incident is an isolated and inevitable cost. But it is well worth the price when weighed against the therapeutic value of the high expectations that we portray to our disturbed and psychotic patients by endowing them with responsibility and dignity in noncoercive, nonpunitive treatment settings.

Continuing our push away from hospitalization toward early care in the community, the pre-hospital-admission home visit program was begun in 1961—as a means of heading off needless legally initiated ("observational") admission to the county hospital inpatient ward. The concept came in part from a community-based emergency service

—the home visiting program established by Querido (1954) in Amsterdam. From private practice, I learned that home visits kept many a mentally sick person out of the hospital. Two of us visited the homes of ten consecutive persons for whom involuntary commitment had been requested. We found that six of these people did not need hospital care at all. Extra funds were soon earmarked for a half-time psychiatrist to visit selected persons for whom involuntary hospitalization had been requested. Ninety per cent of those visited did not have to be involuntarily committed; indeed, only 50 per cent had to be hospitalized at all (Fink, Asbury, and Downing, 1963). This finding affirms the value of early attention by a mental health professional *before* the entangling coils of inflexible legal procedures are invoked.

Our concern for the often neglected severely mentally ill led to meetings with the superintendent of Agnews State Hospital, which serves our county (Rapaport and Downing, 1962). After two years of planning, these discussions bore fruit. Agnews Hospital, in the summer of 1962, established the first of the San Mateo regionalized wards. This highly significant development, influencing a later state decision to regionalize all California state hospitals, is detailed in the next chapter.

After four years, our services, both state and local, were beginning to offer coordinated care. Meantime, partial hospitalization, inserted into the service spectrum in 1961, was being consciously planned as an alternative to full-time hospitalization. This day hospital, in other words, further reiterated a continuing concern for that population formerly consigned to the state. Unquestionably this element supplies one key to the programming dilemma presented by the chronically and severely mentally ill (see Chapter 5). This does not imply that our day hospitals have become receptacles for long-term (or terminal) placement of the seriously impaired. Instead, the day hospitals have been expected to move even the chronically ill individual on to some less inclusive program or back to at least partial independence in the community. Consequently these partial hospital services have been called upon to innovate new dimensions in aftercare and follow-up. Joined to them, as the result of this creative effort by staff workers, are open house programs for discharged patients, ex-patient activity programs of a wide variety, a full range of vocational rehabilitation services, and a vigorous utilization of new and existing community resources, including, above all, the recently established halfway house and the welfare public assistance programs.

These services, when joined to full-time community consultation, constitute the core of the comprehensive program. They carry the largest load with the least cost; they get more people back on their own feet. In a sense, this conviction is the turning point for the mental health administrator. Once he has convinced himself that many of the most costly community mental health problems are most likely to be met not by high-cost, conventionally designed psychotherapeutic elements, but by expedients calculated to draw upon the existing as well as latent strengths of the community, he has taken the first step toward designing what can be legitimately termed a community mental health program. It is only the first step—but it is crucial. Having taken it, one finds it difficult to look back.

Consultation, in particular, is a powerfully educative force. Not only is it an agent for change in the community; it can and should be a fruitful and interminable source of policy and programming cues for the mental health administrator. I can cite my own learning as documentation. The whole indirect service complex, as it has been elaborated by our highly skilled consultation staff, has gone far beyond what I had thought about up to 1958. To it can be attributed San Mateo's attention to the idea of services directed to the non-clinically-defined person, from which we proceeded to the almost inevitable preoccupation with what I have termed broadly *social health,* as contrasted with the much narrower idea of mental health. Community mental health is not primarily a medical issue, a matter of disease identification and elimination. We began looking at behavior in a context that was broader than the simple presence or absence of mental illness. Further, in this endeavor we had long since begun to appreciate the importance of social and cultural factors in addition to the intrapsychic as crucial determinants of human behavior.

I soon discovered the difficulties in persuading nonmedical public administration of the importance of supporting program evaluation and research. Nor did the problem end there. In most other service-oriented settings in and out of clinical psychiatry, these activities stand outside of the normal therapeutic work. Clinicians tend to view clinical investigation, with some justice, as an intrusive element. We found at the New York State Department of Mental Hygiene at

Syracuse, for example, that merely to set up the reporting system required for a given research project often took 80 per cent of our project time. Few clinics have recording systems adequate for their own needs, let alone for investigation. An excellent documentation of San Mateo's adventures in program evaluation and research is presented in Chapter 15; it reveals that even with staff cooperation, we have seldom fully overcome the inherent resistances to research and development activities, even though we have succeeded in weaving excellent data collection and processing into normal service routines. The overall result has been better clinical service and some good evaluation. In some instances we have successfully carried forward projects which included well-done program planning, evaluation, and revision.

To produce the unified service that was so essential, I proposed development of a simplified record system. This, it seemed, held the promise of welding together the diversity of a growing number of individual service elements. Starting in 1958, we executed two comparative studies in the adult and child guidance clinics. The inquiries were designed to compare traditional team intake methods with the simpler intake and evaluation procedure as is ordinarily done by the private office practitioner. One problem, as well, was the reluctance of certain elements to forward their charts to other elements of service. Clearly, the introduction of a system-wide record format would be necessary. Such a record system would help eliminate redundant and needless evaluation and permit the clinical staff to strike a more equitable balance between professional conferencing and time actually spent in patient contacts.

Only a centralized record system that supplies reliable, uniform, relatively brief information, a system that is monitored by clerical staff (whose duty is to alert professionals concerning record-keeping deadlines and to sound an alarm for the service chief and, ultimately, the program chief when these deadlines are missed) can do the job. The system was developed after thousands of professional hours of planning, debate, and review (Blum and Ezekiel, 1962) and is the simplest, most complete, most reliable of any I have encountered. Controlled by a committee of the clinical professionals themselves meeting monthly, it is supervised by a chief clerk responsible directly to the program administrator.

### Administration

Community mental health center administration, at least in urban and relatively well-to-do localities, is generally taken to be a medical responsibility, customarily the purview of a psychiatrist. This decision to allocate to a medically and clinically trained person responsibility for the direction of an expensive and multifaceted public service organization gives rise to certain recognizable problems. Customary clinical schooling provides little, if any, training in organization theory or management. Another problem is the surprising dearth of literature on the subject (now being remedied by freshets of printed advice such as this). Even the bibliographical references in this book are not all relevant, for, as in other aspects of contemporary life, the most prolific authors on this subject are academic theoreticians who have "studied" administrative patterns but have not engaged in the remarkably unscientific and sometimes highly disorderly business of running a community mental health center.

It is a familiar mistake of the clinician to suppose that his experience of training and working in a clinical organization has prepared him to understand how organizations function. The clinician in this instance, of course, is comparable to a schoolboy who supposes that because he instinctively knows how to chew food and swallow it, whereupon digestion occurs, he knows the detailed operation of his own digestive tract. In medicine, the clinically adept physician can be an organizational ignoramus—and nowhere is he more likely to be found than in community mental health, where the administrative tasks include an incredible range of highly sensitive responsibilities. These range from supervision of treatment and training services to the public health and community organization functions that run the gamut from epidemiology to the stimulation and nurturing of an almost endless range of community partnerships.

Of critical importance to this discussion is the identity crisis, seen in psychiatrists and other mental health professionals whose initial identity was that of clinician and who have turned to administration (Levinson and Klerman, 1967). "This process constitutes a major developmental transition not unlike those of adolescence, marriage, or retirement." But "the overlap and the possibility of synthesis of the two identities are greater than is usually imagined. The clinician must deal with his patients' behavior as well as with their private fantasies and feelings. He must be able to set and maintain limits and to take decisive action at crucial points in clinical management. Conversely, the clinical identity retains its relevance for the psychiatrist-executive." For instance, Barton (1967) notes certain attributes, useful in administration, which clinical training contributes to the psychiatrist. These include "an understanding of motivation; the ability to listen with sensitivity to what is being said, to discern what is not said, and to observe the affect that accompanies a communication; an awareness of the impact of change and frustration upon individuals; patience to wait and time interventions to the adaptive capacity of those with whom they deal; and a flexibility in transactions with a wide variety of personality types." However, wise administration demands much more. The administrator, in most modern organizations, is called upon to be many kinds of persons at different moments. Any administrator proves highly talented in responding to certain categories of tasks; without notable exception, he also betrays a certain incompetence in other spheres of his job.

The psychiatrist is more accustomed to being "first among equals" than his medical colleagues who are accustomed to the "ruler-over-life-and-death" relationships of the general hospital. The community mental health administrator combines public health preventive and educational functions with general hospital in- and outpatient services. Often he feels like an opera house manager, beset by disparaging critics, disgruntled customers, primadonnas vowing to quit, and plugged toilets in the women's restroom. Through cajolery, firmness, a strong back, and a deaf ear, the show goes on.

Zaleznik (1967) stresses the primacy for administration of uses of influence, authority, and power, a trilogy of forces he rightly supposes many of us will consider with suspicion and discomfiture. Too many mental health professionals find it difficult to accept that authority has an essential and legitimate role and that the director must exercise it without guilt or apology.

But on the other hand, medical management is not an individualistic endeavor. For instance, Hodgson, Levinson, and Zaleznik (1965) describe the "executive role constellation," consisting of several key figures in the organization. This grouping tends to play a central part in top management decisions. What also needs to be emphasized, however, is the exceedingly intricate pattern by which every participant in the organization influences executive role decisions. Even the janitor influences his own organizational fate and that of the system as a whole. (The wise administrator befriends the janitor, the switchboard operator, and the admitting room nurse, if he wants to know what is happening in his territory.) We are, for better or worse, experiencing an interactional phenomenon. The scientific observer may find it desirable to disregard this complexity, for purposes of evaluative simplicity and tidiness. The administrator, however, had better not fall into that insidious trap. For him the human variables in organizational life must be taken as virtually infinite; he will have to reconcile himself to the perhaps uncomfortable realization that management—which can be aided by the learning of techniques and the gathering of data—is not a science that can be learned. It is an art of human relationships.

Having taken the fateful first steps—a seemingly innocent stroll into the troubled precincts of a social health orientation—I soon found my idea of the tasks to be faced was based no longer upon the individual as delineated by the simplistic functioning of his own psychophysiologic reality but upon the individual as participant in a tremendous problem matrix. It appeared that individual energy patterns engage in reciprocal relationships with larger and wider energy patterns. As an administrator, however, one will postulate some tentative and, no doubt, inadequate paradigm for purposes of considering what will govern the function of a mental health program in such a multi-determined environment. A successful mental health activity, I have concluded, might be conceived of as a network of shared responsibility made up of *reasonably* communicating people with different attitudes and points of view.

Once the import of this discovery has dawned upon him, the administrator will also understand something highly useful about his role when he is introduced into another important community system. Just as the consultant learns to guard against presenting himself to his consultee as an authoritative purveyor of wisdom and advice, the physician-administrator must drop his traditional role of authoritative provider of solutions to problems. He will discover how to join with others and share responsibility in both his own and other community systems in a collaborative quest for answers. He will learn also how to ask for help for the system he represents.

There are, in other words, an endless diversity of relationships in which the community mental health administrator must engage. He will wish to mobilize existing fiscal and personnel resources, under the jurisdiction of other agencies, to paths that offer a heightened probability of positive mental health for the community. His medical reputation hardly carries the kind of weight that will permit him to call the turn for some other community system. He will have to learn how to be a catalyst and a persuader, scrupulously avoiding the Little Caesar stance of community dictator.

In seeking new and expanded programs for his own system, he will be the petitioner rather than the anointed bestower of blessings. Budget justification, a case in point, asks skill in quantifying service needs, explaining the relative importance of various types of specialized personnel, and discussing costs and benefits to be gained from certain courses of action. A grasp of figures, a nimble faculty for interpreting pre-studied material, and a readiness to understand and utilize the give-and-take inherent in any determination of public policy are among the requisites. Because the field of public administration is far from scientifically exact, the mental health administrator may face ethical and personality struggles in discarding cautious clinical habits constraining him to communicate guarded estimates. In the persuasive role of program promoter, he will find it necessary to adopt the linguistic habits of public affairs, stating broad positive affirmation for a proposed course.

In San Mateo, we have never believed there were impenetrable barriers between the public program and private practice. Our activities have not been calculated to carve out inviolable territory or to throw up a fortress of socialized medicine from which the private men would be banished. On the other hand, however, we have been aware that individuals served in public facilities generally are more severely mentally ill and come from disorganized family and social situations. They require more and, often, different services than persons usually seen in private practice.

This, plus the costly records required by any agency that must be equipped to justify its activities to the taxpayer, often means that the cost per patient in a public program is higher than the unit cost in private practice. For some years, I was among those who found this distressing and was disinclined to argue with those who pointed disparagingly at our costs. It was only after we had carried out our three-week time studies (see Chapter 15) that I began to feel I could respond intelligently to these criticisms. It became evident that the patients seen by our staff require a vast number of auxiliary services— telephone calls, letters, conferences with police, with teachers, and with a variety of other caregiving personnel, as well as painstaking and time-consuming attention to after-treatment phases of life, including assistance in making aftercare plans that may involve private practice follow-up for psychotherapy or drug maintenance. Add to this the cost of program evaluation and research, training, and community consultation, and one begins to understand the cost picture in its true perspective.

This apparent lower productivity and higher cost is not real. In fact, we are currently negotiating with two private hospitals which will be picking up major community mental health responsibilities in our projected decentralization of comprehensive services (four regional centers are to be created in the county). One of these hospitals, having received a Public Health Service construction grant, will be jurisdictionally in charge of the north central region of the county. Although we are by no means yet satisfied with the scope and philosophy of care that these facilities (and their private-practice staffs) are prepared to supply, our negotiations have already reached the stage where we can see that anything like truly comprehensive attention to the seriously impaired patient may cost roughly twice what we currently (1968) budget, based upon our careful county cost accounting procedures. This is a serious problem. It is one that should be faced honestly by all who are, today, mouthing glib platitudes about the merits of producing marriages between private and public services. To date, these unions are little more than shotgun weddings, and, if the public doesn't suffer higher tax burdens, then the patient may be destined to suffer by being inadequately served in private facilities that obtain far less funds than are needed to finance the necessary auxiliary services.

Social maintenance and actual treatment of mentally ill by other community facilities and agencies have been an overriding policy in San Mateo. Without going into the philosophical justifications, that policy is an inescapable corollary to the community mental health commitment to serve the total population of the service region. (See Chapter 10 for an excellent exposition of this issue as well as some actual examples taken from our struggles to meet the mental health needs of children.) In doing direct service, we have endeavored to refer as many patients as possible to the private sector (to psychiatry, pediatrics, general practice, and internal medicine, as well as to qualified privately practicing psychologists and psychiatric social workers). Our wide and vigorous pursuit of indirect service has reflected the conviction that many marginally functional individuals can be served —sometimes more effectively—in the context of other human services: welfare, public health nursing, the schools, the local penal and probation agencies, the churches, and in nonpsychiatric rehabilitation and recreational settings. (Chapter 14 offers examples of the patterns this work has taken in the field of adult courts and corrections.) This basic conviction has helped us to make more responsible judgments about how the community ought to allocate its limited money and manpower among the competing human service agencies, including mental health. Sometimes the mental health administrator may find it difficult to operate on the basis of a total community outlook. Nevertheless, it is essential to view the community as an (either actually or potentially) integrated organism, the health of which depends upon the health of each element in its social structure.

In today's technologically-oriented society, mental health may be seen as a higher status and more prestigious service than, for example, public welfare. The former can easily take precedence and gain resources that otherwise might be allotted to the public welfare professional staff. This outcome could actually injure the ability of the social service division of the department to carry its tremendous load of individual suffering and agony, lower its professional morale (often tenuous enough, as it is), and thus do significant and appreciable damage to the mental health of a high risk sector of the community, the welfare clients. Conversely, the respect, understanding, and consistent support of the mental health administrator for welfare by providing consultative services, inviting welfare personnel to mental health staff development programs, consulting with, rather than snubbing, welfare personnel, can be sources of closer collaboration between the two caregiving systems.

In one tight budget year, when we planned to ask for some fifteen new positions (expecting to get two or three to meet our urgent service needs), our administrative staff (the chiefs of services and I) agreed to drop our demands in behalf of an even more desperately needed welfare position. The position sought by welfare, supervisor of staff development and training, seemed to us to be more crucial for the overall mental health of the community. We voiced this conviction to the budget review people, and the position was subsequently authorized.

Workers in the non-mental health caregiving sector of the community may be less adequately trained than mental health workers. However, they will be more expert concerning the realities of their own systems, as well as the realities of the life situations faced by their clients and probationers than most mental health professionals. The stringent regulations and demands of these systems often dictate that these workers behave in what some may consider to be an "unpsychotherapeutic" manner. If mental health personnel take a holier-than-thou—or a more-therapeutic-than-thou—attitude, the possibility of useful partnerships is reduced.

I have learned to acknowledge, respect, and utilize informal systems of communication. For example, at one time each of the many divisions of the Department of Public Health and Welfare had a separate coffee percolator in its own office. When a new wing was added to the building, the director insisted on including a coffee shop that is pleasant and attractive. He arranged with the State Department of the Blind to finance and staff the short-order counter. He then forbade any other source of coffee in the building, and authorized morning and afternoon coffee breaks. There was some grumbling about this being dictatorial, less efficient, less convenient, and so forth, but the order was obeyed. The coffee shop has now become the principal center for informal communication between the various elements which otherwise would hardly ever come in touch with each other. From the standpoint of the community mental health services, contact with the staffs of the public health division, the welfare division, and the other services that are located in this one building has been greatly increased. Consequently, our knowledge of these public services, our ability both to have an effect on them and to be affected by them has been much enhanced.

From the standpoint of administration, there is no substitute for getting out of the office to set the style for the staff. As a role model, the administrator must be an eager initiator of community contacts. His indirect service staff will be doing this kind of thing, also. But his own willingness to meet with other agency executives, to schedule lunch-time meetings and after-hours talks or discussions portray to the entire staff of his organization, as well as to the other agencies of his service region, the value that is placed upon community partnerships. Moreover, even his indirect service unit will look to him for guidance and assistance in priority-setting. He can give this direction only if he has taken the pains to know his community and to assess its variable patterns of resource agencies and their readiness for the indirect services his center can deliver.

### Staff Leadership

I have learned that professionals do not respond well to peremptory administrative edicts. Far more productive in my experience has been giving people as much autonomy as possible. I assumed the only professionals we wanted were those who could accommodate themselves to this kind of norm. Thus each chief of service has been responsible for program development and quality control within his service. It has been my habit and my personal predilection to act as a provoking, stimulating, and enabling element in the organizational formula. Having actively sought highly competent, well-trained personnel, I have tried to excite their imaginations and to elicit innovative solutions to problems. It was my role to participate in the production of ideas, then to seek the necessary budget authorizations to assure an adequate allocation of resources, and to provide support when their programs were unjustly under attack from inside or outside the county bureaucracy.

But the granting of autonomy always poses a multitude of problems. Many want both autonomy and, at the same time, the "secure" feeling of an authoritarian administration; they may complain of a lack of administrative interest and concern. But those who have been most vocal in deploring this apparent lack of concern, have been equally unwilling to recognize that you cannot have it both ways.

On balance, I would judge this has been a modestly successful pattern of administration. Many of our most effective programs were introduced and shaped into viable expressions as the consequence of this sometimes painful process. Lest I be misunderstood, I should add here that my administrative style of promoting change is not inconsistent with the routine exercise of power in the day-to-day operation of a program: insisting that staff observe the designated work hours, requiring adherence to the record and fee systems, dismissing staff when there is no other alternative. I can, however, hazard one observation that I suspect will apply to community mental health administrators in general. Despite the undoubted cogency of the various investigations into the nature of administration, one will usually find that one cannot see himself with the detached and clinical awareness conveyed by a sociologist or industrial relations specialist. What they have to say about our "styles" of administration may be both interesting and useful. It will almost never seem wholly accurate from our point of view. The task is far too extensive to be nailed down or consigned to neat pigeonholes. It is vaguely reminiscent of psychotherapy in being, at bottom, a process and therefore of the nature of a phenomenon that cannot be verbalized.

If I were to draw upon my years at San Mateo to hazard an attempt at saying how it feels to administer, I think I would go a step further than the organization specialists who use the paternal-maternal-fraternal analogies. I would suggest, as the mental health consultants have sometimes done (Haylett and Rapoport, 1964), that there is a similarity between a system and a family; but these "families" are quite different in some crucial respects from the common family we encounter in our culture. They are organized to achieve a different set of goals, and the individual members focus a different set of expectations upon themselves and each other. But like the families we encounter in the homes and neighborhoods of our communities, these "families" are of a magnificent diversity, reflecting many of the special peculiarities that are mingled within our culture. They are systems made up of mixtures of people, just as families are, except that the mixture is somewhat less homogenized.

Each administrator has his own convictions concerning good parenting. But he may not fully appreciate the extent to which he is responded to by his staff as a parental figure. It is all too easy to continue to see oneself as just another worker in the system and not realize that by the very nature of his position and authority he can no longer

be "one of the boys" in the way that he once was. His staff now look
to him for direction and leadership. They may recapitulate with him
their relationship with their own parents, with all that this implies:
dependency, passive acceptance or rebellion against authority or both
together, expectations of omnipotence and infallibility. If the administrator is aware of all this, he is prepared to accomplish one of his
main tasks—helping his staff relate to him in an appropriate way and
not use inordinate amounts of energy reenacting childhood conflicts.
He does not help by being a therapist to staff. Rather, he must act in
an appropriate manner and expect his staff to do the same. When
they do not act appropriately it should be pointed out to them, but
strictly in terms of behavior in the work context. The motivation and
historical antecedents should be left to the person's therapist.

But despite all this, the role of administrator does in many
ways resemble the parental role. The one practical piece of administrative advice that I can give to other program administrators is, be
a good parent to your staff. Nothing else you will do can be so influential in determining how they will deal with community groups, treat
their patients, lift up or cast down the spirits of the people with whom
they deal. When the members of your "family" are secure in their
sense of belonging, they will carry the most weighty burdens of community distress, mentally ill persons' demands, and unsatisfactory working conditions. If they are unsure, afraid of censure or punishment, or
treated distantly and indifferently, there will be all sorts of hell to pay
—disturbed patients prone to bizarre episodes of acting out, angry
community telephone calls, painful and destructive staff disputes, and
other signs of a disturbed family.

As an administrator, look to your own mental health, your
own ability to be supportive when necessary, stern and directive at
other times, and, above all, to be flexible and able to enjoy your own
job. A chronically depressed director will have a chronically depressed
mental health service. A power-based director will have an authoritarian staff, skilled in the petty arts of bureaucratic one-upmanship,
busily passing their grievances on to the lowliest and least defended
person in the entire structure, the patient. No one can force a flower
to bloom, whatever his authority and genius. No director can force
effective service. Set the conditions lovingly, care about your staff,

treat them as you hope the patients and the community will be treated, and good service, sometimes even fine service, will result.

It is true in a very real sense that San Mateo's remarkable distinction of being the first program in the nation to develop and then link together all ten of the so-called essential and supplementary elements of a comprehensive community mental health program (United States Public Health Service, 1964) is a tribute to the staff. This accomplishment was the product of their labor, their willingness to engage in the wearisome give-and-take of innovation and revision.

In the same way, however, there is virtue in identifying the accomplishments that are yet to be achieved. These include a glaring lack of services capable of meeting the needs of alcoholics and their families, as well as inadequacies in serving both emotionally handicapped and mentally retarded children. But even more significant has been our failure to move beyond the relatively conventional indirect service patterns. San Mateo has not, just as so many other community mental health services have not, been able to produce methods and avenues of linkage with the grassroots population. It has been, I think, more versatile than most in linking up with the institutions serving that population; it has come to know the community in a much fuller sense for being able to include many of the perceptions and reality struggles of those manifold caregiving individuals and agencies to which it has delivered its indirect services.

San Mateo has not, however, found consistent and reliable media capable of feeding into its own culture the often-puzzling and sometimes disturbing messages of those population groups that seriously question many of the fundamental assumptions of the middle-class establishment. Nor can this be wholly excused by the fact that in our affluent county these disestablishmentarian spokesmen constitute a much smaller fraction of the population than is the case in the inner city. In my opinion, community mental health has a serious responsibility in such areas as helping dissenters learn how to express their dissenting views responsibly, and in helping the uncommitted middle ground to see how to respond reasonably and sensitively to the often inflammatory and unreasonable criticisms of the frustrated, the disenchanted, and the disenfranchised. We must be helped to understand one another, and to air our all-important differences in a way that will lead to positive growth for all concerned.

Nor have we put a sufficient premium upon the kind of epidemiological research program that would describe why certain people seek our help and others do not. There is little to indicate whether our services are utilized by those who are most in need or only by those who happen to be able to accept our institutional ground rules and scale our bureaucratic barriers. Finally, and most distressing, we are by no means free of the lamentable habits of our medical heritage; it all too often continues to be our categorical imperative to help those who can make a "treatment" contract that includes adjusting them to or integrating them within the dominant norms of what the middle-class professional wishes to define as treatment.

It is undeniable that the professional community exercises a powerful influence upon any administrator's freedom to act. The fact that some of our own professionals were in the vanguard of resistance suggests not only that I may have been a relatively ineffectual persuader but also that there existed some deeply ingrained attitudes about the nature of professional roles and professional ethics. Clearly, we have a long way to go in introducing a creative and positive preventive mental health orientation to this influential group to which we must look to staff our centers.

In San Mateo, I suppose, we have edged closest to this orientation in our North County Mental Health Center (see Chapters 17, 18, 19), which opened in 1965. This regional program has been at the same time the most controversial and the least understood of all our innovative ventures. This staff, too, was given both the responsibility and the authority to deal with those difficulties. Happily, they have persevered, and that program, having painfully evolved into a viable pattern, continues to contain most of the ingredients necessary for a community mental health service that is truly responsive to its total catchment population.

But the community mental health movement generally has affiliated itself with the formal power structure, as it must and as the middle-class background of its professionals makes inevitable. In doing this, it has alienated itself from those minority groups that constitute the informal structure, such as youth, blacks, prisoners, and the disadvantaged. We work with and understand the police and not the prisoner, the schoolteacher but not the pupil, the social worker but not her black client. In my opinion, community mental health runs the grave risk of becoming just one more bureaucratic, self-serving organization that in the long run will no more serve human needs than the state hospital which it replaced.

I must close by sounding one more note of warning. Today, new community mental health centers are being inserted into existing general hospitals, onto the fringes of existing state hospitals, and alongside many of the tradition-guarding departments of psychiatry in schools of medicine. I fear the thrust for our generation is toward stultifying community mental health. It seems destined to be trapped into the traditional psychiatric preoccupation with pathology, diagnosis, and remedy to the exclusion of a far more momentous and creative attention to positive health, community development, and the tasks that would lead potentially to a more satisfying and rewarding culture.

CHAPTER 2

# Liaison With the
# State Hospital

*Norman R. Rogers, H. Richard Lamb,*
*Don Heath*

Regionalization of Agnews State Hospital services was begun in 1962 with the designation of wards to serve San Mateo County patients exclusively. It was the first instance of what was to become a widely practiced procedure, often known as the Unit Plan, in the California state hospital system. It proved the forerunner of statewide regionalization undertaken in 1965. But the success story is checkered with many episodes of challenge, disappointment, and dismay. Most dramatic of these were the thorny issues that confronted the state hospital and the local program, as these two agencies, under different governmental jurisdictions and facing somewhat different kinds of sanctions and expectations from their respective governing bodies, pieced together a viable therapeutic partnership.

Agnews State Hospital, near San Jose, is a thirty-minute drive by freeway south from the San Mateo central county mental health services. It is a twenty-one-hundred bed hospital for the mentally ill and is designated as the receiving hospital for San Mateo and several other counties. Agnews admits approximately four thousand patients a year. Of these annual admissions, about nine hundred are San Mateo County residents, whose impairments cover all types of mental illness. There is an average census of three hundred San Mateo County patients at any one time.

## Liaison and Aftercare

To illustrate the problems and pitfalls facing establishment of the vital and necessary working partnership between the state hospital and community agencies, it will be useful to trace first the evolution of liaison between the regionalized San Mateo unit of Agnews State Hospital and the San Mateo County mental health and welfare services. Kraft, Binner, and Dickey (1967) describe the experience of a progressive comprehensive community mental health center where hard-core chronic patients are accumulating at a rapid rate. We have sought to minimize this phenomenon and also to facilitate aftercare for all patients by actively promoting liaison between the state hospital and the community.

For many years, follow-up services in California were drastically limited. Involuntary patients released on indefinite leave were seen periodically by social workers of the State Department of Mental Hygiene (Bureau of Social Work), who then sent reports back to the state hospital. Following a year's absence from the hospital and reasonable progress, the patient usually was discharged until he again came to the attention of the authorities and had to be recommitted. Voluntary patients, for the most part, received aftercare only to the extent they sought it, either privately or from the various public clinics.

The first attempt at liaison between state hospital and county mental health services was provided primarily by a team from the San Mateo psychiatric inpatient service, consisting of a psychiatrist and a social worker. This team visited Agnews on a regular basis. The ra-

tionale was that the brief-stay county inpatient service sent many patients to the state hospital and, therefore, already had a working relationship with state hospital staff. After a year or so, this liaison had
worked out some of the problems that complicate referrals to the state
hospital. But liaison with a community inpatient service had not really
provided liaison with such aftercare resources as the day hospital, vocational rehabilitation services, and outpatient clinics. What the county
inpatient service had to communicate about patients being sent to the
state hospital was now transmitted in writing and by telephone, and
this initial attempt at liaison was discontinued. The flow of information has worked well, but one disadvantage has been the lack of that
added sense of rapport that develops when two staffs have regular
face-to-face meetings.

Establishing weekly visits by the mental health public health
nurse consultant to engage in discharge planning conferences with
state hospital personnel (Mouw and Haylett, 1967) was an important
step. Public health nurses are able to provide a home visit program
that is vital to the treatment of mentally ill persons who lack motivation to follow through with an aftercare program and are fearful and
distrustful of mental health professionals (see Chapter 7). Such patients need a professional who will reach out to them in their homes.
Lack of aggressive follow-up of discharged patients, it should be
added, is often the principal reason for "patients falling through the
cracks," failing to make the transition from hospital to community
aftercare. Simple referral to an aftercare facility is seldom sufficient
for chronically and severely disabled people who are ready to leave
the hospital. *Aggressive* follow-up services by mental health professionals are frequently necessary to a successful aftercare plan.

A different type of follow-up pattern was innovated by the San
Mateo North County Mental Health Center, which came into being
in 1965, with responsibility for approximately 25 per cent of the
county population. The personnel of that center assumed full responsibility for pre- and post-hospital care of patients in their catchment
area, as well as a full measure of involvement and contact with their
state hospitalized patients. From the beginning, a representative of the
North County Center traveled weekly to the hospital to see patients,
to work with them during the hospital episode, and to arrange for
aftercare services in the center after discharge. A social therapy club

led by the liaison representative himself has been the initial receiving service for these returning patients, and many, in addition, are also referred to the day hospital and various types of outpatient treatment. This bridging arrangement led naturally to a state hospital decision to place all patients from north county in two wards of their own to faciliate visiting and casefinding. This new phenomenon was labeled "subregionalization." In a large county, regionalization may still fail to reduce the number of patients and staff to levels that permit close and individualized liaison. Consequently, subregionalization proves highly valuable.

Another pattern of liaison evolved in the central county. Here, personnel from the day hospital, psychiatric vocational services, and a newly formed halfway house began regular monthly visits to meet with the hospital staff of social workers and psychiatrists from the remaining nine San Mateo County wards (excluding those serving the north county). Following this meeting, the staff from the county mental health services visited currently hospitalized patients whom they had formerly seen in treatment. A social worker from the state hospital also made regular visits to the day hospital and halfway house for even closer liaison. This pattern proved most significant and effective. For instance, during the first year of its operation, the halfway house found that about 90 per cent of the residents it accepted were former state hospital patients. State hospital referrals to the county day hospital and vocational services also increased sharply.

Creation of companion groups was another important development. Real continuity of care dictates this additional dimension— follow-up during the critical period after release from the hospital by therapists with whom the patient is acquainted. In making the hazardous transition from hospital to community, it is extremely difficult for a marginally functional person to form new relationships with agencies and professionals who are strange to him. To eliminate this hazard, three groups were formed in the state hospital, and companion groups were organized in three separate locations in the county. Each of the three separate companion groups had two co-therapists— one from the state hospital, and one from a community agency. Whenever possible, the patient was placed in a group at the state hospital which had a companion group in the community close to the patient's home. When the patient left the hospital, he could continue in that group in the community with the same therapists. If services other than group therapy were indicated, these therapists could serve liaison functions, introducing the patient to other resources in the local mental health program, as well as in the private and voluntary agency sectors of the community. Companion groups were used initially for the treatment of alcoholics but later included all categories of patients.

Liaison by a unit of the welfare division of the county's Department of Public Health and Welfare has become another important dimension of state-local service integration. This unit provides supportive casework supplied by a group of social workers assigned specifically to mentally ill patients. In these cases, Aid to the Disabled financial assistance is handled by the same social worker who provides the supportive relationship. These workers, who receive mental health consultation and help with the prescribing of medications from the Mental Health Services Division, are also active in finding boarding homes and family care homes and in developing vocational and recreational resources for the mentally ill of all ages, including the elderly and senile. Coordination of services is thus much enhanced: many patients have been placed in the community by this unit.

Some important lessons have been learned. For one thing, we have found that after the initial stages of developing a good working relationship between agencies, liaison must be more than good will to be effective. It must be patient-oriented and include both discussion of specific patients being referred to the state hospital and patients being referred from the state hospital to community aftercare facilities. Follow-up information given to the state hospital staff about patients referred to community facilities and reports from state hospital staff about patients still hospitalized are not only clinically helpful but also contribute to rapport between the two staffs. Collaboration on case management and discharge planning between state hospital staff and staff from community agencies is extremely useful. Furthermore, both the state and community agencies should have specific services to offer each other and should have an appreciation of the value and purposes of these services.

A feeling of belonging to a team is shared by the combined staff from the state hospital and the local program, as the result of this experience of sharing responsibility for patients in the San Mateo County wards. However, this was far from true at the beginning. There was an initial lack of knowledge on the part of the hospital staff as to what role the day hospital could play in aftercare and as to how to refer patients to vocational services and why. Many patients in the hospital repeatedly said they didn't want to be patients after leaving the hospital; they wanted to acquire a different, non-patient identity and would, at the most, accept outpatient therapy. In many cases this was not appropriate, since these patients needed a day hospital or a halfway house or vocational services, or perhaps all of these. In many cases, the state hospital staff, having been concerned about patients becoming overly dependent, went along with this thinking and agreed to discharge patients without carefully planned aftercare. A research project concerned with returning long-term state patients to the community by a coordinated program of day hospital, halfway house, and vocational services (supported in part by Rehabilitation Services Administration grant RD-2847-P) began about this time and was useful in demonstrating that these facilities in the community could be very helpful and were often necessary for the rehabilitation of very sick patients.

On the other hand, the staff of the county mental health facilities came to appreciate the value and the quality of both treatment and staff at the state hospital. It came as a surprise to many that the state hospital is not simply a repository for custodial cases. A large number of state hospital patients are short-stay patients. Department of Mental Hygiene statistics reveal that 50 per cent of California state hospital admissions are released in less than six weeks, and 90 per cent remain less than six months.

The state hospital became recognized as a very valuable, high quality resource for patients who need medium- and long-stay hospitalization (three weeks and longer). The value of joint planning for patients also became more apparent. Furthermore, one staff learned from the other. The state hospital staff came to appreciate that patients may appear quite well in the hospital but collapse under pressures of the community and thus require special community resources. The county mental health services' staff learned how to be more selective and sophisticated in identifying candidates for state hospitalization, having found that the state hospital was often a very desirable resource for patients, rather than something to be avoided at all costs.

Liaison meetings between community and state hospital must be institutionalized and on a scheduled basis. This is vital and should be heavily emphasized. Frequently, meetings between personnel of various agencies, including the state hospital and the community mental health services, are held at times of crisis only. Effective liaison simply does not operate this way. The effective relationships between agencies that are required to bridge the gaps between state and local services grow only when time is set aside on a scheduled basis for staffs to meet together.

### Regionalization

State hospitals have long been criticized for being huge, impersonal, and inefficient, for providing poor treatment services, and for giving little thought to post-hospital care—with a resulting high recidivism rate. Unfortunately much of this criticism was justified. However, a number of factors beyond the control of state hospitals contributed to this situation. Often patients were improperly screened or not screened at all before being sent to the state hospital. Inadequate aftercare facilities contributed to the high recidivism rate. The resulting deluge of patients placed an impossible burden upon state hospital staff. Treatment in the hospital consequently deteriorated and lacked individualization because of overcrowding and an ever diminishing staff ratio.

To remedy this situation, a number of significant changes had to be made. First of all, there had to be adequate screening in the community to identify those patients who could be treated in facilities other than the state hospital. Secondly, outpatient clinics, day hospitals, sheltered workshops, and halfway houses were needed to serve as alternatives to hospitalization and to provide effective aftercare.

Changes had to be made within the state hospital itself to prevent patients from becoming just numbers, anonymous figures isolated from their former communities. Modern concepts of social psychiatry assume that the sheer size of large state mental hospitals produces many functional disadvantages. Large groups of patients cannot be housed and adequately treated as one unit. Traditionally, state hospitals were stratified into many wards with particular characteristics and functions—admission wards, acute treatment wards, convalescent wards, geriatrics wards, medical-surgical wards, and the inevitable "continued treatment" or back wards. Manageability of the patient was also taken into consideration, resulting in "disturbed" or maximum security wards, as distinguished from quieter wards with more freedom. Although such relative homogeneity facilitated economical institutionalization of large groups of patients, the chronically ill patient tended to remain hospitalized in an environment lacking expectations for change.

One of the most common and understandable desires of a sick person is to be treated by the same treatment team throughout his illness. In medicine, specialists are called in when specialized procedures such as surgery are required, but the patient usually thinks of his family doctor or internist as the one who will supervise and maintain continuity of his health care. In mental illness, the patient-therapist relationship is, if anything, even more crucial. This is especially true with very sick persons who develop trust and meaningful relationship with mental health professionals only gradually and with great difficulty. Yet, in the public mental health system, this vital canon of continuity of care has been all too frequently neglected and violated. The patient has had to submit to a discouraging and self-defeating system of barriers as he was passed on from treatment team to treatment team or from agency to agency in the community, because of the peculiar organization of the various institutions and agencies that enter into his care. Within the traditional state hospital, it was not unusual for a patient to be transferred from ward to ward many times between admission and discharge. Each transfer would demand that he attempt to synthesize new relationships with a new ward staff, often including a new doctor and social worker as well, as he passed along the assembly line from admission ward to treatment ward to convalescent ward, with an occasional detour to the "disturbed" ward. All too often the process ended with the patient permanently coming to rest on a back ward.

One alternative to treatment in large mental hospitals is to treat patients in small hospital units in the community. However, this is frequently impossible, because of the limited inpatient facilities of city and county mental health services. It is possible, however, to utilize the concept of the small treatment unit in a community setting by the device of regionalizing the state hospital and subdividing the patient population by area of residence rather than by length of hospital stay, phase of treatment, or manageability.

Regionalization, or the designation of one section of the state hospital for the exclusive care of patients from a limited geographic area has proven effective in Iowa (Garcia, 1960), Kansas (Jackson, 1962), Oregon (Rogers and Downing, 1964), Colorado (Kraft, 1965), New York on the Duchess County Unit of the Hudson River State Hospital (Snow and Bennett, 1966), and other states. In this scheme, often called the Unit Plan, the state hospital is divided into units, each one serving a distinct geographic area or region. A patient from a given community can then be placed in the appropriate regional division of a state hospital; each such division endeavors to keep in touch with the community, thereby providing a continuous link for the patient with the community from which he has been removed, it is hoped, only temporarily. This also serves to promote enduring and meaningful liaison with the mental health facilities in the community and thus more effective aftercare for patients returning to the community. Shared responsibility for patient care between local community and state psychiatric hospital is, in other words, a major current trend. Regionalization is a device that permits the patient to remain on the same ward with the same treatment team from admission to discharge, and possibly beyond discharge, as was described above in the discussion of "companion groups."

With this in mind, the county mental health services and Agnews State Hospital embarked in 1959 on a study designed to solve some or all of the problems mentioned above (Rogers and Downing, 1964). A grant from the National Institute of Mental Health enabled a traveling team, composed of three members of the county staff, three people from the state hospital, and a representative of the State Department of Mental Hygiene to make on-the-spot surveys of regionalized mental health systems in Kansas and Oregon. Professionals who had experience with regionalization in other states were called upon for consultation.

The administration of the hospital gave a great deal of thought to the selection and staffing of the building for San Mateo patients and the procedure by which they would be admitted. Reports on regionalization in other states were carefully reviewed to learn about difficulties encountered. Instead of emptying a building completely and admitting a large group of patients at one time, it was, at length, decided to put a "displacement procedure" into effect. Regionalization was a radical departure from the traditional state hospital structure then in effect. A gradual process of displacement, it was reasoned, would cause less anxiety and confusion among staff and patients and a minimum of disorganization of routine hospital functioning.

In July, 1962, the first pilot regionalized ward was started at Agnews. This ward received all female admissions and readmissions from San Mateo County other than nonambulatory and geriatrics patients. In this initial step, female patients from San Mateo County came to the hospital's admitting ward and were examined just as were patients from other counties. (Today, patients are admitted directly to the regionalized wards, and the admission wards have been eliminated.) When the admission procedure was finished, usually within two or three days, the admitting ward notified the San Mateo Unit that patients were ready to be transferred. Non-San Mateo patients were then transferred to different wards to make room for the newcomers.

To minimize bias in evaluating the results, no special procedures were introduced in the unit. No special personnel were selected, and no enrichment of staffing occurred. The wards were selected according to capacity and anticipated needs, and the personnel and treatment program remained unchanged.

Despite efforts to communicate to the hospital staff at all levels the nature and purpose of the San Mateo ward, a certain amount of anxiety, resentment, and suspicion prevailed on the part of staff outside of these wards. This resulted in the inevitable rumors, insinuations, and accusations. For instance, it was said that patients on the pilot ward were enjoying special privileges and were exempt from some of the hospital rules and regulations in effect at the time. There was a tendency to magnify or exaggerate routine administrative errors on this ward.

A characteristic state hospital problem is that of multiple subordination (Henry, 1954; Sanders, Smith, and Weinman, 1967), where lines of authority run from more than one chief to a single employee. In this instance, the nursing staff was responsible to both the director of nursing and the psychiatrists staffing and supervising the ward. This at times led to conflicts in assigning ward nursing staff. On several occasions San Mateo ward nursing staff were abruptly transferred to other wards, much to the dismay of other San Mateo ward staff.

Chronic, hospital-wide complaints of the industrial therapy department that it was receiving insufficient numbers of "good workers" now became focused on the pilot ward, which was unjustifiably blamed for the situation. In part, this may have been a reaction to a program, which, though still limited to one ward, held promise of shortening hospital stay and discharging "good workers." These events highlight the need for continued communication with, and education of, other staff throughout the hospital when such changes are made. It is also important to obtain high-level support and, ideally, active involvement from administration, both within the hospital and in the county government structure.

It was anticipated this first regionalized ward, which began receiving all of San Mateo's female patients on July 1, 1962, would fill up rapidly and, within a short time, would be entirely populated with long-term treatment cases or the so-called chronic cases, who might be expected to remain in the hospital indefinitely for custodial care. This ward had a capacity of forty beds and did, indeed, fill up within a few months, but rather than adding another ward, the patients and staff were moved to a larger ward with a capacity of sixty patients. Again, personnel ratios and treatment program remained unchanged. To the surprise of most staff, it was found this ward was able to take care of all female San Mateo admissions from then on. There had been 250 women admitted to this ward in the first year. At the end of a two-year period, only three of these 250 women remained hospitalized. Thus, the normal turnover in this ward had taken care of almost all patients. The same was true after 1963, when a similar ward was opened for men from San Mateo County.

Success with these wards was instrumental in influencing a decision, in 1965, to regionalize the entire hospital for all counties. The redistribution of all patients scattered throughout the hospital was completed within a few months. The result was that approximately six hundred San Mateo County patients of both sexes were housed on seventeen San Mateo wards. (By January 1969, this number had been reduced to three hundred patients on eight wards.)

At the same time, new admissions and readmissions began to

be assigned to all San Mateo wards in rotation. Consequently, all San Mateo wards were then housing all categories of patients—the short-term and the long-term, the acute, the sub-acute, and the chronic, the mentally ill, the alcoholics, the drug addicts, and the chronic brain syndromes. Each San Mateo ward had now become what is called a *composite ward,* and the back wards had been eliminated.

There had been fears among the hospital staff that the acute patient in relatively good contact would be disturbed by the presence of chronic and deteriorated patients and that the acute patients might begin to behave like the chronic patients. On the other hand, it was feared the long-term, deteriorated patients would not be able to keep pace with an acute, intensified treatment program, perhaps regressing further as a reaction to heightened feelings of inadequacy. Actually, the opposite proved true on these composite wards. The acute patient saw in the deteriorated patients the possible end state of his own illness; he was, therefore, motivated to work harder to get well. There was also considerable gratification derived from being helpful to the more deteriorated patients. Since the treatment program was geared to the acutely ill patient, a long-term patient had the opportunity, in some cases his first in many years, to participate in an active treatment program. He benefited from the increased efforts made on each of these wards to create a therapeutic milieu, and from the increased attention paid to him in terms of individual staff time and planning. In fact, it has been shown that the chronic patient tends to strive to bring his social and vocational performance up to the norms of better functioning of less chronic patients (Fairweather, 1969). The result was that many of these chronic patients improved and were able to be discharged from the hospital. In discussing this heterogeneous grouping of patients that results from regionalization as opposed to the usual breakdown into wards classified by diagnosis, chronicity, or traditional separations of the past, Levy (1965) points out that these changes result in movement toward at least an approximation of a normal community structure.

By eliminating transfers to back wards, regionalization and composite wards erase almost entirely the concept of the back ward patient. Some patients still become chronically hospitalized, but since they cannot be transferred, as in the past, they remain in view. In contrast, when many of the patients transferred from the back wards were first reevaluated, it was found that they were, and in some cases had been for years, candidates for various types of placement in the community. All that was wanting was sound discharge planning. Another aspect is that it is impossible to get rid of a "problem patient" by transferring him. Once a patient arrives on a ward, he remains the responsibility of the personnel of that ward and cannot be transferred. This minimizes the effects of rejection and provides a challenge to the staff.

One of the problems of setting up composite wards is the need to supply facilities for all sorts of patients on the same ward, including some of those that were previously provided in specialized wards. For instance, what would one do with a disturbed patient who needs a seclusion room? The obvious answer is to provide seclusion rooms on all wards. Otherwise one would have to send such a patient to a specialized disturbed ward and thus defeat the composite ward concept. In our case, it was possible to put a minimal number of seclusion rooms, usually one or two, into every ward. These rooms did not have to be of the maximum security type, for the general atmosphere of the ward and the interest of the patients and staff in newly admitted patients reassured most patients in a short time and made extensive use of seclusion rooms unnecessary. It was actually found that most seclusion rooms were not being used, especially during the day. Further, the therapeutic community structure with its patient government, its committee system, its emphasis on self-reliance and interdependence, creates a greater sense of social responsibility among the patients and lessens the necessity for stringent disciplinary or security measures. In addition, we should not minimize the effects of the modern potent tranquilizers, such as the phenothiazines, and the availability of injectable drugs.

In the process of reorganizing these wards, another problem, the open versus the closed door, had to be resolved. Usually the staff accepted a compromise. We found that even the most skeptical staff from a previously locked ward eventually were able to accept the patient door monitor concept and, in fact, ultimately became quite enthusiastic about it, because it not only changed the ward atmosphere but also saved the nursing staff much work locking and unlocking doors throughout the day.

When the California legislature passed the Short-Doyle (local mental health services) Act in 1957, state hospital administrators were somewhat less than enthusiastic. They had waged annual campaigns to secure seriously needed increases in funds for personnel, drugs, and facilities. Suddenly large increases in state mental health appropriations were to be made. But these funds were to be channelled to community agencies on the relatively uncertain assumption that local services might reduce state hospital admissions and shorten length of stay. From the inception of state-supported local mental health programs in California there has been ample evidence that state services and those organized under local jurisdictions held conflicting assumptions concerning one another's functions, operating orientations, and specific mental health missions.

Local programs face constant pressures from home town interests—the local government, which appropriates a considerable part of the annual budget; the various referral agencies, including schools, churches, courts and corrections agencies, and private practitioners, both psychiatric and non-psychiatric; and families and taxpayers. All of these influence the characteristics of the local program, including its service and programming priorities and its decisions concerning the use that may be made of state services. A much different configuration of influential forces is at work at the state level. It is obvious that the jurisdictional differences between state and local entities are actually basic and structural in nature. The two entities clearly possess different and somewhat irreconcilable sanctions and expectations. This does not, however, preclude the possibility that meaningful and mutually profitable work sharing can be achieved, so long as each party recognizes the essential separateness (autonomy) of the other and is willing to engage in negotiation calculated to produce tenable conciliation and compromise of differences. Among the most divisive factors hampering such conciliatory attitudes are the mutually inconsistent mythologies that tend to evolve within any two culture systems that share identical territoriality. Two examples, taken from the Agnews–San Mateo experience, may suffice to indicate this phenomenon.

Professionals within community-based services frequently imagine that closer ties with the state hospital will open up the flood-gates for a deluge of chronic patients who will displace the "good" candidates for intensive psychotherapy. Community personnel express the fear that they will soon be deploying all their treatment time into what they regard as the unrewarding work of "supporting" very sick patients and passing out pills. These fantasies and fears are expressed in many subtle acts and prove to be elusive, shadowy figments which cannot be easily or quickly exorcised. In a sense, it is fair to say that closer linkage with the state hospital does mean increasing the local visibility of the most impaired patients. Although the deluge of chronic patients does not seem to materialize, it is no fantasy to suspect that fewer hours will be available for the more functional and stable patients. The fantasy is twofold: that the community can afford to put its chronic and more severely ill patients out of sight, and that working with these patients is unrewarding.

Clearly, it is not reasonable to offer long-term intensive psychotherapy to most of these patients. Instead, the need is for activity groups, crisis intervention supplied by walk-in clinics, the utilization of regular or intermittent home visits by public health nurses and welfare workers, as well as a wide and still largely unidentified range of non-mental health services—vocational, recreational, social, medical, and religious, among others—that can help to produce an environmental situation within which such impaired individuals enjoy the highest probability of adequate independent functioning.

Education of mental health professionals is, therefore, urgently required, if these needs are to be well provided for in the community mental health era now dawning. This training must begin with the fundamental principle that the state and local programs inevitably share responsibility for every case that cannot be served in the voluntary and private sectors. It must also include an introduction to the new forms of professional gratification that result from achieving creative solutions to the thorny problems presented by these severely impaired groups. Finally, greater emphasis should be placed upon willingness to experiment with innovative demonstration projects that promise new solutions to the challenge of both meeting the needs of such patients in ways acceptable to them, and deploying scarce professional manpower so this can be accomplished.

Our second example of divisive mythology can be discerned

among the attitudes held by state hospital professionals. It is a somewhat different kind of fantasy and one which strikes a curious counterpoint to that harbored by the local program. It is the fear that the local program threatens to supplant the state hospital. Though it, too, is seldom explicit, it permeates certain actions and comments that can be noted by an observer. Nor does it wholly lack credence; indeed, the Joint Commission Report of 1960 recommended the big state institutions be phased out and, in California, a long-range plan for mental health (California Department of Mental Hygiene, 1962) set forth a similar goal of closing state hospitals. Stewart et al. (1968) report that because of a dramatic decline in the patient population of the state hospital at Weyburn, Saskatchewan, there are "strong indications that the hospital will be phased out in coming years."

State legislation enacted in 1968 makes it likely that by 1970 California state hospitals may be largely decentralized in such a way as to bring about a rather close and statutorily enforced union between local programs and the regionalized state services to which they relate. The trend in San Mateo has been (as described earlier under liaison and also in the succeeding paragraphs) to see the state hospital as a vital resource for specific purposes, rather than as a facility to be superseded. The continued operation of state hospitals as mental health facilities is further assured by the fact that they constitute the state's most valuable capital asset for mental health, coupled with the fact that utilization of the state hospitals continues to be high for a variety of categories of patients. Evidently, any reduction in state hospital admissions made by the various local programs has been more than offset consistently by the state's continuing population growth, coupled with the increasingly effective casefinding that inevitably accompanies the development of new local mental health services.

Another concern of state hospital staff is that expanded local programs will "siphon off the cream"—the acutely ill patients—and leave only the chronic and custodial cases for the state hospital. We will describe below the recent increased use of the state hospital for emergency observation cases. What has also evolved in San Mateo has been an appreciation of the state hospital as a high-quality resource for the treatment of those patients who need a longer period of time to reconstitute—and at a more leisurely pace. Further, some patients need a period of asylum, a moratorium from the pressures of family,

job, and society. Workers in community mental health, dedicated to
the principle of minimum separation of patients from their community, need to come to terms with the fact that some patients need a
prolonged separation.

There is still another invaluable function that the state hospital can serve, though it is less glamorous and infrequently stressed.
There appears to be a hard core of chronically disturbed and assaultive
patients who present tremendous problems in management and control. Included are some schizophrenics and patients with a variety of
diagnoses, such as chronic brain syndromes (other than senile) and
mental retardation with psychosis. The kinds of close supervision and
controls required by these patients are much more effectively provided
by state hospitals than by facilities in the community. Further, it is
important that one not close one's eyes to the need for including this
dimension of service in the spectrum of services to the mentally ill.

### Jurisdictional Difficulties

Jurisdictional differences are among the most common causes
of failure in undertakings such as we are discussing here. There is usually a lack of a formal, well-thought-out system of liaison and integration of services. Instead, the linking of state and local services, in many
communities, has been left to a kind of haphazard arrangement based
upon mutual good will and the possibility that people in each jurisdiction will possess sufficient skill, ingenuity, and ability to improvise
to iron out the interminable difficulties that come up.

In the light of the Agnews–San Mateo experience, it appears
that jurisdictional difficulties can be grouped under at least three
headings. Some are of an administrative and geographic nature, having to do with operating patterns and the distance between the two
cooperating entities. A second category of factors concerns the primi-
tive nature of operational statistics and information flow between the
two agencies. Finally, and most fatefully for both parties, there are
sometimes dramatic difficulties imposed upon both entities as the result of changes in federal, state, or local laws, regulations, and policies.

The local program supplies an important screening function
for the state hospital. In San Mateo, local, short-term inpatient and
day hospital services have been functional alternatives for relatively
large numbers of patients who, otherwise, would have been sent to

the state hospital. Beyond this, however, most of those who do go to the state hospital have received some prior local attention; in many cases, state services have been called into play only after a trial period in the local ward or day hospital has demonstrated the need for medium or long-stay hospitalization. In addition, approximately 5 per cent of all patients considered in need of full-time hospitalization are found, for a variety of reasons (but mostly involving issues of need for greater external controls) unmanageable on the county inpatient service. These patients are transferred directly to the state hospital after evaluation on the inpatient service or its intake service, the emergency room.

An evaluative study produced jointly by San Mateo and the State Department of Mental Hygiene (McInnes, Palmer, and Downing, 1964) reported that "for the period 1958 through 1962, San Mateo County experienced a reversal of the generally rising state hospital admission curve, with a net drop of 31 per cent, whereas other Bay Area counties rose 24 per cent. A study of the San Francisco–Oakland area for this period failed to reveal any demographic, social, economic, or judicial factors which might account for this change. We are encouraged to believe that the development of local public psychiatric services, especially inpatient treatment services, can reduce state hospitalization by a worthwhile degree."

Since this study was completed in the early sixties, San Mateo County's population has increased by more than 25 per cent. Although a second day treatment center has been phased into operation (in the North County Mental Health Center), there has been no comparable increase in local psychiatric inpatient beds. Consequently a growing number of individuals have been denied local hospitalization in peak admission periods, simply because all thirty-one beds have been filled. These patients must be sent to the state hospital, often directly from the emergency room, after an initial assessment has ascertained that nothing less inclusive than full-time hospitalization will serve their needs adequately.

This peremptory transfer of "untreated" cases actually violates what can be thought of as the unwritten contract formerly in effect between the two agencies and disrupts a heretofore effective cooperative pattern of service formed by the local program and the state hospital. The latter's work load is increased both by the increased numbers of patients and by no longer having the benefit of the case record and the preparatory evaluation done during a week or two of prior local hospitalization. This change, therefore, subtly modifies administrative flexibility concerning personnel time and work patterns, since the regionalized wards require additional staff hours when workups, formerly routinely available, suddenly become necessary for a growing number of new admissions. Setting up a contract, written or unwritten, is only as effective as the determination and the ability of both parties to live up to that contract.

These somewhat subtle effects, though often basically more important, can be overshadowed by certain more evident problems. Patients sent directly to the state hospital often are placed on seventy-two-hour legal "holds," a temporary involuntary status which can be imposed by law enforcement and public health officials. If the patient is in need of hospitalization but declines to stay after seventy-two hours, court commitment hearings must be held. Fortunately this does not often occur because most such patients will elect to remain on a voluntary basis. Nevertheless, when commitment was necessary, the hospital used to be required to transport patients back to San Mateo County for court hearings and then return them to the hospital. After several years of this awkward and expensive procedure, arrangements were made with the neighboring county, in which Agnews is located, to permit these legal steps to be taken there. San Mateo County agreed to reimburse its neighbor for this service.

Equally distressing are the rules governing eligibility for health and welfare services. It has not been uncommon for the hospital to be told that certain kinds of follow-up resources are unavailable to certain patients. In some cases, the patient was found to have resided in the county for less than one year, a proviso attached to certain welfare assistance categories. Indeed, residence restrictions seem sometime to have been cited by certain units in the mental health center as an excuse for denying aftercare services to "undesirable" candidates (although the local mental health service officially holds only that a person must be able to give a local address and show he is not simply a transient). Thus, the various eligibility factors and attitudes of local agencies can serve to sabotage the state-local relationship, and prove convenient subject matter for ambiguous and conflicting messages.

More realistic is the fact that some returning patients are actually ineligible for the kind of aftercare that has been planned for them prior to discharge. For example, a wife coming back home may seem to require the services of the adult outpatient clinic. However, if her husband's income is above a certain, yet often still modest, level, she would be required to obtain this needed outpatient service from the private sector. Such patients and their families are often only marginally motivated to carry out this kind of aftercare plan. The requirement that treatment be obtained privately often proves a convenient excuse, so the patient eludes the all-important post-hospital phase of treatment and, therefore, becomes a higher readmission risk. Moreover, most private practitioners in San Mateo were unwilling to supply services to such patients, especially when the follow-up needed (and acceptable to the patient) was drug supervision and brief (less than one-hour) supportive contact on a monthly or as-needed basis. Finally, the County Medical Society canvassed its members and compiled a short list of psychiatrists, internists, and general practitioners who were prepared to offer drug follow-up. Even more satisfactory was a sixty-day fee moratorium declared for returning state hospital patients by the local mental health services, so that all such services are now free for two months, regardless of financial status.

In one respect, San Mateo County's relative affluence has proved to be a liability in supplying optimum services to returning state hospital patients. It seems a fairly general rule that protected community living situations are likely to be in more generous supply in lower income neighborhoods. In middle- and upper-middle-class neighborhoods, such as abound in San Mateo County and in much of our nation's suburbia, families seldom wish to convert their homes into boarding homes and to take in ex-hospital patients in return for a monthly fee. In fact, neighborhood objections are often voiced on those rather infrequent occasions when a homeowner seeks the required zoning change to permit his dwelling to be licensed as a boarding home by the local welfare division. Similar objections are heard by local planning commissions and city councils when plans for new nursing homes, sheltered workshops, and halfway houses are announced. Consequently, it is especially difficult to meet the demand for placement of San Mateo County patients who do not need further hospitalization but who do require a protected and supervised setting.

One approach to overcoming this problem was taken by the

state hospital, which succeeded, after considerable negotiations with the local welfare administration in obtaining an agreement that local public assistance funds could be used to pay for placement of these patients in other counties. Even then it developed that the fee customarily paid by San Mateo County was lower than that paid by these other counties. Boarding and nursing home operators frequently refused San Mateo patients until further negotiations with the local welfare administration finally removed this inequity.

Though this solution was certainly a step forward in that it allowed a number of patients to leave the hospital, we regard placing patients outside of their home county and community as far from ideal. We believe middle- and upper-class suburbia should consider a whole new approach such as the satellite apartment program described in Chapter 6.

It must also be added that there is an inherent danger when agencies attempt to provide a multitude of residential, financial, and other services in the community to marginal and dependent persons. Agency personnel may unwittingly or deliberately foster inappropriate dependency and fail to maintain expectations that patients live up to their potential (see discussion of this issue in Chapters 5, 6, and 8). For instance, there may be a tendency to expect little from patients other than reasonably acceptable behavior in a boarding home—which can be like a small replica of a hospital back ward located in the community.

### Statistics and Information

An incredible aura of mystery surrounds state-local patterns of patient flow and service utilization. Data routinely collected from state and local services are not only reported back too late to be used in many day-to-day operational decisions but also are largely irrelevant. The wrong facts are gathered poorly and often with lack of uniformity of data collection and then used to influence decisions upon which they happen to have little or no bearing. This blunt criticism may shock some conscientious biostatistics people; nevertheless, it appears to apply in state after state and is explained in large part by the rapid changes taking place in mental health services all over the country.

Statistics routinely collected purport to indicate utilization of certain specific treatment facilities. They are data modeled after the utilization statistics historically required of individual acute hospitals. These kinds of data are neither complete nor accurate when one needs to know how a complex of state-local health services are responding to shared responsibilities for prevention and restoration, as well as treatment of illness. They are even less useful for mental hygiene agencies, which happen to be dealing with a variable range of chronicity. For instance, collecting mere admission and discharge figures for state hospitals tells one little. If mental illness were always an acute, short-term impairment—similar to a gall bladder problem, capable of being remedied by a surgical procedure—admission figures would be a relatively meaningful measure of the contribution made by the state hospital. Frequently, the most significant contribution that can be made by a modern state hospital may have less to do with actual treatment than with sound discharge planning and a "successful" community placement. Admissions in the abstract will say nothing about this. One must know how many of various categories of patients were admitted, whether these were first, second, or third (or later) admissions, how long individuals in these various categories remained in the hospital for each new admission, and how long—on an average—people in these various categories succeeded in remaining out of the hospital. Success with chronically impaired people is determined by knowing whether they stay out of the hospital longer, whether readmissions are of relatively brief duration and what improvement has taken place in their social and vocational adjustment in the community.

The fact that, for many, the impairment is destined to be a lifelong condition makes absurd any conviction that readmission equals a failure; yet this is precisely the conviction expressed by the idea that a state's goal is simply to reduce mental illness admissions. A state may conclude that a reduction in state hospital admissions is desirable. It must, at the same time, recognize that other non-state facilities will have to cope with a growing number of cases. This may mean that local welfare and nursing homes will provide the needed services. Local jails and relief homes or poor farms may be involved. Local mental health services may be involved. Regardless of which combination is improvised to supply alternative services, and sometimes (as in the case of local welfare services) this depends upon the fact that federal subsidies are more liberally accessible for one than for another, the cost of chronic illness cannot be avoided and mere rates of admissions to mental health facilities tell nothing about many of these costs. Further, state hospital readmission is often more desirable than the community alternatives.

This may seem somewhat remote from the question of jurisdictional conflicts, but, in fact, such conflicts have their very roots in the basic separateness of state and local services. To the extent information patterns can be designed to express the shared responsibility, data collection and reporting will help to minimize unnecessary conflicts. On the other hand, so long as state and local services harbor suspicions and, in fact, can point to clear evidence that one is aggrandizing at the expense of the other, no meaningful collaboration can be hoped for.

An example taken from the San Mateo–Agnews experience may portray the dangers inherent in this jammed communication predicament. In recent years, San Mateo's annual admissions to the state hospital have risen from a low of 86.6 per 100,000 population in 1964 to 147 per 100,000 in 1968. It has been San Mateo's lot to be singled out by a number of state and local spokesmen, who have suggested the county's rising admission rate is at least curious, if not actually reprehensible, in view of the extensiveness of the local mental health services.

During this period of rising state hospital admissions significant changes have been invoked in state operating policies. For instance, many more patients sent home are now officially discharged. Previously, many of these individuals had gone home on an indefinite leave status, and if subsequent rehospitalization proved necessary, they were not, of course, counted as new admissions. Today many admissions may involve repeated rehospitalization of a relatively small number of patients. Another factor has been a greatly increased emphasis on utilization of hospital staff personnel for discharge planning. This, coupled with increased service from community agencies, has resulted in speedier discharge, and of more patients, into the community. This too could be expected to result in higher readmission rates for obvious reasons.

Owing to the incomplete picture provided by the currently available statistics, it is impossible to give reasonable weight for rising admissions to state procedures, to local inadequacies, and to the known population increase in the county. Evidently all three variables are in the equation, but with the available data, one is at a loss to judge whether the condition is desirable or undesirable and, if the latter, where the problem might be eased most readily. Meantime, this lack of knowldge is the fuel from which the conflagrations of misunderstanding and futile debate as to who is to blame are kindled.

As it happens, the mysteries surrounding service utilization and patient flow can be remedied almost immediately. This is one conflict-generating variable that need not exist. Using electronic data processing programmed to fit the requirements of both acute and chronic illness (instead of the more familiar models used to measure acute hospital utilization), and to link all elements of service, whether preventive, therapeutic, or restorative and whether state, local, public, voluntary, or private, it is now possible to channel to all concerned—citizens and their elected representatives, as well as to professionals and their many agencies—the required information. So simple is this task that, under optimum conditions, it could be done nationwide within a matter of months. That it will be done is a foregone conclusion. That it may be delayed for years is an example of the price society is prepared to pay for our apathy and lack of leadership. Most regrettable, perhaps, is the fact that it evidently is destined to be done not by the mental health establishment, which would be likely to give some weight to the humanistic ethics of public service, but by those motivated primarily by dollar economics.

### Impact of New Laws

State and federal legislation may be partly influenced by the federal, state, and local mental health establishment. Often, however, the lawmaking machinery gives equal or greater weight to labor, industry, taxpayers' groups and other special interests; changes in laws, therefore, may impose a more or less unilateral mandate upon the state-local partnership to revise operational patterns, service priorities, and even basic therapeutic decisions. This is a source of difficulty that almost universally results in anxieties and frustrations. Whether or not the new laws are sound from a mental health point of view, major change is, in and of itself, disconcerting.

California is now witnessing the most sweeping changes in laws affecting mental health services since passage of the Short-Doyle Local

Mental Health Services Act in 1957. These laws will have the effect of imposing a fiscal and service union upon the local program and the regionalized state services. For instance, each county will, by law, have fiscal responsibility for all of its patients in the state hospital. Involuntary commitments will be armed with new safeguards, designed to protect the civil rights of the mentally ill.

These modifications will be further complicated by other health care laws, including Medicare and Medi-Cal (as Medicaid is known in California). Adding still other new variables to the complex programming formulas is the growing number of community mental health centers, being built with federal matching funds under Public Law 88-164; often these are under the administration of private hospitals and private practitioners (although they must guarantee to accept all patients within their catchment areas).

Local programs thus face the mandate to link private, voluntary, and public jurisdictions. State programs are evidently to be forced to relate to local jurisdictions in new patterns imposed statutorily. These are extremely difficult mandates, presenting so many new and still barely explored facets that one can only approach the future with grave concern. Clearly the lawmakers themselves are only vaguely aware of the problems these new legal mandates will present. Hopefully, the principles that have evolved through the expensive process of trial and error, as set forth in this chapter, will help state and local programs meet these new challenges.

We would like to close by reiterating what we regard as one of the most important lessons we have learned. Whether linked or not, the local public program and the state hospital serving the community must inevitably share responsibility for every severely impaired person needing treatment that cannot be obtained in the private and voluntary sectors. This basic and seemingly simple truth was recognized early in San Mateo; doing more than paying lip service to it was another matter. Waiting lists, as well as arbitrary decisions calculated to screen out "unsuitable" or "undesirable" candidates, are unacceptable expedients. Too often mental health professionals in local programs have felt that providing treatment for patients coming out of state hospitals is "somebody else's responsibility." We disagree. Local programs can attempt to develop and expand alternative resources in the community; they can become more skillful in utilizing pre-existing re-

sources, they have the option of redirecting or referring some candidates to more appropriate service alternatives. But they can not enjoy
the luxury of sending people away just because they choose to limit
their service to persons whom they find attractive to treat.

PART **II**

﷽

*A surprising number of dominant themes and principles of the therapeutic community recur at many points in community mental health. The very intent of community mental health—to elicit an increasing measure of community responsibility for prevention and treatment of mental illness—is a vivid recapitulation at the societal level of the therapeutic community: to help the individual (in this instance, the community as a whole) take increasing responsibility for himself and others by participating actively in meeting his needs and those of the community.*

*Here in San Mateo County, the local government and the Community Council (a social planning agency) recently published a study of comprehensive community health issues (Heath, 1965) in which the county as a whole was described as having the potential for*

58

# THE DIRECT
# SERVICES

becoming a therapeutic community ". . . which progressively discovers and exploits growing opportunities for strength and well-being. It does not simply prevent illness. It actively promotes the abilities people have for keeping well and for helping each other to do so. Its major investment is in increasing its own capacity as a total community to ward off disability by generating greater strength within individuals, within the various groups that collectively form its society, and within the institutions serving that society."

Clearly, the therapeutic community concept need not be limited only to mental health facilities. In San Mateo County, for instance, a highly successful adaptation of the therapeutic community was set up to meet the needs of the local jail population. The county sheriff's department, in 1962, opened an honor camp for selected jail inmates.

59

*Using consultative and educational services provided by the mental health service, this department soon fashioned a successful therapeutic community, using deputy sheriffs as counselors, employing small groups and the large community meeting to focus on problems and to propagate a helpful milieu.*

*There is certainly much emphasis nowadays upon self-help, coupled with the sturdy conviction that each individual, despite possible impairment, has, for the most part, unexploited potentials for healthy, productive, appropriate behavior. This intention is often expressed in the therapeutic community as working with the "well part" of the individual. Speaking to a San Mateo staff meeting several years ago, Maxwell Jones, the popularizer of the therapeutic community, remarked that when he read descriptions of the Peace Corps and its plans for generating grassroots self-help programs in the underdeveloped nations, he was astonished by the uncanny similarities between this and his own psychiatric treatment orientation. Indeed, the evolving therapeutic community approach shares many of its basic themes with the various movements in our present-day culture—the centers movement in mental health, the poverty program, the Peace Corps, among others. The careful reader will perceive echoes of the therapeutic community within many chapters of this book. This is both accidental and intentional, reflecting the reality of community mental health as it has come to flower in San Mateo; it also reflects a whole new spectrum of problem-solving tools that is slowly emerging from the still tentative marriage of such disciplines as psychiatry, psychology, sociology, and anthropology. Indeed, this new merging of different theoretical frameworks underlies such disparate manifestations as crisis theory, systems theory, family therapy, mental health consultation, research in the epidemiology of mental illness, as well as the therapeutic community.*

*In stressing community responsibility for prevention and treatment of mental illness, one obvious point seems at first glance unnecessary to raise, even paradoxical: mental health professionals share this responsibility. Yet, as the state hospital chapter suggests, there is often reluctance to work with certain types of "less attractive" patients. Moreover, in the chapters on services for children and program evaluation, we shall see that clinging to an evaluation and treatment model, ill-suited to the task of meeting the needs of the community as a whole,* can also result in mental health professionals partially abdicating their responsibility in the total community effort.

The chapters that follow introduce the staff's perception of their work in the various clinical and rehabilitation programs which actually employ therapeutic community principles. These include the inpatient ward, the day hospital, the halfway house, and the areas of nursing responsibility. Working with the healthy part of the individual is also exemplified in the vocational services. In later chapters, some of the same motifs recur—in the chapter on courts and corrections, in particular, but also in the exposition of the North County Mental Health Center, where self-help and responsibility-sharing form the basic philosophy of the total center.

The therapeutic community approach came early to San Mateo, partly because of the consultation of Harry Wilmer since 1955 and that of Maxwell Jones in 1959. At Wilmer's urging, the San Mateo psychiatric inpatient service became, in December, 1956, the first psychiatric ward in a county general hospital to use therapeutic community concepts. The opening chapter in this part addresses itself to some of the practical, specific issues and problems that have arisen in applying therapeutic community principles and methodology to community mental health clinical settings.

# CHAPTER 3

# Using Therapeutic Community Principles

*Harry A. Wilmer, H. Richard Lamb*

The term *therapeutic community,* which at first has an almost esthetic appeal, may wear poorly; like hearing the same poem recited endlessly. On first hearing it may be experienced as a brilliant and well-timed interpretation, but after a while it seems more like a tired cliché. Worse, some of its advocates betray a religious zeal while some of its detractors reveal an equally uncritical, emotional aversion. We hope that an exploration of significant day-to-day issues involved in the therapeutic community will be useful in deciding to what extent and in what ways its principles should be applied.

The therapeutic community has been discussed in detail by a

number of authors (Clark, 1965; Edelson, 1967; Jones, 1967; Kraft, 1966; Schwartz, 1957; Wilmer, 1958); we will not attempt such detail here. As described by Maxwell Jones (1958), the therapeutic community differs from other treatment orientations in that it: (1) is oriented to restore patients to more healthy, normal social roles by so altering the hospital or institutional structure that these roles are expected of the patient while he is still in the institution, by assuming, for example, that patients can help in the treatment of other patients and can share in decision-making with the staff; (2) is committed to the idea that socioenvironmental and interpersonal influences play an important, though not an exclusive, part in the treatment program; (3) is characterized by an atmosphere of intimate spontaneous face-to-face interactions in which lines of communication are relatively free and everyone has access to the total body of relevant knowledge in the life of the institution; and (4) is so designed that group therapy, group activities, and community meetings are essential elements in the propagation of its cultural themes.

The therapeutic community concept has had a profound influence on psychiatric hospitals and other mental health facilities. Just as there is a wide diversity of mental health facilities, correctional, and other institutions where the therapeutic community is used, so there is a great variety of therapeutic communities. Military hospitals, state hospitals, private hospitals, university hospitals, county hospitals, and correctional institutions are all different societies with different subcultures. The physical structure of the unit, the size of the staff, its training and turnover, the social class and status of staff, staff conflicts, and treatment orientation and goals are all significant variables. The age, sex, social class, status, and psychiatric disorders of the patient groups are likewise significant factors. Further, the total environment surrounding the unit, the community relationships, and the involvement of relatives differ from community to community. Consequently, the therapeutic community approach in the San Mateo inpatient service differs from that in the day hospital and that, in turn, differs from the halfway house. Therapeutic community concepts are generalizations which have to be translated into practice differently in each specific situation.

## The Open Door

Symbols are extremely important. The most popular symbol of the therapeutic community is the open door. However, not all open doors are truly open. Some are open only at certain times or under certain circumstances. Some open-door hospitals admit all patients; others are highly selective, rejecting grossly disturbed or violent patients. Nor is it certain that an open door is preferable for every psychiatric patient. Undoubtedly some selection of patients occurs by design or unwittingly in many open-door hospitals, either at intake or in the subsequent transfer of patients elsewhere. However, in some successful therapeutic communities the open door symbolizes free and open communication. Perhaps this is more important than the extent to which the door is in actuality open or locked.

To implement therapeutic community concepts effectively there must be administrative support from the highest administrative levels, including the executive head of the institution. Obviously there must be genuine support from the administrator and key staff of the unit itself. Sympathetic understanding and support must be real, not sham. The program involves inevitable risks, since relaxation of traditional security and external controls results in intermittent crises. Administrative understanding and support are necessary when a patient runs away from the unit, attempts or succeeds in committing suicide, or when personnel from other parts of the hospital or in the outside community react in fear or complain that the open door is, in fact, a dangerous, revolving door. Likewise there must be understanding inside and outside the unit that the community meeting is so vital that neither staff nor patients should be called out of it.

The therapeutic community unit in a larger institution has a more therapeutic potential if all the units throughout the institution share its basic principles. Isolated units may become divisive and engender feelings of envy, favoritism, exclusion, or frustration in other parts of the institution.

A critical factor is the gap between the ideals of a program and its actual operating practices. A blind dedication to the concepts of democracy makes it difficult to see that some situations require a practical, common sense use of staff authority. Likewise, a rigid belief that individual therapy should be totally eliminated from the unit and only group therapy and group process be utilized may blind the staff to the need for one-to-one psychotherapy or individual therapeutic relationships when this is appropriate and needed. In therapeutic communities, rigid rules and unquestioned faith in preconceived methods often produce bizarre results and unnecessarily impoverish cultural versatility.

A social system in a psychiatric hospital cannot function without authority. No society can exist without social controls. Though the goal is to foster self-control, there must also always be available some external controls including that of authority figures. Only with some form of authority and limit-setting do people feel safe or comfortable. This is as true for mental patients as it is for adolescents or children, or, indeed, for us all. Thus, a mental health unit, like any system of social organization, depends on finding ways of controlling, within limits, the impulses and drives of its individual members. The therapeutic community, in part, grew out of the need to create a social system where excessive and repressive external controls could be removed. However, today we often see a serious problem in therapeutic communities at the other extreme, where staff leaders for personal or ideological reasons are reluctant to use authority when it is clearly needed. This results in considerable staff and patient anxiety, and often needless and damaging patient regressions.

The examination of patient and staff roles and role conflicts is inherent in a therapeutic community where all persons are considered co-equals. But this means co-equals in sharing a sense of human dignity and worth, not co-equals in function or status. There must be in the therapeutic community, as in society, a reasonable division of labor. Social therapy is often the equal treatment of unequals. The concept of blurring of roles is useful and permits the relaxation of the rigid differentiation and hierarchy among the various disciplines and between staff and patient. In many cases, roles should and do overlap and hence are properly seen as blurred. But excessive role blurring makes for confusion as to who is responsible for what. In our experience, staff and patients function best when their basic roles are defined. Staff members need pride in their own disciplines—their own identities—and respect for the unique contributions which their specific training enables them to contribute to the total treatment process. This is important, for example, when nurses are co-therapists with social workers and psychiatrists in small group therapy or when social workers and doctors participate to some extent in the activity program normally executed by the nurses and activity staff.

A leader is essential, and difficulties arise when the leader, himself, or the group diminishes his leadership role. Although some communities minimize the personal factor of the physician or other professional in charge, he cannot abdicate crucial leadership functions without adversely affecting the community. In other communities, through some technical legerdemain, it only appears that his role is minimized. A wise leader is in command or clearly in charge when he feels that the situation demands such direction, as, for instance, during brief interludes of crisis or unexpected danger. This may involve revoking, temporarily, authority normally delegated to other community members. Of course, other community members may see it differently and question the need for him to impose his authority in this way. In such instances he must be willing to listen and sincerely consider all opinions and feelings and not listen in pretense or as a ritual. Thereafter, he must be willing to change his opinion or, on the other hand, adhere to it despite total opposition if he is convinced this is necessary. If either leader or staff or both believe that all members of the community have an equal voice in all decision-making, then certain responsibilities which properly rest with the leader are abdicated.

Delegation of responsibility to the group or to other individuals is extremely important, but the leader can delegate no more than that which he is strong enough to possess. If the leader delegates responsibility to others not because it is appropriate to do so but because he is weak or indecisive or depressed, he has abdicated his leadership functions. Anxiety is generated within the community of patients and staff when there are doubts as to the leader's capacity for leadership. Paradoxically, when staff sense a lack of appropriately strong leadership, they often complain not that the leader is abdicating his responsibilities but rather that the leader is too authoritarian. This same paradox is more familiarly encountered in the way many patients ask for limits and leadership. Both the staff and the leader must recognize that a complaint of too much authoritarianism may be a valid complaint, but on the other hand it may express the direct opposite of what the community of patients and staff really wants and needs.

## Democracy and Patient Responsibility

The concept of democracy in the therapeutic community is not necessarily the same as political democracy (Binner, 1967) and does not mean that staff elect their leaders nor that every patient and staff member has an equal voice in making every decision. When a unit is working well, many decisions can and should be made by consensus of staff or sometimes of the entire community of staff and patients. However, many decisions must be made by the leader of the community or by members to whom these decisions are delegated. The concept of democracy in a therapeutic community should mean that all members of the community are given an opportunity to voice their opinions and that the people making the decision will listen to and consider these opinions. Any deception in this area may have serious consequences. Furthermore, as described by Edelson (1967), the therapeutic community, and in particular the community meeting, "provides the opportunity for those who are directly responsible for making any decision to consult with those who would be affected by it and whose support is required to implement it." Thus, it makes possible as wide a base of consent as is needed to support the decisions of those whose responsibility it is to make those decisions.

Perhaps no problem in a therapeutic community is more vexing than deciding what responsibility should be delegated to patients and how to do this. In considering this problem, we find it useful to recognize at least three different kinds of situations, each of which requires a different approach. First an acute inpatient service which serves both as a receiving ward and an acute treatment ward with a rapidly changing patient population: an example is the San Mateo County inpatient service, where there are approximately a hundred admissions a month to a thirty-one-bed unit with an average patient stay of about seven days. Here the amount of responsibility that patients can take varies from group to group and from day to day. At times, a number of patients are able to assume responsible leadership roles, and the ward seems stable. At such times a considerable amount of responsibility can be delegated to patients. A week later these patient leaders may have gone home and the ward may be full of acutely psychotic or passive patients unable to assume such leadership. Then the staff must feel free to intervene and assume responsibilities that had been delegated to patients quite successfully a week before. Unless this flexibility is present, the patients may never be able to assume responsibilities or the ward may disintegrate into psychotic chaos. The staff at all times must be honest and straightforward about what they are doing. For example, if, either because of lack of leadership potential or because of the disruptive leadership of a sociopathic patient, patients are about to elect some very psychotic patient as patient chairman, the staff must be able to intervene forthrightly, frankly stating what they are doing and why.

The second general kind of situation where therapeutic community principles can be utilized is in a day hospital or a less acute and crisis-oriented ward. Here slower patient turnover and longer patient stay make for more continuity of patient leadership, and patients are more significant culture carriers of the institution, assuming more ongoing patient responsibility.

Yet even here, contrary to the experience of some where patients are allowed, or at least are said to be allowed, to make what are commonly known as "medical decisions" or "treatment decisions," we feel that treatment decisions such as when a patient is ready for discharge, or when a patient should have a pass to return to a highly charged family situation, generally must be decided by staff. This is due, in part, to the swift pace of the treatment programs, the constant need for rapid reevaluation of appropriate goals for each patient (a process in which the patient himself participates with staff), and the extensive knowledge of the community resources which is possessed by the staff and not shared by the patient group.

Patients may be asked for their advice, and this may be invaluable. But relinquishing these decisions totally to patients often represents an abdication of responsibility for decisions which even experienced professionals may have difficulty in making. This can be a manifestation of ambivalence, passivity, or inadequacy on the part of leader or staff or both. For instance, a patient may have received what is believed to be maximum benefit from an institution, but has become very dependent on the institution and is afraid to leave. He may be able to evoke guilt, shame, or uncertainty in both patients and staff when his separation from the institution is considered. Suppose, in this situation, the staff feels unable to take definitive action and move the patient on to the next step in his rehabilitation program. It is even less likely that the patient group could do better if the decision was delegated to them. Staff inability or unwillingness to act is detrimental to both the patient, by fostering dependency, and to the other patients, by giving them the message that they can also avoid leaving the institution and rehabilitating themselves if they, too, can succeed in making enough people feel guilty. Moreover, it may subtly diminish the respect for the competence of the staff. Perceiving the staff as weak, patients may as a result regress in various ways.

What kinds of decision-making and responsibility can be delegated to patients? We find that patients can often deal effectively with disruptive behavior in a group situation, especially if the disruptive behavior directly affects other patients. The group can examine such behavior and help the patient understand and better handle the situation. Cultural norms invoked by patients serve as potent means of limit-setting and the normalizing of behavior within the group. Patients are able to plan for their recreation and make suggestions or even changes in the administrative structure of patient government.

A halfway house is a third general kind of situation where therapeutic community principles can be used. Here residents should be able to handle most of their day-by-day household affairs—meal planning and preparation, cleaning up, assigning and monitoring housekeeping tasks. Again, it is crucial for staff to make clear what responsibility is and what is not being delegated to patients. For instance, giving them responsibility for meal planning does not mean that the patients have the power to decide to no longer plan and cook the meals. In our halfway house, patients vote to recommend suitable sanctions and restrictions and in some instances may even recommend that disruptive patients be ejected from the residence. These recommendations, it should be noted, involve problems of daily living of all residents rather than individual treatment decisions which may not directly affect other patients. Staff reserves the power of veto but uses it sparingly and only when patient recommendations are grossly inappropriate. It should be mentioned that staff experienced considerable uneasiness until they finally came to terms with the fact that the halfway house resident group could not be completely self-governing— that it was necessary to carefully delineate what powers should be delegated and in which areas staff should retain the power of veto.

We have found that an extremely important part of delegating responsibility to patients is consistency as to how much and what kind of responsibility is actually being delegated to them. If powers are delegated, they should not be withdrawn or changed even if staff does not agree with the patients' decisions. Patients, like anyone else, will avoid painful decisions such as might be called for in dealing with the disruptive behavior of guilt-provoking fellow patients, if they feel staff will step in and get them "off the hook" whenever the patient group falters. (As noted above, the rapidly changing treatment milieu of the brief stay, acute inpatient service is an exception to this principle.) Knowing that the staff will not rescue them, the patient group will feel the commitment to deal with the situation themselves and take the responsibility for making appropriate decisions.

Because of the emphasis on the power of the socioenvironmental and interpersonal influences in the therapeutic community, the importance of drugs is frequently underestimated (Fleishman, 1968), especially if one's ideology is that therapy without drugs is better than therapy with drugs. The therapeutic community concept could be effectively utilized, we believe, in a community mental health setting without the use of drugs, but such a policy would greatly restrict the number and type of patients who could be successfully treated in a day hospital, an open-door inpatient service, or a halfway house. The liberal use of the phenothiazines, in particular, makes it possible to treat many acute and chronic schizophrenic patients who would otherwise need the controls of a locked ward. The introduction of thorazine in the mid-fifties played a leading role in making the therapeutic community a widespread success for acutely disturbed patients in settings with minimum external controls.

### Community Group Meeting

A community group meeting where all patients and all staff (insofar as possible) attend and participate is a central part of most therapeutic communities. Although this meeting has a ritualistic significance, it is in addition a very powerful and effective way of translating the concepts of the therapeutic community into action. Our experience, like that of most others, has led us to believe that the community group should focus on "here-and-now" reality issues. To classify the purposes of the community group meeting, we list four points:

First, the meeting deals with patient resistances to making optimum use of the community. These defenses or resistances may be
manifested as disruptive behavior of psychotic or sociopathic individuals or the formation of cliques. The group may be overwhelmed by
a number of new patients either because of the frightening nature of
their illnesses or the sheer number of new people to be absorbed into
the group. Anxiety over the disappointing outcome of treatment when
a patient is transferred to the state hospital or has had an exacerbation of psychosis may lead to reactions of depression and guilt, in the
community of patients and staff, about the treatment that failed. If
these issues are brought into the open and freely discussed, there is
usually a considerable sense of relief in the group. Further, if the
treatment failure was related to the patient refusing to take his medication or follow other treatment recommendations, this can be an
opportunity to educate the patient group by pointing this out.

Patients are relieved to see that the staff is not too threatened
or frightened by these issues to allow them to be discussed and to examine both staff and patient behavior and reactions. This is especially
important when implicit or explicit criticism of the staff is involved.
Many patients come from families marked by faulty communication
where it was hardly ever safe to freely discuss crucial issues. Free discussion constitutes a new experience for these patients and is therapeutic for them over and above its contribution to the welfare of the
group. Getting the resistances and conflicts out in the open and clarified usually makes it possible to resolve them in a way which is understandable to both patient and staff. On the other hand, if the staff
is truly threatened or unable to act because of staff conflict, bringing
this conflict into the open can be therapeutic. Patients may be dumb-
founded and horrified, but then patients usually sense the staff's problems anyway. Moreover, the patients may be relieved to see that the
staff can be anxious and human, too. However, the staff should not
use the community meeting to try to resolve serious intrastaff conflicts.

Second, the community meeting may be extremely valuable in
promoting an *esprit de corps,* a sense of belonging coupled with pride.
A group of people who have had the experience of discussing difficult
subjects together and resolving them feels a greater sense of closeness,
a greater sense of being a group.

Third, the community group meeting can be used as a way of

establishing and consolidating the culture and philosophy of the unit. Patients may catch on very quickly to the culture of the unit. However, their impressions may be distorted or they may not understand what seems distasteful to them or what they do not wish to understand. A frank exposition by staff, and hopefully by patients, as to the group's expectations of the individual, of the purpose of the program, and how patients can best make use of the institution is important. This is particularly so in the development and evolution of a new treatment program. Staff should remember, however, that occasional or perhaps even frequent reinforcement and reinterpretation of the treatment philosophy is necessary as long as the therapeutic community exists. In San Mateo, for instance, the treatment philosophy varies with the service, but each service generally expects patients to involve themselves in the treatment program, to take as much responsibility as they are able, to be active rather than passive, and to make full use of their potential. As this philosophy is put into action, frank discussions in staff meetings as well as in the community meetings are essential to firmly establish these concepts as part of the working culture of the unit. Daniels and Rubin (1968) point out that this use of the meeting for indoctrination of treatment philosophy is often not frankly acknowledged.

Fourth, sometimes when there seem to be no major resistances or interferences in the community, when *esprit de corps* is high, and the culture is understood and accepted by both patients and staff, when patient leadership is effective and the staff is working in harmony, the group may approximate the more traditional forms of dynamic group psychotherapy. Issues such as fear of leaving the institution, anxiety about the "outside world," and dread of recurrence of illness can then be freely and meaningfully discussed. Members of the group are able to feed back to each other information and feelings about their interpersonal relationships both in and outside of the community meeting.

Caution has been expressed by some (Edelson, 1967) against using the community meeting as a decision-making body. We agree in general, but feel that it is a mistake to impose this restriction as an absolute prohibition. From time to time there are issues that can and should be decided in the community meeting. For instance, an urgent issue, which would ordinarily be resolved by a decision by the patient government, may come up at a time when this decision cannot wait for the next patient government meeting. Some crises arise during a community meeting. In such instances, avoiding a here-and-now review and decision may be evasive and deceptive. Some issues should not be decided without total community consensus. For instance, a club from a local high school of students who aspire to be doctors and nurses may want to visit the unit and see it in operation. The staff may agree, but if permission is given without consultation with the community, the patients may feel used and exploited by the staff. Such topics must be discussed at the total community group meeting with the staff's unequivocal position that the patients are free to say no. After all, it is primarily their community.

The conventionally trained mental health professional often feels lost in large groups because he does not know the histories of individual patients. Of course, knowing the history and specific conflicts of individual patients is extremely useful in understanding what is going on, but what takes precedence is awareness of what is going on in the current community history. It is important to know what happened in the previous community meeting and before the present meeting. A staff meeting just before the community group meeting for a review of the events of the past twenty-four or forty-eight hours is a useful technique. Attention may be directed then to specific incidents on the unit and to individual and social behavior patterns, such as dominance, passivity, aggressiveness. It is important to learn who are the group leaders and how they are functioning, what cliques are present and how they are affecting the group. Is there a feeling of closeness in the group, or are the patients operating as isolated individuals? Is there tension between various individuals or cliques? Is the tone of the group active or passive, with the patient group looking to the staff for dependency gratification, guidance, and limits? How and what limits are being set and how effective are they?

Rapoport (1960) has provided a useful way of understanding the community in his description of the phenomenon of oscillation: the fluctuation or phases of a social organization from integration to disruption to reorganization. This is characteristic of the natural history of groups of all types. In the phase of integration, the unit is cohesive and relaxed; the members of the community actively participate in the program and strive toward therapeutic goals. In the phase

of distintegration, the opposite is found. Assessing a unit in these terms
can lead to staff decisions as to how various situations should be handled. For instance, staff may need to be more authoritarian and directive in a period of disorganization than in a period of integration.
Oscillation is caused by a combination of factors; among the more important are turnover in staff, staff dissension, such crises as a suicide
or patients relapsing into psychosis, and the influx of new patients,
especially when they are persons who are disruptive or difficult to
integrate into the group.

Lack of appreciation of the phenomenon of clique formation
within a community can lead to considerable difficulty in understanding community behavior. Cliques, as described by Wilmer (1966),
are usually composed of three members and form by attraction around
one dominant often highly popular, high status, verbal individual
whose behavior or belief system is deviant from that of the leader or
the emerging group norms. Cliques may include staff when the staff
is in conflict. Cliques tend to be unstable, to oppose the therapeutic
aims of the culture, and hence, they are social elements of resistance
and defense. They may be perceived and analyzed in a large group
meeting in this context. Not all small subgroups are cliques. Many
free-forming small subgroups, usually of four to six members, are primary groups whose behavior and belief system establish the group
norms. These subgroups may be based upon mutuality, and the relationship of these subgroups with each other or with other individual
patients can be dominant cohesive forces in the larger group. These
free-forming small subgroups tend to increase group morale, cohesiveness, and effectiveness. Against this force are set the cliques. What fosters cliques fosters disorganization. Ignoring, denying, or punishing
cliques tends to facilitate their growth. They represent the real and
symbolic aggressive, destructive elements in group life and the nidus
of vicarious acting out of impulses for the rest of the group. Because
of this—and especially when group tension is high or aims are frustrated—they are fostered and encouraged by the more passive patients. It is better to discuss these cliques freely and identify them in a
large group meeting. Occasionally one or more patients of the clique
may need to be excluded from the community. Such a need would
occur when, for example, a sociopathic individual consciously tries to

disrupt the group, and group pressure or staff intervention is unable to modify or set limits on his destructive behavior.

The group is most effective when the staff is active and spontaneously participates. In our experience, patients find it difficult to understand and accept a stolid, reflective staff which limits itself to well-timed interpretations. Though it is desirable that important issues be brought up by the patients, if they are unable to do so then the staff should feel free to take the initiative. Equally important is the staff's ability to express their own feelings. But there is an element of balance here, since staff must not talk too much or be meddlesome. Above all, the staff must not use the meetings for their own group psychotherapy to resolve serious intrastaff conflict. Most arguments between parents are best resolved away from the children, especially when these are neurotic conflicts concerning the management of the children. This applies to the therapeutic community as well. Nor is this the same as hiding intrastaff conflict from the patients, because, if the patients sense such conflict in the group meeting, it is wise to acknowledge it. As we have observed, direct statements acknowledging staff conflicts and anxieties can be anxiety-relieving and therapeutic. The point is that to the extent that such conflict can be resolved in staff meetings without patients present, to that extent the staff is free to devote their energies in the group to patients' problems, and patients are not burdened by the problems of staff.

What sort of feelings should the staff feel free to talk about? If a significant staff member or patient is leaving, the staff can talk about the sense of loss, and the concern about who will take that person's place. If a patient has disappeared, it is helpful if both staff and patients express their concern. The staff should serve as mature, healthy models for the patients. The staff's active participation and ability to express feelings and thoughts openly free the patients to do the same in the group meeting and outside of it.

What kinds of interpretations should the staff make? Perhaps the word *interpretation* is misleading, since it implies a technical intervention in a psychotherapeutic process that leads to the clarification and resolution of unconscious conflict. This is not the primary purpose of the group meeting. The staff activity in the group meetings is aimed at a resolution of ward problems and of whatever resistances are hindering free communication. It is aimed at facilitating psychological thinking so that patients can begin to understand themselves and others, individually and in group relationships. This type of staff activity also serves an educational function in the creation and maintenance of the philosophy and culture of the unit.

Although mental health professionals should be trained to be alert to unconscious processes, it is important to emphasize to all students of group therapy (and individual therapy) the simple statement that the *unconscious is unconscious*. This artless and deceptively obvious statement of fact is commonly unappreciated. Failure to appreciate this homely statement accounts for some of the mistrust of psychiatrists and mental health professionals. For example, in a community meeting in a prison, a patient recounted a series of unhappy, broken marriages to older women who dominated and frustrated him. Finally he married a woman who, in fact, was a prostitute and, unable to dissolve the marriage, he attempted to murder one of her occasional lovers and was sentenced to prison. In the group the inmates quickly perceived the pattern of his marital wayfaring, and the leader made an interpretation that this was an "unconscious search for his mother." Whether this interpretation was correct or not is beside the point, for to focus the group on this dimension moved it into an intellectualized "expert land." It was useless though interesting. The group simply ignored it as clever but irrelevant. Further, the patient's search for his mother was not even unconscious to him. It was simply an abhorrent thought that he himself already knew consciously. What was unconscious was unconscious and not even known to the therapist. It could not be fully known unless the therapist were able to explore this man in depth. Otherwise, this dallying with the unconscious is at best a clever guess, a bit of pleasurable reassuring talk for the therapist. But its danger is that it makes the group suspicious and resistant, or they latch onto the jargon and talk "psychologese," and avoid real conflicts which they could comprehend.

In "uncovering" psychotherapy, the therapist presumably aids the individual to gain insight into his unconscious conflicts by helping him to unlink the early influences from the contemporary reenactment. In this kind of resolution, the therapist is concerned with helping the patient recognize at both the conscious and unconscious levels that today's reality and circumstances are necessarily different from that highly charged and painful reality of childhood which occasioned the maladaptive behavior pattern.

The therapeutic community focuses upon the group and its contemporary history and does not delve into antecedents or intrapsychic aspects of impairment. Instead, the life experience within this special kind of supportive community supplies recurring incidents in which individual members of the community are led to the testing of old behavior patterns and, through what might be thought of as experiential learning, come to a heightened awareness of their inappropriateness and lack of value in making productive or positive adaptations to one's contemporary life predicaments. We would guess that this experiential process is at the heart of what is actually therapeutic for patients in any form of psychotherapy, irrespective of the therapist's theoretical orientation or the extent to which he attempts to reconstruct the past by interpretation.

Staff should feel free to set limits on inappropriate or uncontrolled behavior, preferably in collaboration with the patients. There is much to be said for patients' influencing each other through group pressure as a means of social control. However, when a patient is too psychotic or utterly out of control or excessively disruptive, then the staff must institute definite measures to prevent the group from dissolving into chaos.

Occasionally a topic of discussion can be too threatening for the group to handle. For instance, one of the authors (H.R.L.) once led a group on an acute inpatient service to which had recently been admitted a woman who had thrown her eighteen-month-old baby off the Golden Gate Bridge. She told how the child had fallen down a flight of stairs and was, according to the mother, dead when she found the baby at the bottom of the stairs. She had not called a doctor to examine the child but instead had rushed to the bridge with the body and thrown it into the bay. The body of the child was never recovered. She then made a bizarre suicide attempt and was brought to the hospital. When her situation was openly discussed in the group, it led to a morbid discussion of death wishes toward children and the brutal treatment some patients had received as children. The intensity of the anxiety and guilt that were generated in the community was never resolved despite attempts at talking about it in subsequent meetings. The mother, who presumedly had killed her child, could not be integrated into the patient group and became increasingly isolated following the meeting. On succeeding days, meetings were silent and unproductive until the mother was transferred and the rapid patient turnover resulted in an essentially new group. In retrospect, a well-timed staff intervention could have kept the group discussion within the bounds of what the patient group could tolerate and would have been an appropriate, therapeutic way of handling this situation. For instance, at the moment when the group moved from the tragic event to a discussion of their own childhoods and death wishes, the leader could have shifted the focus to the social-cultural level: "Let's talk about how one accepts strangers in our midst who arouse almost unbearable anxiety." Even with this intervention, the community might not have been able to cope with this matter. In that event, the better part of wisdom would have been for the leader to acknowledge that the community could not deal with it and move on to something else.

### Community Group Leaders

Just as the community as a whole needs a leader, so also does the community group meeting. Leaders must feel comfortable about leading and not feel that if a particular group is in need of leadership, there is something wrong either with the group or himself. To be a leader, one must be able to set limits on behavior. Problems arise, for example, when a leader cannot end the group at a definite prescribed time (a social limit) and rationalizes his ambivalence and inability to act as "therapeutic permissiveness" or as a means of fostering patient "responsibility." In fact it may be symptomatic of a therapist's passive-aggressive neurotic conflicts, his fear of responsibility, or fear of not being liked—all of which must be projected onto the patients. A variation on this theme is the often bizarre ending in groups in which leaders are seduced at the "end" of the meeting by manipulative patients who take over and continue the group. Patients learn the leader can be "had" by the simple expedient of introducing "interesting," "important," or "significant" contributions in the closing moments of the group. But if he were to adhere to a definite stopping point, patients would be compelled to bring things up within the allotted time.

Jones (1967) points to the importance of skills and experience in group work on the part of the leader and his consultant if the meeting is to be effective. The leader should use his psychotherapeutic skills to help focus the group on the crucial issues at any given time. At the same time, he should make the staff feel comfortable in participating in the meeting and help them to understand they are not intruding upon his province when they speak.

To reiterate, it is vital that neither staff members nor patients be called out of the group or be unnecessarily absent from the group, and that interruptions of any sort be kept to a minimum. To do otherwise devalues the group in the eyes of both the patients and the staff and gives a mixed message as to the importance of the community meeting and the principles of the therapeutic community itself. Both the staff of the unit and the people in positions of higher administrative authority must agree about and cooperate in this matter.

A perplexing problem for therapeutic communities is that of announcements. If an announcement is made at the very beginning of the group meeting, it is apt to influence the total hour. If it is made at the very end, when there is no time for discussion and reaction, it may be seen as autocratic or as diminishing the significance and emotional impact of all that happened during the hour. It is preferable to bring up announcements while there is still time for reaction in the group meeting—so that no more dust is raised than can be settled. However, the timing ultimately depends on what is happening in the hour and announcements should not intrude into an important flow of material. Perhaps the most important aspect is that, whichever way announcements are made and at whatever time, there be general agreement in the staff and a consistent policy.

## Staff Meetings

A therapeutic community, we believe, includes staff meetings that exclude patients. If held, as recommended by Jones (1967), immediately after the community meetings, these meetings become an exercise in social psychotherapeutic learning and training. Such staff reviews or critiques should direct the attention of all levels of staff to any distortions, misunderstandings, misapprehensions, or technical errors.

We have observed therapeutic communities whose policy was that all staff review meetings should include the patients. But we noted that when the patients were in the staff meetings, the staff subsequently had their own "secret" private staff meetings under the guise of a luncheon chat or a social gathering in the evening. Since these discussions are informal, not all staff are present. Further, a sense of uneasiness or guilt is felt in the staff, who sense or are aware that they are doing something that they say they should not be doing. Moreover, lack of consensus in the staff about including patients in staff meetings may lead to a covert power struggle which undermines the whole community.

Perhaps in the ideal therapeutic community there would be no need for staff meetings without patients present, but in actuality we have never seen such a therapeutic community. We believe that staff need a place where intrastaff conflicts can be candidly aired and worked out, where they can give each other mutual support and where they can speak without the inhibitions which professionals feel in the presence of patients. By having staff meetings without patients, one avoids the sham of professing one thing while secretly and unconsciously doing something else.

The staff often need to be able to talk about important issues themselves before they can help the patients to do this. For instance, if a highly respected and important member of the staff is about to leave, and the staff have not yet come to the point where they themselves can talk about it, they cannot be of much help in assisting patients to talk about it. In the staff meeting the staff should strive to talk freely about feelings toward other staff and patients. It is a place where the roles of the staff can be further defined and explored, where staff can determine who is responsible for what.

As already described, therapeutic communities fluctuate in their stability, tension, and strife and go through periods of oscillation, social disintegration, reconstitution, and restitution. When the cycle is lived through and talked through, not only by the entire community but also by the staff meeting separately, there is an increase in the group's and the staff's confidence in their ability to manage dyssocial, neurotic, and psychotic behavior.

It is important that the staff not analyze each other's character defenses. Trying to analyze what is unconscious in another staff member may be devastating, especially in a group of his co-workers. Staff members ought to feel comfortable about discussing aspects of their work—raising questions as to whether another staff person was defensive in the group meeting, whether he should have responded to or perhaps ignored a certain point or suggesting that he became over-involved at one stage and, at another, completely missed a significant issue. This can and should be done without attempting a character analysis of that staff member, questioning his motivation, his personality, his problems with men, women, or authority. When people get to know each other and feel comfortable with each other they can comfortably hear and benefit from comments based upon the reality of the situation and the straightforward issues of human relationships and technique. Character analysis in a staff meeting usually provokes a negative response in not only the person to whom it is being directed but the rest of the group as well; it is an effective way to silence meaningful discussion. In short, a staff critique meeting is not a staff psychotherapy group.

Therapeutic communities have been frequently described by many writers. They have become commonplace in community mental health. Yet each one tends to take on characteristics which, in certain respects, diverge from the descriptions found in the literature. Indeed, some of the least successful therapeutic communities are those that seem to have followed the templates obsessively, declining to admit the need for idiosyncratic mutations in response to unique local factors.

There appears to be no one "right" way to apply therapeutic community principles. We in San Mateo have felt free to adapt these principles to our particular setting and patient population and to our own personality styles, both individually and as a group. The therapeutic community, in our view, need not be a specific program or doctrine; it can simply be an orientation out of which programs may be evolved in response to local realities and in accordance with the unique attributes and needs of each community and each institution.

# CHAPTER 4

# Inpatient and Emergency Services

*Richard J. Levy, Dorothy M. Asbury,*
*Gerald Lutovich*

ʃ❋ʃ❋ʃ❋ʃ❋ʃ❋ʃ❋ʃ❋ʃ❋ʃ❋ʃ❋ʃ❋ʃ❋ʃ❋ʃ❋ʃ❋ʃ❋ʃ❋ʃ❋ʃ

In San Mateo, the inpatient service provides twenty-four-hour hospital care and certain services closely affiliated with that type of care, specifically, pre-admission services, emergency services, and legal commitment procedures.

The county hospital in California has statutory responsibility to provide detention for persons on mental illness, inebriate, and habit-forming drug petitions, pending examination by court-appointed physicians and a court hearing. Further, a person felt to be mentally ill and a danger to the person and property of himself and others can be signed into the hospital on an emergency basis for a seventy-two-hour period of observation by a peace officer or a deputy health officer. In either case, there is no requirement that the person receive treatment, and in the years prior to 1956, mere detention was the primary function of the hospital experience. If the allegations of a petition were sustained, commitment to a state hospital was effected. Similarly, a person on a seventy-two-hour hold was either released or placed on a petition.

In San Mateo, the opening of a new thirty-bed inpatient unit in 1956 closely coincided with several major trends in psychiatry. These included: (1) the recent development and medical acceptance of potent tranquilizers which made early treatment in local hospitals practical and effective; (2) a renewed interest in dealing with the ambient factors of the institutional approach to mental illness to maximize the therapeutic potential inherent in a treatment experience; (3) passage of state legislation subsidizing local voluntary psychiatric care (Short-Doyle Act, 1957). These events led to the emergence of the psychiatric inpatient unit as a resource for the care of severe psychiatric problems within the community where diagnostic and therapeutic efforts could be applied without delay, where family and local resources were readily available to aid in evaluation, resolution, and disposition of problems. Voluntary hospitalization was emphasized. Involuntary status, when it existed, became a part of the treatment problem rather than simply a basis for disposition.

The San Mateo unit was opened as a therapeutic community. Use of a psychiatric receiving unit in a county general hospital as a therapeutic community with an open door was no small innovation in 1956. It was necessary to enlist complete support of local authorities at the same time that the staff explored much difficult and unknown territory. When the trial was first reported (Young, 1959), mention was made of the work necessary to educate hospital staff, local police departments, and the community at large to the meaning of the effort. The endeavor was considered highly successful, with favorable response from most persons involved. Young makes several interesting observations in his report. He notes that much effort was required to reorient professionals to modify their role relationship with patients to mobilize the maximum active participation of the patient in his own care and in assuming responsibility for others as an essential element in maintaining an open-door program. Personnel without specific psychiatric training who were mature and could be comfortable in a setting which made great psychological demands on them were preferred. No untoward events were reported, although many "unauthorized absences" were mentioned; he claimed 99 per cent of the potential patient population could be successfully handled in an open unit. A later description of the program was made by Newton (1963).

As the inpatient care program developed, alternatives to hospitalization were being expanded. These further changed the role of the county hospital in the care of the mentally ill. The inpatient staff had little involvement in cases prior to their admission, and the disposition of court cases was out of the staff's jurisdiction. More effective service would be possible in a situation in which staff had more involvement in early intake and discharge process. As a result, in 1959, by arrangement with the district attorney's office, staff social workers began screening all involuntary petition requests. In 1960, a home visit program was established. These efforts were effective in developing alternatives to hospitalization and in improving staff's ability to work with cases hospitalized. Ward psychiatrists, in addition to the court-appointed physicians, appeared in court to report their observations and to make recommendations. This close working relationship with the court produced a climate of growing mutual understanding, in which each party came to a greater appreciation of the other's role in the handling of involuntary problems. This, in turn, led to important innovations.

Alternatives to commitment for involuntary cases were actively utilized. A judge can "continue" a case without acting on the petition. Patients on continuance can be further evaluated or treated and alternatives to commitment explored with ongoing supervision of the case by the court. With the problem evaluated in all respects and alternatives to commitment presented, the court is in a position to make an informed decision specific to the needs of the patient. The judges in San Mateo, realizing they were not dealing with hopeless situations with little choice, took an exceptional interest in their work. A hearing, instead of being a confused and painful ritual, became an important means of defining for their patient and the family the issues involved in his illness and of providing for all a chance to participate in the decision-making process. Legal and clinical issues could be clarified and dealt with as appropriate.

The program was further enriched in 1959, with the development of a residency affiliation with Stanford University. This increased staff coverage and made possible the development of twenty-four-hour psychiatric staffing of the emergency service. The appearance of the other community mental health service elements resulted in further advantages. A separate day center was opened in 1961 (see Chapter 5); outpatient services were expanded; public health nursing became an available resource. Increasingly, hospitalization became a means rather than an end.

A developing complexity of services can be a mixed blessing. Though it increases the alternatives available for care, a complex spectrum alone does not insure effective service. Communication and information problems increase; the tendency of professionals to assume a parochial point of view in operating exclusive or competing domains is ever present. A major effort to combat this was made by establishing efficient record and information systems. Wherever possible, ongoing interservice liaison meetings were established. Maintenance of such liaison requires a continuous effort, since time is always short and such meetings are easily canceled, permitting liaison to fall to attrition. With rare exceptions, it has been possible to maintain monthly meetings with mutually interdependent services. However, geographical separation has posed a real problem; the North County Mental Health Center, being an inconvenient distance from the hospital, has never had the satisfactory liaison that has existed with the on-site resources. Responsibility for state hospital liaison, maintained actively by the inpatient service for several years, has been shifted to other elements of the program (see Chapter 2).

Overall we have gained much from our efforts. Many patients, still ill, but stabilized, are returned to the community with referral to local services. While this may be done, in part, in response to pressure for beds, it is more importantly in accord with the San Mateo philosophy that inpatient care is a drastic intervention and is best kept as minimal and specific as necessary. Transitional day and night care are extremely valuable supports for such an approach. Another practical device to support such cases is to guarantee readmission if a discharge plan does not work out in view of the patient or the professional involved. This reassuring pledge provides strong psychological support for the patient and the treatment personnel asked to assume responsibility for difficult cases. It is rarely misused. Our guess is that with such support, community resources may well overextend themselves to carry difficult cases. Similar arrangements are available for geriatric cases sent to nursing homes in lieu of state hospitalization. This single article of the San Mateo policy has made nursing home staffs much more willing to work with such cases. Thus, through evolution of this program and the development of multiple alternatives to hospitalization, San Mateo now provides an average acute inpatient stay of seven days, with a range of overnight to one month. Approximately one-fifth of all discharges are to the state hospital for longer than acute care. Transitional day and night care are also available. In considering this average stay, it is important to emphasize the strong conviction that time factors should not become an end unto themselves. The more correct measure is determined by balancing the patient's needs and compatibility with the resources and limits of the facility. In any case, the San Mateo experience seems to confirm the principle that when diagnosis and treatment are offered promptly and alternative treatments are available, need for extended twenty-four-hour hospitalization is significantly reduced.

## Emergency Services

An effective emergency service is essential to an effective community mental health program. Yet it is probably safe to say that emergency services are one of the weak links in the whole chain of mental health services. Several factors are contributory: programming of such services tends to be an extension of medical models, with little adequate definition of the problem, critical analysis of need, or measure of effectiveness; there is a sustained lack of interest on the part of professionals to work in such services on an ongoing basis; and a resultant lack in continuity of service and decision-making with responsibility assigned to the least experienced professional psychiatric residents. These patterns have been noted in the literature, particularly by Chafetz, Blane, and Muller (1966; Blane, Muller, and Chafetz, 1967). Also noted is the public's accelerating utilization of such services.

These, indeed, have characterized the problems in San Mateo. Full-time psychiatric coverage for psychiatric cases began in 1960, when psychiatric residents were first available for such activity. In 1963, with increasing utilization, part-time psychiatrists were employed to cover busy afternoon periods. Increasing utilization of this service has been an unvarying trend. Between 1963 and 1967, there was a 150 per cent increase in emergency room psychiatric discharges.

For many persons, an emergency service is a first contact with mental health personnel and a first admission or recognition that such contact may be appropriate. To peace officers, it may also be an only point of contact with mental health professionals. To professionals and caregivers in the community, it is a resource for the critical problem, a backup support for the difficult case being kept in the community. To established patients, it is likewise an important source of support. In San Mateo County General Hospital, the emergency unit is also a hospital admitting service, which undoubtedly establishes a set of expectations about the care which will be available within. It has been the intent of the psychiatric inpatient service to develop a program to meet the responsibilities and exploit the opportunities inherent in these facts.

Foremost has been a policy of availability. At the risk of overuse, we actively encourage persons to feel free to use the service. No fee is charged, partly because collections would not be worth the expense, but primarily to avoid a barrier to the seeking of assistance. Where overuse is a problem, staff attempt to limit contact on an individual basis. This is not altogether satisfactory, owing, in part, to the inexperience of the staff on this service. Some residents may spend too much time with such persons or, on the other hand, dismiss them abruptly, often with unnecessary medications, which undoubtedly eases the doctor's conscience more effectively than the patient's problem.

In the emergency room, the physician is asked to develop a concept about the type of service to be rendered in the setting and to maintain an ability to adapt to rapidly changing circumstances. A slow, time-consuming interview may be interrupted by the simultaneous arrival of several crisis cases which demand prompt attention. The doctor has to shift orientation from the detailed problems of a single patient to a problem of psychiatric triage, and make rapid decisions with a minimum of available information. This calls for special skills that generally are not taught in school. Ability to elicit the most pertinent information in a brief period and to utilize ancillary personnel is essential.

Effort is made to give priority to cases brought in by peace officers. Two factors affect this policy. It is a major conviction in San Mateo that law enforcement personnel are a critical first-line mental health resource. Too often, they are afforded little positive feedback of the importance of their role. Prompt attention to their presence can be a simple but valuable statement of our attitude and can lay important groundwork for further contact. Beyond establishing a positive collaborative relationship, our efforts can have an important educational effect. In substance, this can help significantly to dissipate the peace officer's stereotyped attitudes toward psychiatric cases.

By demonstration, the psychiatrist can convey to the officer an understanding of the problem he is dealing with. If the doctor brings a patient under control in a dignified manner, this can serve as a model that the peace officer can apply in the future. By providing feedback on disposition, within the limitations of confidentiality, the doctor can help the peace officer make better use of the emergency services. We have had complaints from the police that persons brought in after suicide attempts were often back in the community before the officers were. The police questioned the value of bringing in such subjects, expressing the feeling that discharge was a repudiation of their judgment or a measure of the incompetence of the doctor. We have tried to clarify that suicide attempts are appropriate referrals but that we assumed responsibility at the emergency room and that hospitalization is not necessarily an outcome of all suicide attempts.

Education is a two-way situation. The officer can be an important source of data about the problem, helping the doctor extend his awareness beyond the confines of the clinical setting in which he works, making possible common-sense judgments that sometimes elude us in the rarefied clinical setting. The practice of community psychiatry demands this extended orientation of professionals. Principles that apply to peace officers are also applicable to the other care-providing collaterals with whom the emergency room psychiatrist deals.

We use the emergency room not just for evaluation and alleviation of symptoms but also to prepare a patient for his inpatient experience. An attempt is made to establish a working relationship with the patient in this setting and to define the purpose of the hospitalization. In addition to explaining what will be done for him, his role in the experience is emphasized. To the extent possible or appropriate, we identify his responsibilities, the limitations of the unit, the means of solving problems. This very early establishes a treatment compact, which can be the basis for future discussions; it lays excellent groundwork for a trusting relationship. Appropriate medications are given to allay anxiety, and nursing staff escort the patient to the unit. The total effect of this approach is to mobilize the effective coping resources of the patient. Not only does it protect or restore damaged self-esteem but it sets into motion restorative adaptive patterns. We attempt to offer the same type of service to patients who are discharged (that is, seen in the emergency room but not admitted to the ward), depending on their needs and the availability of resources. Here, we are less certain of our total effectiveness.

The workload of the emergency service has reached a point that exceeds our staffing ability. We foresee the development of a drop-in service for elective cases. Set hours of service at the convenience of the public will permit better allocation of professional time and, hopefully, provide better service to the patient.

### Inpatient Treatment Program

Our clinical program is eclectic. This is both by choice and in response to the very diverse functions and responsibilities we have. Clinical problems and syndromes seen on an acute receiving service are extremely varied. Age groups range from early adolescence through the extreme senium. Cases cover all classic psychiatric syndromes, both functional and organic, and encompass the fullest possible range of acuteness to chronicity. The psychiatric aspect of the problem may be relatively small, secondary to crucial situational, social, or legal issues. Patients are simultaneously being detained, evaluated, treated on a first admission or multiple admission basis. Only the flexibility of an eclectic approach aimed at practical problem-solving can offer a means of providing effective service in such a setting. Eclecticism is often seen as a last resort for the uncommitted or inadequately trained. Our opinion is to the contrary. Eclecticism characterized by ongoing and honest self-criticism is a means by which disciplined professionals can deal meaningfully with the complexity of the human problems that present themselves to a community-oriented patient care program and is applicable to theoretical models used to conceptualize cases, as well as to practices and procedures used to carry out diagnosis and treatment. In San Mateo, this eclectic approach has involved considerable application of the therapeutic community concept, particularly as discussed by Jones (1953, 1962) and Wilmer (1958). It has undergone continuous modification through the years.

When our unit was opened as a therapeutic community, there was a rich mixture of sound thinking and naive assumptions. Sound thinking was manifested in a determination to minimize the depersonalizing effect of the institutional environment, to develop a comfortable and supportive atmosphere to bring about the patient's active participation in his own treatment, and to open communication between and among staff and patients. To achieve this, patients were given maximum access to ward areas—locked rooms were kept open, and the unit itself was unlocked, the door monitored by a patient or staff member. Food service became a patient responsibility, with meals self-served and free access to the kitchen at all times for snacks. Numerous other significant responsibilities, such as light cleanup and gardening, became rotating patient responsibilities. An extensive program of off-ward activities, planned by the patients, was established. Patients kept their possessions, wore their own clothes, and had their own pay telephone for incoming and outgoing calls. Liberal visiting hours were established, from 12:30 P.M. to 8:30 P.M. (excluding the dinner hour), with restrictions only when specifically indicated. Since 1964, there has been no age limit on visitors, and there is rarely an afternoon when children or infants are not on the ward. We have been extremely impressed with the beneficial effect on parents and children when early visiting is permitted, and can report not one untoward incident arising out of this policy. The presence of children has a remarkable effect on "softening" the atmosphere for all persons, patients and staff. Some of the design limitations of the facility were actually useful in realizing a comfortable environment. Patients needed laundry facilities, but the only available space was in the medications room. As a result, this room is used for both functions. In addition, it is where women patients can use a hair drier and where new patients are checked in. We would not recommend such space limitations to anyone, but we found the sharing of facilities increases contacts between patients and staff in highly natural activities. The nursing station is open and central; doctor's offices are all located on the ward, also increasing the frequency of informal contacts. The result is a stimulating, active environment which encourages socialization of the patients and permits simultaneous staff observation of and interaction with patients in a highly beneficial manner. It is a demanding setting, which does not permit staff to hide behind institutional privilege, except when appropriate and essential to carry out responsibilities.

The abandonment of these essential responsibilities is among the early, naive assumptions mentioned above. We do not believe the therapeutic community concept implies a fully egalitarian relationship between staff and patients. The responsibilities inherent in running an acute inpatient unit cannot be effectively carried out unless staff is able to differentiate those spheres where it must act solely on its authority and expertise from those spheres where mutuality of decision-making and information sharing is possible and desirable. For example, patients initially attended nursing reports and, at the daily community meetings, voted on issuing passes. We would not argue that such innovations would never be useful—they might be in a setting with a stable chronic patient population—but in an acute treatment setting they are inappropriate; they are not comprehended by patients as making sense but seen as a pointless abdication of basic staff responsibility. Further, they were misleading, since inappropriate decisions had to be overruled. In the rapid scheme of things, this was often done behind closed doors and probably repeated some of the ambiguous and duplicit life situations which contributed to the patient's illness. Our most refined notion about patient decision-making is that responsibility should be limited to those situations where staff are prepared to abide by the decision. Negotiations for a pass are between patient and the doctor who bears responsibility for the case.

Another notion which has been discarded is that a select group of patients should be kept for extended treatment—up to three months —and function as carriers of the ward culture. Such a group was felt to be essential because of the rapid turnover. The error of such a practice should be obvious. Further, we have found it is not necessary. Our present experience is that patients rapidly assimilate the ward culture —often on the day of admission—through their immediate, close contact with fellow patients and staff, and we have no need to maintain the culture artificially. Staff do have to exercise considerable flexibility in the way they offer leadership—directive, if the patient population lacks capacity to carry responsibilities, and informally supervisory, when strength is clearly there.

A word about innovations is indicated here. Our present philosophy is that innovations should not be undertaken for their own sake, but because they hold promise of leading to desirable goals. Staff are encouraged to try new approaches or programs, to participate in their evaluation, and to retain them or agree to discard them as their usefulness is demonstrated. The rewards in terms of participation in a creative program clearly outweigh the difficulties entailed. This approach tends, also, to minimize interdisciplinary conflicts that may arise regardless of the program.

At times people justify a new approach for other than its actual merits. For example, early in our program development, it was decided to have nurses wear street clothes instead of uniforms. It was felt this would help reduce the institutional atmosphere and break through the symbolism of the uniform to the extent that it inhibited or limited "therapeutic" interpersonal transactions between patients and nurses. Undoubtedly it has done this, but it has also become a mark of status on the part of nurses to have escaped their uniforms. Suggestions that occasionally arise from patients that nurses should wear uniforms so they can be better identified are met with considerable resistance by the nurses. Although we feel that the advantages of working without uniforms have been demonstrated, one might wonder whether all the arguments used to justify the practice in terms of patient care are as conclusive as the desire of the nurses to preserve new professional status. The same observations can be made for other professionals in their valued new roles, as well as for all program innovations.

Such professional foibles are not a problem unless they dominate a program. A staff willing to examine its program in a realistic and ongoing way will get sufficient reward from its efforts that it will not need to invent program justifications. Quite important to note, also, is the probability that this type of programming establishes a service "culture" that is otherwise independent of its leadership. The inpatient service at San Mateo has had four different clinical chiefs and a considerable staff turnover in the course of its history. Outside observers who visit over the years tend to be impressed with the consistency of the program. Each chief adds the stamp of his own personality and modifies the program along his own lines of preference, but the "culture" has remained consistent.

It would be difficult to demonstrate here the manner in which we attempt to employ the structure of a multitude of activities to maximize intrastaff exchange of information and planning about each case. Information exchange at a very high level of effectiveness is essential, we believe, to competent decision-making in a fast-moving program such as this. Although our training program also requires this information exchange, we would work toward the same goal even in the absence of training responsibilities.

This is one of a combination of factors that seem to be important elements in maintaining therapeutic effectiveness despite the rapid pace of the unit and the fact that many of the more than one hundred monthly admissions include individuals who are acutely psychotic. Preparation of the patient in the emergency room, careful and constant attention to the milieu of the ward, involvement of the court in the treatment process, and intensive work with both patients and families are among the other crucial ingredients.

This work is done at a time of special receptivity on the part of the family, often at the culmination of a crisis that has brought the patient to the hospital. In the course of a few days, the patient may be seen daily by his psychiatrist; he will have participated in a wide range of ward activities (see Table 1); one or more family members will have been interviewed by the social worker; and a joint conference, involving the doctor, patient, social workers, and family, may have been held. All of this is done against the backdrop of interdisciplinary team planning.

The individual case management model on our unit has emerged as an amalgam of traditional and new approaches. Clinical treatment teams consist of a supervising staff psychiatrist, two residents, and two social workers. To simplify communication, one social worker is assigned to work with each resident psychiatrist on a regular basis. The residents, under full-time psychiatric staff supervision and in collaboration with the social worker, carry basic responsibility.

A social worker is assigned to each patient admitted to the hospital, but the role to be taken by this worker is decided by the treatment team at its daily meeting, when information about newly admitted patients is presented by the resident, and initial case man-

# Table 1

## Weekly Schedule: Patient Activities

| | Mon. | Tues. | Wed. | Thur. | Fri. | Sat. | Sun. |
|---|---|---|---|---|---|---|---|
| 9:00 A.M./ 9:45 A.M. | Community Meeting | | | | | → | 9:00/ Protestant 10:00 Catholic Services |
| 11:00 A.M./ 11:45 A.M. | Small Group | | Small Group | Patient Steering Committee | Small Group | → | |
| 1:00 P.M./ 3:00 P.M. | Occupational Therapy on Ward (first day after weekend) | Outings ---------→ | | | | | |
| 1:00 P.M./ 5:00 P.M. | Visiting Hours | | | | | → | |
| 7:00 P.M./ 8:00 P.M. | | | | Family Group | | | |
| 6:00 P.M./ 8:30 P.M. | Visiting Hours | | | | | → | |
| 8:30 P.M./ 9:30 P.M. | Patient Steering Committee | | | | Sing Along | Ward Movies | Patient Orientation Meeting |

# LIST OF OFF-WARD ACTIVITIES

| Sports Participation | Sporting Events | Outings | Special Events |
|---|---|---|---|
| Miniature golf | S.F. Giants games | Parks | County fair |
| Bowling | Stanford games | Beach | Ice Follies |
| Volleyball | Polo games | Museums | Plays |
| Croquet | Soccer games | Tours of industrial plants | |
| | | Colleges | |
| | | Airport | |
| | | Boat harbors | |

Doctors see individual patients daily; length and goals of contact determined individually. Doctors are encouraged not to pull patients from organized activities, but this is ultimately at their discretion. Occupational therapist, who also serves as recreational therapist, works in close collaboration with the nursing staff in the total activity program. Space limitations and duration of stay dictate a program of one-day projects, in general, although special projects can be developed, when desirable. Off-ward activities (always at the discretion of the responsible staff member) are emphasized.

*Table 2*

WEEKLY SCHEDULE: MORNING STAFF ACTIVITIES

| Time | Activity | Mon. | Tues. | Wed. | Thur. | Fri. | Sat. |
|---|---|---|---|---|---|---|---|
| 8:00– 8:40 | Team Meetings | | | | | → | |
| 8:40– 9:00 | Nursing Report | | | | | | → |
| 9:00–9:45 | Community Meeting | | | | | | → |
| 9:45–10:15 | Staff Review | | | | | | → |
| 10:00–10:45 | | | Case Review | | | Case Review | |
| 11:00–11:45 | | Small Group | | Small Group | | Small Group | |

96

agement planning is done. A series of team meetings, community meetings, a daily staff review of the community meeting, and formal staff meetings induce total staff participation in the ongoing evaluation, treatment, and planning for cases (see Table 2).

Nursing functions are discussed in detail elsewhere (see Chapter 7). As do the physicians, social workers, and the occupational therapist, nurses, too, participate in the daily community, staff review, and case review meetings. In addition to activities listed in the schedule, there is a weekly case conference and a staff business meeting.

Clinical social work services are directed, for the most part, to collaterals, since the patient is seen regularly on an individual basis by the doctor. In cases in which the patient is being actively treated by a therapist in another unit of the mental health service division, efforts are made to coordinate the hospital treatment with the ongoing therapy, rather than to involve additional hospital specialists. The same practice prevails for staff of other agencies, such as family service, juvenile probation, or the welfare division of our department. Social workers occasionally work directly with individual patients, if the problems are primarily social ones. More often, the social worker may act as the resource person or a consultant to help the resident deal with the social problems presented by his patient in the context of the total treatment.

A common referral to the social work staff is to see family members for additional information needed to formulate the treatment goal or to plan for discharge. Social histories, as such, are not taken routinely, and when such information is obtained, it is usually shared verbally at team or general staff meetings. Once the social worker has become involved with the family, this contact often develops into a natural entrée for beginning collateral treatment. We frequently alternate individual sessions with four-way conferences between the social worker, a relative, doctor, and patient. When the admission rate is high or the case is very complex or changes rapidly, it is sometimes necessary for a particular resident and social worker to talk together more frequently than during the daily team meetings. All personnel on the inpatient service are readily accessible by telephone. We long ago abandoned the idea that interviews are sacred and cannot be interrupted. Common courtesy and consideration are exercised, so that interruptions are avoided as much as is reasonable, but we believe the needs of the department and of the public are not well served by constantly uncompleted phone calls.

Social workers are paired with nurses as co-therapists in the small group meetings three mornings a week and in the group of patients and relatives which meets one evening a week. The small group consists of all patients assigned to a given team, one of the social workers on the team, and one of the staff nurses. The social worker has more detailed information obtained during the daily team meetings about the patient's problems, whereas the nurse is much better acquainted with the patient from having worked directly with him in ward activities. The co-therapists are assigned on an ongoing basis, and other staff nurses assist at the meetings on a rotating basis. Pertinent information from these groups is fed back into other staff deliberations about individual patients or about the community as a whole.

A reader who works in a more leisurely setting may well wonder what, if anything, can be done for patients in a setting such as ours. Our answer would be that the pace of our program, while partly a response to admission pressures to what is, after all, a receiving unit, is also an appropriate response to the rate of reconstitution we see in our patients. Under such a program, patients with severe psychotic decompensations can return quickly to a sufficient level of functioning to return to the community. We try to use the hospital experience as specifically as we can. There is no delay in undertaking active treatment on admission, and our intensive staffing minimizes administrative delay when inpatient care is no longer needed. If we felt someone would benefit from three months on our unit, we would offer such service. Our general experience with persons requiring long-term inpatient care is that the rapid turnover of patients is dismaying—either too stimulating to handle or too depressing, serving only to accentuate the patient's own lack of progress. Such patients are generally sent to the state hospital where the pace is slower. If such a setting were available in the community, they could be treated there.

Certain types of patients do poorly on our unit; these include persons with manic syndromes, in particular, as well as those for whom no local resources at all can be found. Indeed, we must acknowledge that, while an open unit can indeed serve about 92 to 95 per cent of our population, there remain a small but difficult group of patients, mainly psychotic, who are assaultive and require a secure setting, and those who will not remain on an open unit regardless of cause. Over the years, our regionalized state hospital service has been extremely helpful in accepting such cases on referral.

## Social Work Services

As the inpatient program has grown, social workers have been largely freed from administrative duties, such as eligibility determination and statistical reporting. A clerk now performs these duties, interviewing patients and their families and setting fees according to a mental health division formula. This person also processes insurance and disability claims and assists patients in filing for Medicare benefits.

It became possible for social workers to assume new functions. These activities fall into the pre-admission and intake phases of the inpatient service program. Generally, if a patient comes voluntarily or is brought to the hospital, he is seen in the emergency room by the doctor on duty. All non-emergency room referrals are routed through the social service office. If someone other than the patient telephones or comes in to arrange for admission, he is directed to the social work office. Frequently, the patient in question is not aware that inquiries are being made in his behalf, or he may have refused to consider himself a candidate for psychiatric treatment. In a large number of the cases, the presenting request is to sign petitions for state hospital commitment, and in the majority of instances, the caller believes the matter is urgent. One social worker is assigned each day as intake worker, and incoming requests take precedence over other work. It is possible to offer appointments the same day or the following day. Personal interviews have been found to be more satisfactory than telephone screening, because a constructive working relationship between the social worker and the client can be established. The fact that relatives often have delayed taking action until the situation becomes so serious as to be regarded as an emergency makes it very hard for them to think in terms of alternatives which may be suggested over the phone. Too often, this is perceived as refusal of service or a discounting of the pressing need of the patient and his family. An immediate response to telephone callers and to unscheduled clients does much to allay anxiety. When we make it clear that we are available to help, clients become amenable to considering alternative solutions.

The guiding rule for social workers is that our intervention should be as minimal as possible and that active client participation should be developed to the greatest possible extent. Many factors determine the success with which this goal can be achieved, and the ability of the intake social worker to diagnose the problem effectively and evaluate the strengths and weaknesses in a given family situation is very important. Availability of community resources which can be mobilized is also a realistic consideration. For example, the lack of detoxification centers for alcoholics in the community has probably resulted in many petitions for commitment to state hospitals, when the real wish was to have the person admitted somewhere for a few days for "drying out."

Often people do not know that one may enter a psychiatric hospital voluntarily. The term *commitment* is used interchangeably with *admission,* and often a court procedure is not sought at all. Not infrequently, we also find that families have not told the patient directly that they think he is mentally ill, nor have they consulted their family doctor about their concern. In the first instance, it is useful to convey information about private and public treatment centers, inpatient and outpatient services, and to describe the service of the emergency room.

When a family is reluctant to involve the patient in the plans for treatment, the social worker must identify the factors that may be preventing them from allowing the patient to participate in his own care. Fear that the patient may be hurt or angry, that he will run away or retaliate in some fashion, or that he may become even more belligerent are common inhibiting concerns. It may be necessary to see relatives on more than one occasion, in order to decide the best action to take. Assurance that the worker, the emergency room doctor, or the local police department are available, if the situation deteriorates further, helps to support family members in dealing with the patient. If it appears the family has tried unsuccessfully to deal with the patient, a home call by the visiting psychiatrist can be arranged.

There are cases where alternatives are not possible or are inappropriate, and it is in order for the social worker to initiate court intervention. We view the court as an import adjunct to the total treatment process. There are many persons who cannot voluntarily seek treatment yet who never challenge an involuntary admission or contest a court's decision, even though there is full opportunity to do so. In San Mateo County, patients have access to an attorney at all stages of involuntary proceedings. Some attorneys see their role as an adversary when they become involved in a commitment proceeding; others will relate to the proceeding as being in the best interest of their client and will use it to help solve clearly acute social-psychiatric problems. A clear delineation between the medical treatment requirements and the legal rights of the patient enhances the opportunity for providing effective solutions. Difficulties occur primarily when any of the parties involved fails to understand or to represent his position effectively.

### Home Visiting Service

The precommitment or "home visiting psychiatrist" program was started in 1960 to provide an even more effective screening prior to hospitalization. It was felt a significant number of persons bound for inpatient psychiatric care probably could be handled adequately and safely by measures other than hospitalization, if evaluation and referral to an alternative method of care was offered before the patient reached the hospital doors.

A basic assumption of this program has been that the alternatives to hospitalization are to be found within, or can be developed from, already existing family or community resources, supplemented by already existing professional facilities and techniques. The program thereby affirmed the community mental health concept that instead of removing the mentally ill from society, the community can be helped to assume greater responsibility for the well-being of these individuals.

By allowing for psychiatric evaluations in the home, opportunities were opened for a quick and accurate method of evaluating patient-family interactions, for establishing a working relationship with the patient on his own ground, and for intervening in the movement toward hospitalization before the process became irreversible. If and when hospitalization was necessary, the psychiatrist could supply to the staff valuable information about the patient and the precipitating circumstances of his illness. If treatment in a state hospital was indicated, the patient could be routed directly to such a facility without going through the procedure of admission to the unit in San Mateo. The service could be of particular help to those (for example, chronically withdrawn and paranoid persons) whose symptoms often force families to resort to petitions to have them evaluated. It could also offer a new avenue to those with serious mental illness who are either unmotivated to seek treatment or else incapable of actively managing their own way into treatment, even if they are willing to do so.

When this activity began, it was also believed these alternative measures would cost no more and probably cost less in time, money, and personnel than hospital admission. This assumption has now been amply confirmed here, as well as in similar programs elsewhere (Fink, Asbury, and Downing, 1963; Friedman, Becker, and Weiner, 1964; Greenblatt et al., 1963).

The program provided that a diagnostic home visit by a psychiatrist be offered to relatives who request a mental illness petition for court commitment of a designated person. As originally conceived, the service applied mainly to patients who were unwilling or unable to be brought into the adult clinic or emergency room for evaluation. As the program has evolved, and within the time available, the service has also become available to other families considering hospitalization, where, for instance, even though the patient might willingly come in for evaluation, it is sometimes evident that a home visit would provide a more meaningful picture of the total situation and lead to a more appropriate dispositional solution.

The psychiatrist's prime function at the present time is to evaluate the appropriateness of hospitalization in the San Mateo inpatient unit, albeit with an operating assumption that treatment outside the hospital, if feasible, is to be tried before resorting to inpatient treatment. This differs somewhat from the attitude at the inception of the service; at that time, initial enthusiasm and the need to prove the value of the service led to the bias that treatment at home, in almost any case, was preferable to hospitalization. It was possible, by maintaining this attitude to demonstrate in a study covering 1964–65 that 60 per cent of hospital-bound patients could be kept at home and adequately handled for long periods of time, that is, two years and more (Lutovich, 1967).

Other programs (Meyer, Schiff, and Becker, 1967) have achieved comparable results, and Pasamanick, in a research program, has reported even more impressive figures by following a strict policy of avoiding hospitalization in spite of extreme difficulties (Pasamanick, Scarpitti, and Dinitz, 1967). Our attitude has been modified by the observation that when extreme efforts are necessary to keep someone out of the hospital, the cost to family members and the question of the ultimate benefit of such measures, makes the justification of such a rigid program questionable. Hospitalization is viewed as a useful disposition, when appropriate, and is not considered an indication of failure on the part of the home visiting service. The essence of the program remains, however, that if the visiting psychiatrist, after evaluation, decides hospitalization is unnecessary, or that an alternative plan is worth trying, at least, he then has at his disposal a rather wide range of community resources to choose from.

As originally conceived, the visiting psychiatrist was providing a limited range of psychiatric services: diagnosis, evaluation, and referral to an appropriate resource. As the service has evolved, his functions have become much broader. They encompass various aspects of treatment, environmental manipulation, consultation, and follow-up, which he now finds himself providing selectively.

### Referral

The staff of the home visiting service includes a psychiatrist, currently available for twelve to fourteen hours weekly, divided between two days. He makes all the home visits. Inpatient social work staff members do initial screening and intake from complainants and petitioners, collect pertinent data from all available sources, and consult with the home visiting psychiatrist regarding appropriateness of intervention by means of home visits. They are available for supportive or therapeutic sessions with family members who can come to their offices; they take petitions and provide continuity with the case should hospitalization come about. Being more continuously available than the psychiatrist, they also provide a ready source of contact for patients and families of patients being managed outside the hospital.

It is during the period of information gathering and evaluation for mental illness petitions that relatives can be informed that a home visiting psychiatrist is available and that, if desired, a home visit could be made before the petition is actually signed. The worker exercises some discretion in declining to offer this service to families in a state of panic, where the emotional resources of the family and the patient are obviously totally exhausted or in circumstances in which the patient's potential for violent or self-destructive behavior seems high.

Although it is ready to respond to urgent situations, it is not an on-call service geared to meet "emergencies" in the home or elsewhere in the community.

A state of "emergency" is taken as a sign that there has been such a depletion of resources in the family constellation or in the patient himself as to militate against the probability of successful home treatment at the moment. Other programs have also come to the conclusion that community management in the midst of this type of extreme turmoil has small chance for effectiveness (Friedman and Weiner, 1965). In these circumstances, patients are brought into the hospital without recourse to the home visiting service. On the other hand, we have noted that many so-called emergencies turn out to be less than that, and if the family is adequately reassured by the prospect of a home visit within a day or two, the case is referred for home visit. Nearly all cases are seen in less than five days. If arrangements to meet in the home become complicated and if it appears the home visit will be further delayed, telephone contact is maintained by the social worker during the waiting period.

The collected case material, including any information obtained by phone from other involved family members, the family physician, or other agencies, is discussed with the home visiting psychiatrist. The consultation with the social worker serves to underline the unknown or questionable areas and points to considerations which should be explored during the diagnostic home visit.

Frequently a good deal of further groundwork is done by the psychiatrist before he actually makes the home call. For instance, if there is a private physician in the picture, he is always called. This informs him of our wish to help; it also gives us his view of the situation and permits us to gauge his willingness to become or to stay involved.

The home visit is usually made in the company of a responsible family member or the referring professional. Our policy emphasizes the desirability of informing the designated patient about the planned visit prior to the arrival of the psychiatrist; yet some flexibility is exercised when the family feels the patient will be too disturbed by the prospect of a visit. There is, however, rigid adherence to the policy that the psychiatrist never assumes a false identity, despite strong pressure from the family to pass him off as someone else less threatening. The initial reaction of the patient needs to be handled gently but firmly, and the psychiatrist is prepared to absorb a certain amount of angry abuse directed at him or the family members. The initial interview may take place in any room of the house or even outside, with the patient alone, or with family members present, as seems appropriate. Attempts are also made to provide an atmosphere devoid of such time pressures as might exist in an admitting room setting.

The diagnostic home visit often results in a quick, accurate picture of the family interactions. Conclusions can be reached from this as to the adaptive ability of the family, its ego resources, and which manipulations might be attempted within the family to benefit the patient. In some cases, it reveals evidence that the wrong family member has been labeled the "sick one." This general evaluation of the family strengths, attitudes, and flexibilities, as well as those of the patient, is the essence of the home visit, heavily influencing the decision whether the patient can be treated at home.

If treatment is deemed necessary and treatment without hospitalization seems feasible, an alternative is suggested; this may include any of a number of plans, from instituting a drug regimen with family or public health nurse assistance to referral to a socializing experience, such as a senior citizen activity.

The patient's attitude toward and willingness to rely upon the family physician, where there is one, is usually explored. As the program was originally conceived, the local nonpsychiatric family physician was to be a key resource. Having an established relationship with the patient, he was expected to be in a highly strategic position. He could continue the prescribed treatment within a medical framework, maintaining psychoactive medications once appropriate dosage was established. His support of the patient and family would be backed up by the home visiting psychiatrist who would serve as an ever-ready consultant. At times, the response from family doctors is surprisingly cooperative and effective. For the most part, however, this resource has not proved to be as valuable and reliable as we had anticipated. Lack of established involvement in the case, a desire to be relieved of a difficult patient, lack of proficiency in the use of psychotropic drugs, fixed ideas about the need for hospitalization, or mistrust of the psychiatrist, often lead physicians to rule themselves out as resources. Even more disappointing, indeed, are instances in which they cooperate superficially but subtly undermine the program suggested. Establishment of a workable psychiatrist–family doctor relationship still remains one of the more challenging aspects of the program, however, and our experience should be taken, perhaps, as a clue to the kinds of factors we must consider in developing this potentially valuable collaboration.

Public health nurses have been of greater practical value in the operation of the program. Although they generally have no particular psychiatric training beyond that given in nursing schools, they have proven extremely adaptable and helpful in fulfilling the requirements and goals of the home visiting service. (For further details of the mental health program's relationship with these nurses, see Chapter 7.) Usually they are contacted after an initial home visit and evaluation have been made and the feasibility of home treatment has been decided upon. The psychiatrist ordinarily accompanies the nurse on her first visit to the patient. Depending upon the needs of the patient, the nurse may supervise the management of medication, work with the family in a supportive capacity, or work with the patient to improve self-sufficiency and reality testing. The psychiatrist serves as an informal consultant to the nurse and makes periodic return visits to the patient with or without the nurse, as the situation requires. He carries medical responsibility as long as the nursing visits are provided.

If the evaluation results in a recommendation for boarding home or nursing home placement instead of hospitalization, the psychiatrist is in a position to modify existing unacceptable behavior, as well as reactions to a new placement, by prescribing tranquilizers before the move is made, asking for public health nurse help, and remaining available to the nursing home as a consultant. If the request for commitment originates in a nursing home, the psychiatrist attempts to convert this demand for hospitalization into a consultative relationship with the nursing home staff, attending physician, and family.

Church and volunteer groups, as naturally existing agencies in the community, have been helpful in some cases. They have, for instance, provided increased social contacts at home and have performed well in doing essential errands for organically deteriorated or intractable phobic patients.

## Home Treatment Program

As the program developed, it was found the psychiatrist himself was handling an increasing number of cases by a series of home visits, often without the assistance of a community resource. On examination, the majority of these cases proved to have certain common characteristics: the situation required rapid establishment of a medical regimen; the family needed emotional support; the need for supervision was obvious; but the patient remained highly resistant to referral to any other source of help and would probably lose interest or get lost during the process of transfer. In these cases, because of the relationship established during the first visit, the home visiting psychiatrist appeared to be the most logical person to return and handle the critical period. As a result, the precommitment service began to broaden its scope to include "home treatment with minimal use of outside resources" as a treatment modality, in addition to its diagnostic-referral services.

Medication regulation was a frequent focus of these return visits, especially if the family physician was not in the picture. They have, however, evolved into a type of therapy-in-the-home, involving both patient and family in an intervention which seems particularly well suited to the tasks of handling crisis situations, keeping chronically psychotic patients in the community and out of the hospital, and managing those who would not accept conventional modes of psychiatric treatment or be much helped by them.

In evaluating the factors which contributed to this development, we would probably have to include such pragmatic considerations as the failure of some community resources to fulfill their anticipated roles, as well as the difficulties entailed in getting through the administrative policies of some agencies quickly enough. While greater effort might have been devoted to the task of obtaining smoother cooperation from these agencies (with unpredictable results), the fact remains that this inconvenience has helped to compel us to develop an effective mode of treatment which fills a void in the range of services previously available in the county. On further reflection, we might support the idea that the time and effort spent in motivating patients to accept more conventional modes of treatment or trying to negotiate administrative barriers to referral could be better spent in offering short-term treatment at home. However, this facet of the program remains feasible only so long as it does not drastically limit the psychiatrist's availability for the higher priority responsibilities: diagnosis, evaluation, and referral.

To a large extent the effectiveness of a home visiting program depends upon the flexibility of the psychiatrist and the participating agencies in adapting themselves to the particular requirements of each patient's situation. A basically pragmatic but by no means unsophisticated approach is used. Above all, there must be a willingness to assume the roles and perform actions that will be most helpful to the patient rather than unyielding observance of rituals dictated by overspecialized professional training. In part, the home visiting methods are those used in brief, crisis-oriented therapy, where a wide variety of techniques is available. These techniques are used freely, depending on the requirements of the particular case. Crisis psychotherapy and, to an extent, home treatment, require an expediency approach. From the beginning everything is used that can achieve the goal of restoring the premorbid or precrisis level of functioning. It should be emphasized, however, that although attempts are made to enlist the cooperation of important family members, and some work is done in making members aware of how their problems may be affecting the patient, family therapy, as such, is not offered.

As might be expected, treatment in the home appears to work best when there is an overtly ill person within a functioning family that contains a minimum of grossly disruptive interactions between the family members. Limits are imposed, of course, by the willingness of family and community to live with the problem (plus our own judgment as to the desirability of this); yet, for example, we have successfully handled cases with several other family members being frankly psychotic.

The geriatric population represents a significant proportion of the home visiting case load and presents a continuous dispositional problem because of the insufficiency of resources that may be called into play. Physicians confronted with aberrant behavior in the elderly are often reluctant to try appropriate or adequate medication and tend to think more about hospitalization than may be their habit when treating younger age groups. Suggestions made by the consultant psychiatrist regarding the elderly tend to be thought of by the physician as "holding actions" or as delaying the inevitable; as such, they are passed on to the patient or family in an ambivalent manner. This is an example of the undermining mentioned above.

If nursing homes are considered, the geriatric patient's symptomatology is often evaluated by the nonpsychiatric physician in the light of how it would be tolerated by the nursing staff of the given home, with a bias toward saving himself and the nursing staff as much as possible the prospect of repeated calls regarding aberrant behavior, initial adjustment reactions, or drug dosage adjustment. In some cases, a lack of close contact with the nursing home leads physicians to underestimate the capacity of a given home to handle a prospective boarder and trial periods tend to be frowned upon. Because the home visiting service can offer consultation to nursing homes, it sometimes is able to effect modifications in these processes.

In essence, then, professional evaluation, consultation, and treatment have been delivered to a segment of the population that previously would, of necessity, have gone through the process of hospitalization to obtain these services.

When the home visit reveals that treatment outside the hospital is not possible, the psychiatrist's energies are directed toward bringing the patient in voluntarily. In our inpatient service, we have found that even though the patient comes in grudgingly, the fact that he has entered voluntarily significantly increases his ability to benefit from the experience. In many such cases, we encourage a patient to come in accompanied by relatives, thus keeping the family involved and permitting them to see themselves as being helpful rather than as those who have banished the patient via "the authorities." If this is not workable, the psychiatrist is willing to bring the patient in his own car, with the relatives agreeing to come in at a later time.

If the need for hospitalization is immediate, and efforts at voluntary admission have failed, the psychiatrist, as a deputy health officer, is empowered to sign a seventy-two-hour observation hold; police aid may be obtained, if needed. In most cases that come to this point, however, it has been found satisfactory to rely on ambulances and ambulance attendants, who generally are quite proficient in handling such situations. Our figures indicate that approximately 20 per cent of the initial home visits result in hospitalization being expedited by the psychiatrist. About half of these admissions agree to come in voluntarily.

## Special Considerations

A public psychiatric receiving and treatment facility is confronted with a set of circumstances that may not be shared by other kinds of mental health programs. These demand a reexamination of some assumptions and convictions that are commonly accepted in other psychiatric settings. There are, in particular, seven considerations that have a special relevance to this discussion. Some have been referred to previously, but they deserve more detailed comment.

Having accepted responsibility to serve the needs of a total population, one is no longer in a position to ignore gaps in the service spectrum or to overlook certain needs that are met marginally, if at all. Alcoholism is perhaps the most significant example of this, so far as this service is concerned. Moreover, this same basic community mental health responsibility, coupled with the conviction that long-term institutionalization of the mentally ill is undesirable, leads to a new set of attitudes. Readmission offers an excellent instance; one can no longer confidently equate readmission rates with therapeutic effectiveness.

An open unit can be unusually versatile in meeting crisis situations; nevertheless, it has some distinct limitations. There has been a temptation to express overenthusiastic promises concerning new community treatment methods. To avoid the danger of overstating our capacities, it is useful to delineate these limits realistically. Problems of role definition seem characteristic of programs in which milieu techniques have been utilized in creating a new division of labor within the treatment team, as well as between staff and patients. The extent to which training activities influence the program patterns is still another sphere that must be reassessed in a community treatment context.

Finally, there are two potential sources of major ethical and philosophical dilemmas for a program like ours. One is the problem inherent in collaboration with legal institutions of the community in sharing responsibilities for the confinement of certain individuals. The question of collaboration versus collusion is an ever-present one that must be reexamined in each case in which it arises. The other dilemma, equally difficult, though less frequently encountered, stems from the possible effects of new laws that may subtly or drastically revise basic operational assumptions of a tax-supported, public enterprise.

*Alcoholism.* Although the problem of alcoholism is of major proportions, we have developed very little in the way of effective services. Separate medical units under our supervision are available in the hospital, but many of these cases are treated on the psychiatric ward. Regardless of his location in the hospital, the patient receives the same overall collaborative services as are provided for psychiatric patients. Our staff is also active in working with the court on petitions and working out dispositions for these cases. As was observed earlier, lack of effective local alternatives frequently leads to reliance on involuntary methods and commitment. It is our feeling that an effective program for alcoholism needs to be developed independently to the specifically psychiatric services. The psychological difficulties of the alcoholic are fundamentally different from those of the person who usually ends up on a psychiatric unit. This is demonstrated most clearly by the participation of the alcoholic in group activities. When first admitted, he commonly is antagonistic and provocative, but once relieved of his unpleasant symptoms, he becomes the most glib speaker in the group, reciting the litany of therapy to the exclusion of participation by depressed and psychotic patients. He often becomes patient chairman and dominates ward recreational activities. A few alcoholics on a psychiatric unit can be part of a total mix which is quite stimulating. However, if their numbers increase, we find the program takes on a semblance of a twenty-four-hour testimonial-inspirational program.

We have tried to make constructive use of the involuntary program to deal with the alcoholic whose "denial" keeps him from being able to admit the severity of his problem. Very few alcoholics in our program are directly committed to a state hospital. Practically all of them not clearly physically ill are given a continuance by the court, if they can demonstrate any ability to mobilize themselves or resources in the community. Judges show varied interest in these problems; some have been willing to carry such cases for a year with monthly reports. Many individual cases responded quite favorably to this approach.

We must also report limited success with the other addictive problems, unless they happen to be symptomatic of more malleable psychiatric syndromes. In recent years, we have seen a sharp increase in the number of habit-forming drug users, but these individuals tend to return to previous modes of adjustment promptly after discharge, often being readmitted in a very short time with the same problem. The low incidence of narcotics addiction in our county makes this a very infrequent problem. We have successfully withdrawn some persons from narcotics, but because of the open unit with free access to visitors, most have not been manageable on our ward.

*Readmissions.* When we discuss our rapid turnover and short average stay, we are often asked about readmissions. A large percentage of our patients are people with severe chronic problems who, in the past, tended to spend years in state hospital settings. The essence of our program is to provide prompt and effective support to keep such people in the community. Need for rehospitalization is not necessarily seen as a treatment failure but as part of the inevitable consequence of the illness that certain patients have. Sometimes we actively encourage readmissions. Persons who have displayed a prior pattern of destructive or suicidal behavior are often encouraged to apply for hospitalization before they reach such desperate straits. If by readmitting a person, one can avoid a serious suicide attempt or its equivalent, then the readmission can be considered a positive achievement, rather than a treatment failure.

It has been mentioned earlier that a number of patients are discharged with psychic compensation recent and still tenuous. Part of the discharge plan includes our willingness to readmit, if adequate adjustment cannot be made. We do not consider such a readmission an indication of our failure. When patients see that we take such problems in stride, they, too, can handle readmissions without a sense of disgrace or failure.

We would not want to give the impression here that we explain away all readmissions as inevitable and, therefore, do not use them to evaluate the efficacy of our earlier efforts. This is a necessary discipline, and staff must work very hard to be honest in evaluating the effectiveness of their earlier efforts.

*Crisis Situations.* We have described in some detail our open unit and our staff approach to patients. We would be less than honest if we did not discuss very frankly the limitations of an open unit. In our opinion, a number of patients cannot be handled suitably on an open unit. Some patients, out of confusion or determination to leave, will not remain on an open unit in spite of all reasonable supervision and persuasion. If it is necessary that they remain in the hospital, such individuals must be kept on a locked unit. Patients who are assaultive also cannot be handled on our unit. Part of this is a staffing problem, but it is also an expression of our program. Because of the size of the ward, we have not had available enough male attendants to handle physically assaultive patients. Further, in an attempt to encourage staff to be maximally available to patients as empathetic, helping persons, we discourage reliance on physical control methods. An assaultive patient leaves us no choice but to transfer him to a facility where he can either be secluded or handled in such a way that he is not a danger to himself or others.

An unusual innovation that we have developed in such situations is to call the local police to help us bring such problems under control. Although one might question such a practice on a psychiatric unit, we have found it to be surprisingly effective. The police disarm themselves before they come on the unit and attempt to deal persuasively with the patient just as they would out in the community. Only when persuasion will not work do they physically restrain a patient. We have on a number of occasions asked for patient opinion on this practice, after such crises have occurred. The usual response was one of relief that the problem was brought under control, and on no occasion has anyone expressed the feeling that this was not a suitable practice. An unexpected benefit from this practice, in our opinion, is the way it communicates to the patient how close, in fact, he is to the community at large. We handle situations very much as they would be handled anywhere else in the community. We think this decreases the sense of the hospital being a special place for special people.

We have found we can operate quite well without formal suicide precautions. On an open unit they are thoroughly impractical. If any staff members are concerned about the possibility, the matter is discussed. If indicated, a note of the concern is made in the patient's chart to call staff attention to the problem. Staff then increase their overall direct supervision of the patient but take no other steps. Under such an approach, suicide attempts have been a rarity.

*Maintaining Definition of Roles.* This is a complicated problem that affects both staff and patients. Earlier we alluded to our efforts to design program and environment to elicit the best patient-staff interaction. We would consider it a disservice to patients, if we did not maintain some of the basic distinctions of the professional role that we play. We are frank about discussing the differences, and, in fact, actively attempt to define the extent to which we will function in a purely professional sense and the extent to which we are available personally. We make no effort to have patients call doctors by their first name as a way of suggesting a peer relationship which does not, in fact, exist. Nurses, however, are quite comfortable in relating to patients on a first-name basis.

Our collaborative approach often creates conflicts for staff who may have established a particularly close role with patients. Sometimes there develops a sense that a particular communication is confidential and cannot be shared with the rest of the staff. The staff, of course, are free to use their discretion in communicating such things to fellow staff, but it is our impression, more often than not, that this represents a problem of staff over-identification. A great deal of staff effort is spent defining these issues.

*Collaboration versus Collusion.*   A fundamental problem in community mental health programs concerns our ability to arrive at a comfortable position regarding the doctor's relationship with the patient, particularly regarding confidentiality. Working as we do with police, district attorney, judges, and other official and nonofficial professionals, and with families, who are often seen as adversaries, we constantly have to be aware of the difference between collaboration in a patient's behalf and collusion in imposing upon a patient our collective notions of what is best for him. This problem is the subject for a full chapter of discussion and will not be developed here beyond observing that a philosophy and a policy must be worked out and continuously reviewed. As professionals, we are trained to recognize that our first responsibility is to our patient or client, and we certainly subscribe to this. However, we often find ourselves in very complex and critical situations where we represent official agencies, the community at large, or are working at the request of relatives. Some people choose not to do such work, rather than have to make these difficult decisions. We can only say that it is a matter of choice, but once one makes his choice, one has to be willing to take clear and definite positions on these matters.

*Training Program.*  The training of psychiatric residents and student nurses is a major undertaking of the program described in this chapter. Although this provides us with very special opportunities and resources useful in the conduct of our work, we do not feel that it changes the basic thrust of our program, which would be maintained in its present format if trainees were not available. Trainees both add to and make demands of a program. Much of the work that is done by residents would be shared, in a non-training setting, by the psychiatric staff and the social workers. Social workers would undoubtedly carry more direct case responsibility, and the psychiatric staff would deal more specifically with medical and case administrative problems. We invite the reader to separate out the different role distinctions that would apply in another setting.

*California's New Mental Health Legislation.*  The California Legislature in 1967 and 1968 passed major reforms in public mental health programs, changing criteria, procedures, and responsibility for the care of the mentally ill. These reforms, in many respects, are an outgrowth of much of the pioneering work carried out in San Mateo in developing techniques to deal with mental health problems on a local and voluntary basis. They are oriented, also, toward severely restricting the means by which involuntary services can be provided. The commitment system will be terminated, and a system of short-term (fourteen-day) medical certification will be substituted. Long-term cases involving persons who are "gravely disabled" will be handled under local supervision through conservatorship laws, rather than through commitment procedures. Involuntary treatment for inebriates is eliminated entirely, unless a person who is a criminal defendant is ordered into treatment by a judge. This legislation will have a major effect on the program in San Mateo. It is our hope that the principles which have worked well in developing our present program will continue to apply.

We have attempted in this chapter to describe the evolution and development of a complex set of services that, overall, have been effective in providing psychiatric intervention in severe problems. The underlying pattern at all levels of the program involves adapting professional skills to the needs of the patient and expanding alternatives of all types that are available. This approach has made necessary considerable modification of what had become traditional professional roles; it has been our impression that the benefits greatly exceed the disadvantages. We encourage innovation and continue our own innovation. Our experience has been that program innovation is best when balanced by thoughtful program preservation. We heartily recommend the challenge and opportunity to all.

# CHAPTER 5

# The Day Hospital

*H. Richard Lamb, John Odenheimer*

The concept of a hospital where patients go home at night and on weekends was embraced enthusiastically in San Mateo and elsewhere in the late 1950s and early 1960s. The advantages of continuing contact with family and community during a period of hospitalization was easily recognized by the professional community. What was not fully realized in the early period, however, was the lack of clarity as to who should be treated, and how, and for what purposes. In retrospect, the initial enthusiasm for the day hospital obscured the fact that a clear formulation of goals specific to the day hospital was lacking. The present philosophy of our day hospital places a heavy emphasis on the early formulation of specific and limited goals and the maintaining of expectations that patients will strive toward realizing their full potential. This chapter traces the evolution of these and other aspects of our treatment philosophy and identifies the problems that one may expect in the establishment and development of a day hospital.

Initially it was assumed by both those referring to and those working in the day hospital that one of its important functions would be to serve as a sort of repository for chronically ill persons who would remain for indefinite lengths of time and thus be maintained so that they could be kept out of the state hospital. Indeed, many of the first referrals to our day hospital fell into this category. However, without the benefit of a clearly-defined treatment and rehabilitation philosophy, the staff soon began to develop a sense of frustration and dissatisfaction with the lack of movement which characterizes the chronic patient when "baby-sitting" is the only goal.

Another general type of referral was the patient who was thought to be in need of moderate or long-term outpatient treatment but where the referring professional also felt that the patient "needed more than one or two hours a week of treatment." The purpose of the referral then was to provide a background of support for the patient while the main work of outpatient psychotherapy went on. Here again the function of the day hospital was seen as a place only to gratify dependency needs, frequently for indefinite periods of time, and, in many cases, with patients for whom this was inappropriate and unnecessary. A clear conceptualization of how the day hospital itself could specifically be of help was lacking. When pressed, professionals would say that the patient could benefit from the day hospital by "improving his social skills." Though in a general way this may have been a legitimate goal for some patients, such a statement lacked specificity and often served as a cliché to close off further meaningful examination of how the day hospital could best be utilized.

A related notion saw the day hospital as a place where, by means of intensive psychotherapy from therapists on the day hospital staff, character change and insight in terms of a true resolution of unconscious conflict could be achieved. Such goals were explicitly or implicitly stated for both severe character disorders and schizophrenics. Again all other aspects of the day hospital were seen as supporting psychotherapy and gratifying dependency needs. It soon became apparent to us, as it has to others (Meltzoff and Blumenthal, 1966) that if we were taking a patient into the day hospital with the goal of resolving his core problem (that is, "curing" his schizophrenia or effecting some radical change in his character), we were attempting more than could be accomplished in a day hospital setting within a reasonable period of time. Frequently the net result of such overambitious therapeutic efforts was that a year or sometimes two years had elapsed with very little working through as far as the core problems were concerned. On the other hand, a great deal of dependency had been fostered in a setting where such long-term care was unnecessary and inappropriate.

There began to develop a group of "professional patients" for whom the goals of the staff were character change and insight. The goals of the patients, on the other hand, were consciously or unconsciously to remain dependent on the day hospital. These professional patients became adept at saying what the staff wanted to hear, being "good" group members and verbalizing the psychiatric "party line." Progress was continually noted by staff both in individual and group psychotherapy, but a closer examination revealed that it was a steady progress to nowhere. The patients attempted consciously or unconsciously to defer discharge by reacting to the impending discharge by the recurrence of old symptoms or the development of new ones. These patients in many cases were attempting to set up a symbiotic situation almost paralleling that in their own earlier life experience.

Another common type of referral was the patient being discharged from the inpatient service who was felt to need a period of transition from the ward to the outpatient psychiatric clinic. Experience showed, however, that if a patient were truly in need of only a week or two of transition, such transition could be more effectively and efficiently accomplished by making such a patient a day patient on the inpatient service for this brief period. This arrangement offered the advantage of remaining with the same staff that had treated him on the ward through the acute phase of his illness (and whom he regarded, perhaps, as his rescuers). It obviated the necessity of getting to know a whole new staff in the day hospital for such a brief period of time. This offered many advantages to the inpatient service also by bringing the community more into the ward and having more continuity of care and continuity of the ward patient group and culture.

## Treatment Goals

Out of these experiences gradually evolved our present philosophy of specific and limited short-term goals for patients in the day hospital. It has been our experience that it is important to think in terms of goals and to remember to ask ourselves and our fellow staff members and the patients, at all phases of treatment from intake to discharge, "What are the goals of day hospital treatment?" We have come to think in terms of limited goals, for we have found that by having our goals limited, we accomplish a great deal more in the long run. We may not have effected any basic change in the patient's personality structure, but often we have restored him to a productive, satisfying life in the community. Some examples of limited goals are: the resolution of an acute psychotic break or depression with return to premorbid adjustment; the resolution or beginning of resolution of a marital conflict; helping a patient develop a sense of trust in mental health professionals so that he can and will follow through with psychiatric outpatient treatment; the development of social skills and vocational rehabilitation. Sometimes the goal for a patient is mostly evaluation, so that we may refer him to another facility more suitable for treatment. There are many goals in the vocational area which are specific and important. These include: vocational evaluation, vocational counseling and preparation for work placement, sheltered workshop placement, and vocational training.

At first some felt that an emphasis on short-term and limited goals would rule out the treatment of the chronic patient in the day hospital. We have found, however, that the day hospital may undertake the treatment of many chronically disabled patients and still be seen as a short-term treatment facility for such patients (Lamb, 1967). We have taken patients with severe and long-standing disorders into the day hospital with very definite, limited, short-term goals. The fact that a patient is chronically ill does not mean that the day hospital's commitment to him must be indefinite. An example of this can be found in a chronic schizophrenic with a history of many years of poor functioning at home or in the state hospital, who is admitted to the day hospital for a period of evaluation including vocational, social, and family assessment, and resocialization. After a month or two, there follows half-time referral to a sheltered workshop, with discharge and full-time sheltered workshop a month or two after that.

We have come to accept many patients on a trial or evaluation basis of, say, one month. This is especially so with patients who are chronically disabled by their illness. Doing this helps make clear to the patient that formulation of goals is important, and that treatment is time-limited. Too often both the patient and his family are consciously or unconsciously seeking a permanent place of asylum and haven from the pressures of the world or each other, and want to see any institution, including the day hospital, as offering this asylum. Thus, the evaluation period, with emphasis on (1) treatment being time-limited and (2) early formulation of goals, helps to remind the patients and their families that the day hospital is a place where one is cared for temporarily while one actively works on his problems, rather than being a place where one receives eternal care.

The day hospital can offer treatment for a wide spectrum of psychiatric problems ranging from acute psychotic episodes and depressions in usually well-functioning members of the community to chronic and long-standing psychiatric disorders in patients who have not functioned for many years. The treatment of the acutely and chronically ill can proceed side by side in the day hospital. Mingling of acute and chronic patients has many advantages, for it has been shown (Fairweather, 1969) that the chronic patient tends to strive to bring his social and vocational performance up to the norms of better functioning of less chronic patients.

We find it useful to think in terms of two general categories or phases of treatment. The first phase emphasizes the resolution of the acute problem, and the second phase is that of rehabilitation in which the more long-standing problems, if any, are the focus of attention. Many of our patients have a chronic long-standing disorder with an acute problem superimposed, and for them both phases of treatment are indicated. For patients who normally function well in the community, only the acute phase of treatment involving resolution of the acute episode and precipitating stresses is necessary. Many patients come to the psychiatric day hospital with the acute problem partially resolved on an inpatient service, or with no recent history of an acute problem at all but with a chronic, severe long-standing adjustment as an ill and disabled person. For these patients only the second phase of rehabilitation is needed.

The resolution of the acute phase is in many ways similar to what would be done on an inpatient service and indeed it has been shown that the day hospital can serve as an alternative to twenty-four-hour hospitalization (McDonough and Downing, 1965; Odenheimer, 1965; Wilder, Levin, and Zwerling, 1966). Intensive work with both the patient and the family in this time of crisis, an attempt to understand and resolve the precipitating stress, and a structured program of activities are all part of our therapeutic armamentarium. Because of the relative lack of controls inherent in a day hospital setting as compared to an inpatient service, liberal use is made of tranquilizing medications, and emphasis is placed on limit-setting, especially with patients who have problems with control. Thus, with cooperation from the family and intensive work on the part of the day hospital staff, acutely ill patients can be helped through the period of crisis without separation from their families and the community.

Although experience in our own day hospital as part of a research project showed that the day hospital could serve as an alternative to twenty-four-hour hospitalization for many acutely ill patients (McDonough and Downing, 1965; Odenheimer, 1965), our experience since the research project ended has been enlightening. The number of acutely ill patients referred to the day hospital has decreased markedly. Though staff in the day hospital remained committed to the idea in principle, in many cases they too have become somewhat less than enthusiastic about accepting acutely ill patients. Likewise, Hogarty et al. (1968) found that their sample of day hospital patients did not resemble their samples of inpatients. For instance, "The hostile, belligerent, negative patient, as described by the family, is more likely to be admitted to a hospital, than to the day center."

Some reflection on these observations has brought us to the following conclusions. Because of the inherent lack of structure of a day hospital as compared to an inpatient service, the acutely psychotic and in particular the aggressive and out-of-control psychotic can be much more easily handled by an inpatient service than by the day hospital during the day and the family at night. These patients require a tremendous amount of energy and attention from the day hospital staff, which is of necessity diverted from the rehabilitation of less acutely ill patients. Furthermore, the patient's psychotic behavior may be frightening and even destructive to the family who may themselves need some relief from the patient's illness. In some cases the anger of the family directed toward the patient, the day hospital, and the referring therapist for not meeting their hopes for twenty-four-hour hospitalization and relief from the patient's illness may result in a nonsupportive family situation and more than offset any advantages of day hospitalization. Similarly, referral from the emergency room to the day hospital of an acutely psychotic patient may be a much more difficult procedure than simple admission to an inpatient service in terms of preparation of both family and patient. This may be a factor in making the emergency room psychiatrist reluctant to refer to the day hospital.

In retrospect, we feel that only staff dedicated almost exclusively (either philosophically or because of research or both) to the admission of acutely psychotic patients to a day hospital can successfully carry out a program with so many built-in difficulties. It is also far from clear that the day hospital offers clear-cut advantages in the treatment of such acutely ill patients. For instance, Wilder, Levin, and Zwerling (1966), in a two-year follow-up study of 189 patients admitted to their day hospital and 189 patients admitted to the inpatient ward, found little difference in the clinical course of both groups two years after admission.

What has evolved then in our setting is that most acutely ill psychotic patients, especially those who are aggressive and out of control, are admitted first to the inpatient service for a brief period and referred to the day hospital when they are in at least partial remission. Whether or not this is the ideal arrangement we are not prepared to say at this point, but our experience has shown that it is the most workable one.

### The Chronic Patient

The phase of rehabilitation that attempts to deal with the problems of chronic and severe mental illness, chronic poor functioning, chronic regression, and chronic dependency, requires the development of what is in many ways a new philosophy, alien to the usual thinking of many mental health professionals. First of all, we have to recognize that we are dealing with borderline, marginal people—both socially and vocationally—for whom life is a constant struggle. Their tendency is to regress. They are skilled at evoking guilt to get people to gratify their dependency needs. They have done this with their parents, with their spouses, and with social agencies. Since this has been, at least in some ways, an adaptive, problem-solving device for them, they attempt the same approach with us. The results are not surprising; we feel guilty. Before we can work effectively in rehabilitating these chronically disabled psychiatric patients, we must come to terms with these feelings in ourselves. We must be convinced, and not just intellectually, that pulling a patient in the direction of rehabilitation and away from chronic dependency may be painful for the patient, but in the long run beneficial to him in terms of heightened self-esteem and self-concept and greater ability to enjoy life.

In our own day hospital and in our observations of other agencies in varying stages of development our experience has been that overcoming feelings of guilt evoked by patients who attempt to manipulate us into allowing them to remain dependent and regressed is a major step in creating an effective rehabilitation process. Guilt may prevent us from discharging patients when they are long past being ready to move on; it may cause us to make them more dependent when their need is to become more independent. It may make us hesitate to suggest vocational planning.

One example of a guilt-provoking maneuver (though one which is less subtle than most) is the suicide gesture. It is, of course, not limited to the chronic patient. On occasion the suicide gesture may be a communication to us that we are expecting too much of a patient, but even in such a case it is certainly a faulty form of communication. More often the patient's intent is to evoke guilt and prevent us from putting into operation a much-needed therapeutic maneuver. It has been our experience that if such gestures are not dealt with quickly and firmly we put ourselves at a serious handicap in dealing with both the individual patient and the patient group. If the suicide gesture results in the patient getting what he wants (postponement of discharge or referral to a vocational placement or not involving a certain family member) then this mechanism may become "contagious" and other patients may use it. Furthermore, suicide gestures make those around them, including staff, angry and resentful. If these feelings are not openly conveyed to the patient, the staff's resentment may take the form of separating the patient from the agency for "other therapeutic reasons." Where possible the staff should see to it that the manipulative suicide gesture results in disadvantages to the patient which outweigh any advantages that might accrue, and this should be done directly and firmly.

Before one can make inroads into the thorny problems of rehabilitation of the chronic patient, one must first involve him in treatment. One must get him "hooked." Again the day hospital is well suited for this purpose. In a day hospital patients are taken care of, they are given a structured day, and are fed both literally and figuratively. Many patients who have little interest in rehabilitation are attracted to the day hospital initially by the prospect of receiving gratification of their dependency needs. Only later do they begin to become interested in the goals of rehabilitation.

Many chronic mentally ill patients have histories of social and emotional deprivation and chaotic family environments with resulting ego defects causing inadequacy in coping with the everyday stresses of life. In addition, cultural and superego deficits are all too frequent. For example, these patients may not have incorporated the values of work and responsibility. This is in contrast to many motivated outpatients in both clinics and private practice where we take such values for granted, and need not concern ourselves with the issue of whether or not we make demands of our patients to take responsibility, both for their treatment and their role in society. Much of our training has led us to believe that we should be non-judgmental and not make such demands. With the chronic psychiatric patient, on the other hand, the absence of motivation, both to "get better" and to work is often the first major obstacle that must be overcome in trying to effect their rehabilitation.

### Maintaining Expectations

Our experience, like that of others (Freeman and Simmons, 1963), has been that it is important for mental health professionals entrusted with the rehabilitation of chronic patients to maintain expectations of them that they will fully realize their potential, to make these expectations very clear to the patients and to use whatever influence that can be brought to bear to motivate them in this direction.

If we are to successfully maintain expectations of our patients these expectations must be no less than the patients can handle, but also they must be no more. To expect more than our patients can realistically do is to guarantee failure. In fact, there are some patients whose unconscious motivation for having unrealistic goals appears to be so that they will fail, and thus again be taken care of by a welfare agency or institution. Furthermore, it is important not to impose our own values or goals on our patients unrealistically. For instance, a very frequent goal that the staff might have for a patient is that he or she go to college or take a course to be a registered or licensed practical nurse. Patients, too, will often have these goals because of identification with us, and will strive toward these goals in order to please us. Though going to college or becoming a nurse is appropriate in some cases, in many more of the cases with which we work it is inappropriate and results only in another failure. We have to learn to be pleased if a patient with above normal intelligence but limited ego strength becomes a janitor if this is the realistic extent of his total social capabilities. Though perhaps this might, at first glance, seem like a limited achievement, it can in fact represent a great advance from a previous adjustment of institutionalization or chronic dependency.

Experience in the early stages of operating our day hospital made us realize the importance of community and family supports. The less the patient's ego strength, the more important are these external supports. We have learned that it is important early in our contact with the patient and his family, and preferably at the time of intake, to ascertain the interest, involvement, willingness to cooperate, and any tendencies to undermine the treatment on the part of the family. We have tried to deal with these problems before admitting the patient to the day hospital. In some cases we have postponed admission or if a patient is already in the day hospital, discharged him with the understanding that admission or readmission could be arranged at such time as the family was able to be more involved and cooperative with the patient's treatment.

The family's attitude in many cases helps to determine what the goals, if any, of day hospital will be. The family may want the patient to become more stabilized and less overtly psychotic, but not want the patient to be independent, to work or to increase his social life outside of the home. If the patient has similar wishes or does not have the ego strength to proceed with his own goals toward even partial independence, then any attempts at rehabilitation will be fruitless and we must settle for a partial reintegration of the patient up to a point within the family's tolerance. Sometimes the family can be worked with in resolving issues threatening to them, but we have learned that it is important to recognize when the family's psychopathology is more powerful than our therapeutic efforts.

We were often hard put, especially in the beginning, to decide whether a patient could live alone and still possess sufficient outside resources to support his treatment in the day hospital. Initially some sick patients living alone suffered rapid exacerbations of illness, and we became extremely hesitant to accept any patient living by himself. Our experience since has shown that one should judge this issue on an individual basis, for some patients have sufficient ego strength to be able to live alone and survive in the community during the hours they are not in the day hospital. Other patients do not have sufficient ego strength to live apart from their families or a resource like a halfway house. Thus, although one needs to evaluate a patient's living alone very carefully, this fact alone need not exclude him from treatment in a day hospital.

Although seemingly very obvious, mention should be made of the importance of arranging transportation prior to admission to the day hospital. Our experience has been that lack of a clear understanding between the patient and his family and the staff as to just how transportation is to be arranged has often given family or patients a readily available rationalization for their resistance to treatment in the day hospital. We have also found, especially with sicker patients, that having the family bring the patient for the first few days, even when the patient can drive, can be very supportive to the patient during the initial difficult period of adjustment and integration into the day hospital.

### The Sociopath

Few issues are as perplexing in the day hospital as those raised in trying to formulate goals for treating patients with sociopathic tendencies. One aspect of the problem is the expectation on the part of the referral source or the day hospital staff, or the patient, that the day hospital experience will result in character change. As described above, this is seldom a realistic goal for a short-term treatment facility. Our experience with patients with severe character disorders, including those with sociopathic tendencies, is that they become very dependent, and that so much of their efforts and energies become channeled into maintaining themselves in the situation where their needs are met that very little energy is left over for the work of therapy and character change. Furthermore, these are people who tend to act out or live out their problems rather than internalizing. Close, meaningful relationships are extremely threatening to them; as they become involved with staff and other patients, their tendency is to revert to some of their sociopathic and acting out kinds of character defenses as ways of warding off the threat of intimacy. Thus disruptive behavior, excessive drinking, undermining of the staff and patient leaders, and the like, become obstacles not only to their own treatment but to the treatment of the total day hospital group. Moreover, schizophrenic patients with poor ego strength are impressed by the charm and what seems superficially like the relatively healthy ego strength of the sociopath and are easily involved and influenced by the patient who uses sociopathic defenses. Sometimes the non-sociopathic patient with poor ego strength and poorly fixed identity is manipulated into acting for the sociopathic patients while the latter sit innocently in the background. Moreover, schizophrenic patients are often frightened by the lack of impulse control of the sociopath and even more frightened when the staff seems unable to cope with them. Conversely, the schizophrenic who himself is unable to rebel may vicariously enjoy watching the sociopaths act out their conflicts with authority and for this reason further encourage the disruptive behavior.

Here again our own experience has led us to keep in mind the concept of limited goals. For instance, a patient with sociopathic tendencies may be treated in the day hospital for a depressive episode and then leave to continue his life as before without the day hospital staff feeling compelled to alter his life style. We have also learned that the day hospital can tolerate only a few patients with sociopathic tendencies at any given time. When there are more than two or three such patients, then the staff's problem of setting limits on their behavior and the patient leadership's problem of coping with them become such that the therapeutic goals for all the patients in the day hospital may be compromised. We have also concluded that only rarely can the "hardened sociopath" (the heroin addict, the habitual criminal, and the like) be helped in a setting as unstructured as the day hospital unless all the patients there are "hardened sociopaths" and thus able to understand and handle each other.

## Day Hospital Program

Early in the history of our day hospital, many of the staff, and in particular the psychiatrists and social workers, tended to downgrade the importance of occupational therapy and recreational therapy, and to see individual and group therapy as the cornerstones of treatment. This attitude was detrimental in at least two respects. For one thing, it reduced the effectiveness of the activity program, for these attitudes could not help but be communicated in subtle ways to the patients. Further, the nurses and activity staff felt left out and devalued and began to compete with the psychiatrists and social workers for a place in the therapy limelight. These problems were resolved in two ways. First, nurses were included in small group therapy, a plan which will be further discussed below when the team approach in the day hospital is described.

Secondly, we came to recognize that, in addition to setting the tone and establishing a therapeutic atmosphere, the activity program played fully as important a role as any of the other treatment modalities. This is especially so in a setting where group and individual psychotherapy on the one hand and art lessons, discussion groups, and recreational activities on the other have been assigned almost equal status by virtue of a treatment philosophy which stresses short-term limited goals and restoration to functioning rather than a resolution of unconscious conflicts or change in character structure. We found it extremely important to make this explicit to both patients and staff in both staff meetings and therapeutic community meetings. In the same vein we have found that it is extremely important to stress the philosophy and purpose of occupational therapy and recreational therapy in general, and the specific activities in particular to both patients and staff. For instance, one should point out to the women that their grooming sessions are for the purpose of helping them become more attractive and well-groomed to enhance their success in both social and vocational activities outside the day hospital both before and after discharge. Recreational activities became more meaningful as we explained that the purpose was not to kill time in the day hospital but to help our patients learn how to play and how to use their leisure time. Explaining the purpose of each activity helps the patient to approach these activities with a more enlightened enthusiasm and helps staff to support the activities and encourage their patients to participate in them actively.

As in the Brooklyn day hospital (Carmichael, 1964), we emphasize activities which impart to the patient skills that can be translated into his life beyond the day hospital and into the community. Our stress on translatable skills emphasizes the ultimate goal of productivity rather than dependency, activity rather than passivity, and early return to the community. Thus, after the patient has passed through the acute phase of his illness we aim to provide in the day hospital, insofar as possible, a setting in which he can assume his normal social role. For instance, if the patient is normally a wage earner, vocational goals and the development of skills are emphasized. If a patient is normally a homemaker, activities involving cooking, sewing, and the like, are emphasized. If the patient is a student, we might arrange to have a home teacher come to the day hospital so that the patient can continue his studies while still a full-time patient. By the same token, we are concerned with helping patients to learn how to play and use leisure time. We gear many of our activities to interesting patients in hobbies and activities which hopefully can be continued after discharge. While some patients find it all too easy to play, others are constricted and guilt-ridden and find it difficult to indulge themselves in any way.

It is sometimes not realized that patients can become institutionalized in a day hospital just as much as they might on a twenty-four-hour inpatient service. Even though patients go home in the evenings and on weekends, they are still involved in a treatment program that occupies their full day, five days a week. Not only does this provide a tremendous amount of dependency gratification, but also establishes their full-time occupation as that of patient. If continued for extended periods of time, this can be a very powerful environment for fostering dependency and an identity of full-time patient. From these considerations has come the emphasis on active treatment and movement in the day hospital. We have learned that we need to ask ourselves continually, "Are patients making good use of the day hospital rather than remaining static? Are they actively participating rather than passively being taken care of?" We must constantly translate into action the concept of maintaining expectations that patients will realize their potential.

With this concept of active treatment in mind, we expect all of our patients to arrive on time, stay for their full assigned time, and participate in the program as if it were a job. As a matter of fact, we try to get across to our patients that they should consider the day hospital as a place of employment where they are to work on their problems. The day hospital begins each day with a meaningful structured activity—either small group therapy, the large community group meeting, or the activity group meeting where the patients plan some of the activities and much of their recreation during the week. In this meeting they also participate in some of the administrative functions of the day hospital. Beginning each day with a group meeting points up the importance of arriving on time, and makes arriving late something that is noticed and discussed by the group or individually with the staff. In contrast, at one time we attempted to start the day hospital day with a fifteen-minute period allotted for coffee. If a patient was late, it was difficult to discuss with him meaningfully why it should matter that he was late for coffee. We still offer coffee the first thing in the morning, but we offer it a half-hour prior to the start of the group meeting. Attendance at this coffee time is elective. But whether or not they come for coffee earlier, all patients are expected to be present at 9:00 A.M. when the meeting starts.

Friday afternoon can be a difficult time in a day hospital. Patients may be anxious about the weekend—because of increased interaction with family or lack of sources of support outside of the day hospital. Problems may arise on Friday which cannot be resolved before the weekend. With this in mind, we instituted a social hour for the last hour on Friday afternoon, in which all patients and staff participate. Patients choose the activity, which may be any of the regular day hospital activities. Table games are the most frequently chosen. The social hour has provided an informal, relaxed ending to the week, and Friday afternoon is no longer the hectic time it once was. Staff schedule nothing else during this time; if a crisis should arise, they are available to take care of it. Participating in a social gathering with staff also furthers patients' development of social skills.

One of the major problems in working with chronic patients

is lack of motivation. Much is to be learned about remotivating chronic patients, but some methods can be cited. The day hospital culture, which emphasizes that the day hospital is a place to work on one's problems, and not simply a place to be taken care of, is one. Such a day hospital culture needs to be initially fostered for the most part by staff, but once in operation it can be maintained by both patients and staff. The effects of group pressure, especially from one's peers, are very important in fostering maturity, independence, and responsibility. Identification with the staff is another powerful tool. Patients, as they get to know us and to like us, want to be more like us and attempt to perform not only as we expect, but as we ourselves perform. Thus staff become models for the patients.

An important concept in this area of remotivation is *leverage*. For most of our patients life is a constant struggle. Because of limited ego functioning, even the everyday stresses of life seem difficult. For these patients the path of least resistance is often to regress rather than to continue to grapple with their problems. In addition, superego defects frequently complicate the picture, and the pressures from within to strive toward maturity and responsibility are lacking. Therefore, most chronic patients are in need of some kind of pressure from the staff and community. In order to exert this pressure, one has to have some kind of leverage. In some cases leverage can be provided by the authority of the court where the judge presents day hospitalization to the patient as an alternative to commitment. The patient realizes that if he does not involve himself in treatment he will, in fact, be sent to the state hospital. The family can be encouraged to place pressure on the patient. In many cases we acquire leverage only gradually as the patient gets to know us, to like us, and to become dependent on the institution. He gets to the point where the fear of being excluded from the day hospital becomes greater than the fear of attempting some vocational or social task. At this point one can say to a patient, "You must take this step if you wish to remain in the day hospital," and this is frequently a very powerful motivating force. In all these ways one hopes to compensate for the patient's deficient superego development and fear of even partial independence, and help him ultimately to develop his own superego and provide his own motivation. Frequently leverage needs to be applied only for a short time until the patient has gotten into the situation and found that he is able to master it. At this point, fortified by his new-found self-esteem and self-confidence, he needs little or no further leverage exerted by day hospital staff to continue.

Another aspect of motivating the patient and helping him to overcome his fear of a step forward is structuring the situation into which he is moving in such a way that he is partially protected from some of the normal pressures of society. Examples of this might be a sheltered workshop, a job placement with an understanding supervisor, a social therapy club run for ex-patients, or a halfway house.

### Treatment Teams

A day hospital program hopefully evolves into a well-functioning group program with an emphasis on integrating patients into this program so they can realize benefits from group therapy, the activity program and the resocializing milieu. As our program developed, we found that, in addition, our patients were very much in need of an individualized treatment plan taking into account the patient and his family's psychodynamics, their strengths and weaknesses, and their individual and collective motivation to determine what problems could most effectively be resolved and which were most important to resolve. Decisions were needed as to the extent and nature of family involvement; should staff contacts be with one particular relative or with several, and should these contacts be with relatives alone or relatives and patient together? Collaboration was needed between day hospital staff who knew the patient well and the vocational counselor so they could pool their knowledge of both the patient's psychodynamics and his vocational potential to formulate a workable vocational plan as part of the overall individualized treatment plan. Formulation of specific day hospital treatment goals was closely linked with setting up an aftercare plan tailored to the needs of each individual patient.

An interdisciplinary approach was needed, but at the same time the total staff was unable to formulate a detailed plan for each and every patient in a day hospital with an average daily census of over thirty patients. Our solution to this problem was to divide the staff into three treatment teams, each team consisting of a psychiatrist, a social worker, and a nurse, having responsibility for all of the eleven to thirteen patients on their team.

We have tied the use of small group therapy into the team concept by having the treatment team be co-therapists for small group therapy in which all of the team's patients participate three times weekly. This has also resolved the problem of patients and staff being excluded from small groups, for all patients are included and the nurses are brought into group therapy as co-therapists. In many ways each team and small group of patients re-enacts within itself the pattern of a family with all of its rivalry, sharing of accomplishments and concerns for its members. When properly utilized, this has been a very powerful therapeutic tool for our patients, many of whom have come from chaotic and pathological family situations.

We have found that using teams in this way works best when the staff of each team is given considerable autonomy in the planning, decision-making, and treatment of their patients. But this, too, leads to problems. Each small patient group becomes a simulated family unit which then must in turn interact and function within the larger context of the total day hospital which in this sense represents the community. This arrangement provides a fertile field for therapeutic interaction for the patients. However, the staff on each team also finds itself in a similar situation with regard to the total staff. Thus there may be a conflict between team staff autonomy and the total institutional interest. An example might be found in a referral which is borderline acceptable in terms of the usual day hospital admission criteria but where the referral source is an agency with whom it is important for the day hospital to have a good working relationship, such as the state hospital or the county inpatient service or family service. Obviously an inappropriate referral should be turned down, but in borderline cases the treatment team may not see the need for maintaining such good working relationships as clearly as, say, the chief psychiatrist or supervising social worker. The result is that the treatment team may hesitate to give other agencies the benefit of the doubt on borderline cases and not accept the patient on at least a trial basis. Another example would be where the team wants to treat a patient in a way which runs counter to the philosophy of the day hospital and which would give other patients a mixed message as to what we are really expecting of them. It is in situations like these that the team can feel that their autonomy is being threatened. Our experience has been that most professionals can at one time or another, depending on the issue, feel that team autonomy is more vital than the welfare of the day hospital as a whole, especially when the small group and treatment team morale becomes strong as it can in such a simulated family.

We have come to deal with this problem by impressing on the teams that limitless autonomy when not properly used can compromise the needs and image of the total institution (which of course includes the teams) and as a by-product penalize unnecessarily those patients who become innocent victims of inter-team and team-administration conflict. In short, administration must be free to grant autonomy to the teams but must also feel free in setting limits on this autonomy when necessary. Frank discussion in total staff meetings has been very helpful in getting these issues into perspective.

Another problem has been conflict in deciding who should lead the teams. Our day hospital has followed the medical model of having the psychiatrists (both staff and resident) assume medical-legal responsibility and leadership on each team. However, we recognize that this way of running a team is not the only way nor even necessarily the best way. For a period of one year an experienced psychiatric social worker assumed the role of leadership on a team with a psychiatrist handling only medications and being available for consultation when necessary. There was some initial negative response from patients who felt deprived at not having a doctor for their primary therapist, and there was also some doubt on the part of the staff as to the effects of a social worker assuming what had always seemed to be a medical responsibility. The results, however, showed that a team led by an experienced nonmedical therapist can be fully as effective as the medically led teams. As a result of this experience, we feel we would not hesitate to assign gifted, nonmedical therapists to all of the treatment tasks now assumed by psychiatric residents or staff psychiatrists—with the exception, of course, of those functions which legally can only be performed by a physician. We realize that this arrangement is not unique, and that many day hospitals are administered by physicians but actually run by nonmedical personnel. One unique aspect of our situation was that treatment teams led by social workers or psychiatrists could function side by side without undue feelings of differing status.

### Blurred Versus Defined Roles

The question of blurred, overlapping roles versus well-defined roles is one that every institution must resolve. Our day hospital has resolved this question by a combination of the two concepts. Our experience has been that blurring of roles has been very helpful to our treatment program. For instance, nurses participate in group psychotherapy and are expected to contribute to the decision-making processes of both individual treatment plans and total day hospital policy. Psychiatrists and social workers are expected by the total staff to attend and be active at many of the social and recreational activities in the day hospital.

We have also seen the importance of each staff member feeling that he or she has a specific contribution to make and a specific and unique skill based on his own training and experience. As an example we would like to describe the role of the social worker as it has evolved in our day hospital.

In addition to being a co-therapist in small group therapy, an active participant in the large community meetings and in decision-making both in the team and at total staff meetings, and a participant in some of the social and recreational treatment modalities, the social worker is seen and sees himself as having a specific contribution to make from his own training and background. Social workers have primary responsibility for contact, and, if indicated, treatment for family members or other collaterals. Without family contact or if the family is not effectively drawn into the total treatment effort, attempts at successful treatment may be sabotaged by family members who see treatment as a threat to the family equilibrium. It is also recognized that little, if any, feedback from the patient's life situation would be available to the team if the family were not involved. The information gained in such a way is essential for a sound treatment plan. The social worker's contact with the relatives and evaluation of the family dynamics may show, for example, that a particular symbiotic bond between patient and collateral exists which, although pathological, may be one which either the patient or the collateral or both are unable or unwilling to give up at that point in time. Thus, the social worker's evaluation may prevent a fruitless and possibly even antitherapeutic attempt on the part of staff to separate the patient from his family. Therefore, in keeping with good casework practice, it has become the task of the social work staff in the day hospital to examine the family interaction patterns that enhance or impede individual or family function and have direct bearing on treatment goals.

A knowledge of cultural values is a necessary part of the social worker's armamentarium, for cultural factors need to be considered when diagnoses and treatment plans are formulated. In addition, the social worker contributes his experience in collaborating with other agencies. In many cases, even when a psychiatrist is on the team, the social worker's expertise in casework and psychotherapy enables him to be the primary therapist for many individual patients. Thus, the social worker has the feeling that his specific skills and training can contribute to his value and effectiveness as a part of the total treatment team.

Consideration was given at one time in our day hospital to "legislating" against one-to-one psychotherapy. We also know of other day hospitals and inpatient services where this has been done. We observed in our own and other institutions that such a situation leads to a form of bootleg psychotherapy. A patient and staff member appear to be playing checkers but in actuality they are busily engaged in a form of individual psychotherapy. We have concluded that individual psychotherapy does have an important place in the day hospital.

Many issues can be more meaningfully and effectively dealt with in a one-to-one situation than in a group situation. We have found it necessary, however, to consider some special problems when using individual psychotherapy in a day hospital setting. The patient's stay in the day hospital is time-limited. If one uses outpatient intensive psychotherapy as a model, in most cases one has barely reached the opening phase of such treatment by the time it is appropriate to discharge the patient from the day hospital. At this point, either it is decided to keep the patient longer, which is inappropriate and fosters dependency, or the patient feels cheated and angry in that he has been seduced into opening up painful areas which he then must leave unresolved, and is now perhaps further confused and more conflicted than before.

Another problem that frequently arises with individual therapy is the establishment of too close a relationship between the therapist and the patient when this cannot be continued as an ongoing aftercare relationship. Thus at the time of separation from the day hospital, which is at best difficult and painful, the patient finds himself further burdened by having to give up a very meaningful and important relationship. The net result of this inappropriate use of individual psychotherapy is, therefore, a more painful separation at the time of discharge and a heightened feeling of anger and resentment, which make more difficult his shifting over to needed aftercare on an outpatient basis. Equally important is the diversion of the patient's attention from one of the primary goals of day hospital treatment, namely improvement of his social and vocational skills, and return to functioning in the community. These pitfalls can be avoided by keeping the subject matter of the individual therapist-patient relationship oriented toward reality here and now, and by attempting to deal with issues which can be resolved in the time allowed in the brief course of day hospital treatment. Such subjects might include the precipitating stresses which brought the patient into treatment and their resolution, patient's feelings about giving up a life of dependency and attempting again to compete in the world, and interpersonal problems in the day hospital which may typify the patient's interpersonal problems with people in general. We have tried to maintain sufficient rapport between the patient and his individual therapist so that the goals of treatment can be accomplished, but sufficient distance so that the patient's separation does not become more painful than need be.

Employment and vocational services have come to be an important aspect of our day hospital program for both acute and chronic patients. Vocational services and work not only help persons toward the goal of employment, but also can be an essential treatment modality in the overall rehabilitation of patients. This will be described in more detail in the chapter on vocational services.

### Day Hospital Aftercare

A number of studies (Fairweather et al., 1960; Freeman and Simmons, 1963) in recent years have shown that the patient's success or failure of adjustment in the community after hospitalization is related not so much to the kind of treatment that he received in the institution prior to discharge, but is related almost entirely to the treatment and support that are available to the patient in the community.

Likewise, it has been our experience that fully as important as rehabilitating the patient in the day hospital is our role in providing him with an adequate aftercare plan and having the resources available in the community to carry it out. For most patients with problems severe enough to warrant day hospitalization, discharge from day hospital should be simply a point of transition to another phase of ongoing treatment of which day hospitalization was only a part, albeit a very important part. To put these concepts into action we have initiated a program where our day hospital is closed for one afternoon a week to current day hospital patients in order to devote itself exclusively during that afternoon to the aftercare of ex-patients (Lamb, 1967b).

Most of our patients have come to our day hospital because of problems, both acute and chronic, of psychotic or borderline psychotic proportions. As described above they, in general, are not candidates for intensive, uncovering psychotherapy. Many are from the lower socioeconomic classes, and are relatively nonverbal and nonpsychologically minded (Carlson et al., 1965). Many of our patients tend to drop out of treatment prematurely because of their need to deny their dependency, or because of elements of obstinacy in their character, or inability to trust, or fear of closeness, or a combination of some or all of these factors. Thus they need active pursuit by mental health professionals who will reach out to the patient in spite of poor motivation and help him return to treatment.

In these characteristics they are unlike the so-called good patient who seems to get priority of outpatient treatment from many mental health professionals (Hollingshead and Redlich, 1958). Indeed, we have found it difficult to "sell" most of our patients to other mental health facilities for outpatient treatment. Furthermore, many patients have strong feelings of rejection when they are referred outside of the day hospital for aftercare. Fears of meeting new treatment staff also contribute to the difficulty of making the transition to a new agency.

For all these reasons our attempts to refer day hospital patients to other treatment resources frequently resulted in no aftercare at all. We therefore gave much thought to ways of providing aftercare within the day hospital itself, utilizing the day hospital staff. Ex-patients have always been welcome to return to visit in the day hospital since it opened in 1961. On one afternoon a week, which was set aside as open house, ex-patients were invited to come to the day hospital, join in the activities with patients currently in the day hospital, talk to the staff and other patients, and in some cases receive psychotherapy or medications from the day hospital staff. This was a source of considerable support for many ex-patients, especially in the period of readjustment following discharge from the day hospital, and at times of crisis.

But problems gradually became apparent. The staff found it difficult to divide its time between the current day hospital patients and the aftercare patients. There was competition between these two groups for the time and attention of the staff. Most importantly because of limitations of staff time, we were able to offer meaningful aftercare services to only a limited number of our ex-patients. It was with this background that we evolved our present aftercare program, which has been under way in its present form since March of 1966.

Our day hospital is now closed for one afternoon a week to current day hospital patients in order to allow the entire day hospital staff to focus on aftercare without distractions from the regular business of the day hospital. The same staff members who treated the patients in the day hospital provide a social therapy program as well as individual and group psychotherapy, couples therapy, casework with families, occupational and recreational therapy, and medications for whatever period of time is indicated. In some cases it appears that this may be a long-term or even lifelong contract, either continuously or intermittently. With this new program we are now able to offer aftercare services to almost all of our patients after discharge. We are also able to capitalize on the patients' familiarity with the setting and transference to the institution and can give them all the advantages of continuity of care. Initially, there was much staff concern that cutting our program for regular day hospital patients to four and one-half days a week would have an adverse effect upon them. To our surprise, even acutely ill patients have seemed to do as well.

The afternoon begins with a twenty- to thirty-minute meeting of all aftercare patients and staff. The group assigns tasks for the afternoon such as cleanup, plans activities, and sometimes discusses problems that are of concern to them. A different patient acts as chairman each week, which permits many patients to take a position of leadership before a group of people (at this point about fifty persons on the average, including staff). This meeting has been successful in helping the group become more cohesive. Such questions as "Who will clean the coffee pot?" have become standing jokes shared by both patients and staff. This meeting also sets a tone of informality and encourages easy mingling.

An activity period follows the meeting. The activities chosen by the patients are usually ones familiar to them from the day hospital program. As happens in the day hospital the patients often want the staff to plan the activities, leaving the patient's role in planning one of passive compliance. Or the patients may choose activities in which they can be passive, such as movies and lectures. However, with some gentle urging by the staff, especially in the beginning, we have been able to get the patients to assume responsibility for planning a balanced program. Most popular are table games (which provide a vehicle for social interaction in many social groups), socializing over coffee, and volleyball. These three activities have become part of the regular weekly schedule. The patients also select other activities requiring active participation, such as holiday parties, a personal grooming program for women, and occupational therapy.

Food is an important part of the program. There are refreshments each week—coffee provided by the day hospital and cake and cookies brought in by patients and staff. Potluck picnics, where again the responsibility for supplying the food is shared by both patients and staff, are also extremely popular with the patients and, we feel, therapeutic. One chronically schizophrenic young man, who at one time was quite resistant to treatment, was heard to say as he left the buffet table with his plate laden with food, "This is the kind of therapy I like!" It is important for the patients to be fed. It gives them a feeling of being taken care of, which makes treatment more acceptable and attractive. At the same time, bringing in some of the food themselves helps them gradually become more able to feed others. As would be imagined, this whole question of feeding and being fed is a core conflict with many patients in our group.

We usually let the patient himself decide how often he should attend the activity program. We believe that the informality of the program and the familiar faces of the staff and other patients make it fairly easy for the patient to return to it in times of crisis. However, for some patients who appear reluctant to come and for whom we feel attendance at the activity program is especially important, we may "prescribe" regular attendance and participation especially in the period of transition immediately after discharge from the day hospital. For those who attend regularly, the program is like a half-day a week day hospital.

We attempt to tailor the specific services made available to each individual patient to his specific individual needs. For some patients medications and the activity program seem to be the therapy of choice, with more intensive treatment and intervention at times of crisis only. This group includes a number of patients whose relationship is primarily with the institution. Several patients who in the past developed "transference psychoses" in more intensive individual psychotherapy, which could not be worked through and led to reinstitutionalization, have done extremely well in such a program. For those patients for whom we feel group therapy is indicated, groups meet for an hour every other week. Some patients and their spouses are seen in couples therapy.

We emphasize employment and vocational services as an important part of our program both in the day hospital and in aftercare. Many of the patients in our aftercare program continue to be seen by our vocational counselors. Many are involved full- or part-time on work placement or in our sheltered workshop.

Despite the large amount of emphasis on group and social therapy we feel that individual therapy on a regular ongoing basis is extremely important for many of our patients. As in the day hospital itself, we feel that the group and social therapies on the one hand and individual therapy on the other are not mutually exclusive but rather that they complement and supplement each other if an individualized aftercare plan takes into account the patient's particular needs and problems. Individual therapy, we should add, need not be a fifty-minute hour, nor weekly; it may be twenty minutes every two weeks, or once a month. For many patients there is no substitute for the one-to-one relationship with a therapist who understands the dynamics of the case and who can apply this knowledge in a practical way by helping patients work through current and past conflicts and by giving specific kinds of advice. Again, this is not working through the core conflicts in an attempt to "cure" schizophrenia, but rather a more reality-oriented therapy or ego-building therapy geared to handling situational and interpersonal stresses which might, without help, overwhelm the patient. We consider this more than supportive therapy; we hope that the patient will learn how to better cope with his problems and in time will need less help from us in handling stressful situations.

We have described earlier our belief that the activity program plays fully as important a role as any of the other treatment modalities in the day hospital, and in many ways sets the tone and establishes a therapeutic atmosphere. In our aftercare program, too, we aim to place emphasis on occupational therapy and recreational therapy. We see our program as one where all the treatment modalities, individual and group psychotherapy, occupational and recreational therapy, social therapy and medications, play an important role.

We have come to know our patients and their individual patterns of reaction to stress quite well during their stay in the day hospital and subsequent participation in the aftercare program. Thus, staff members, while chatting informally with patients or observing their participation in activities, can often readily identify the early signs of exacerbation of illness. Frequently, patients are unable to ask directly for help. The early recognition of illness has enabled us to avert crises or to readmit patients while the problem can still be easily managed and resolved.

All patients in aftercare are assigned to both a psychiatrist and a social worker. If the psychiatrist is the primary therapist, the social worker usually is called in only when the family must be involved. If the social worker is the primary therapist, then the psychiatrist may only write prescriptions and not be involved otherwise except in special circumstances. The patient is aware that both a psychiatrist and a social worker are assigned to his case; we feel this knowledge is very supportive to him, even though he may contact the secondary staff member infrequently or not at all.

The philosophy of our aftercare program is an extension of that of our day hospital. We want our patients to be able to take responsibility and to give to others and to the program. When they become able to do so, they frequently then are able to apply these attitudes in their lives outside the program with a consequent improvement in their level of functioning and rise in their self-esteem. We work to make the culture of our aftercare program one in which the attitudes of active participation and taking responsibility are taken for granted and communicated to patients not only by staff but also by other patients. Sometimes these issues are explicitly discussed in the group meeting.

Our aftercare program provides considerable support, but not on the scale of a full-time day hospital which over long periods of time would foster dependency to an unnecessary and unhealthy degree. At the beginning the staff was concerned that the half-day a week program itself might foster undue dependency. But we have found that only about a fourth of our active aftercare patients come regularly, stay the full afternoon, and appear to be permanent aftercare fixtures. Considering the neediness and the degree of illness of this group, a half-day a week of ongoing day hospital appears to be quite appropriate for them. We have found that some patients tend to attend less than they should or drop out prematurely, but for the most part patients do not tend to overprescribe for themselves in terms of treatment in our aftercare program.

At first, staff also feared that they might be overburdened when the responsibility for a multitude of needy, dependent aftercare patients was added to their regular caseload in the day hospital. But this has not been the case. We feel that our patients make good use of our program, but they do not drain us—perhaps partly because we emphasize active participation and acceptance of responsibility, perhaps because our support helps them make better use of their own strengths, and perhaps because of the ongoing collaboration with psychiatric vocational services and the sheltered workshop.

It is too early to evaluate fully the results of our aftercare program. Nonetheless, we feel that we have been able to provide most of our patients with a meaningful continuation of their day hospital treatment, a continuation that helps them maintain and, in many cases, improve their level of functioning and sense of well-being in the community. Furthermore, the staff had found it very rewarding to participate in the ongoing treatment of patients, rather than simply catching a prolonged glimpse of them in the very specialized situation of the day hospital.

CHAPTER **6**

# Transitional Housing

*Charles Richmond*

ᒫᒷᒫᒷᒫᒷᒫᒷᒫᒷᒫᒷᒫᒷᒫᒷᒫᒷᒫᒷᒫᒷᒫᒷᒫᒷ

**H**alfway houses, as we now know them, are a distinctive new development, still in an early stage of evolution. Despite a growing literature, many of the theoretical and operational assumptions are destined to receive much more research and evaluation in the years ahead. In San Mateo County, the appearance of a halfway house in February, 1967, after two years of community organization groundwork, marked an important new stage of interest in sheltered transitional placement of the mentally disabled. The current thrust of the San Mateo halfway house program is two-pronged: toward evolving a high-expectation, performance-oriented culture for residents within the halfway house, on the one hand, and toward utilizing existing housing in the community in creating post-halfway house living accommodations with built-in provision for follow-up and aftercare. For some individuals, the halfway house will

145

lead to fully independent living; others will require continuing supportive living arrangements and therapeutic social group contact while
residing semi-independently within the community. This latter trend
is exemplified by our satellite apartment program and social club,
which will be described later in this chapter. These aspects of the El
Camino House program appear to depart from operational patterns
reported elsewhere in the literature. In recounting the experience of
this program, the focus will be upon these twin concerns, each of which
is highly relevant for any community trying to innovate methods by
which large numbers of disabled individuals can be maintained locally
without creating huge new institutions in the community.

### Varieties of Halfway Houses

It is significant that what might be considered a halfway house
movement did not begin until the early 1950s—approximately coincident with the early birth pangs of the community mental health movement. In one of the early papers on residential halfway houses, Reik
(1953) proposed the following rationale:

> It is conceivable that some [patients], if carefully selected, would do
> well in an environment in which the emphasis was placed on health
> rather than on disease. . . . It seems logical to think that an en-
> vironment intermediate between the hospital and outside world—
> a "halfway house"—would make an important contribution to the
> rehabilitation of properly selected patients. . . . Having moved
> from the restrictive and dependent existence of the mental hospital
> to the more independent, but still relatively simple, . . . life at
> "halfway house," he would logically be better prepared to take his
> place in his own community again.

The definition of what constitutes a halfway house has undergone constant change since the beginning of the movement. Reik (1953) initially defined the halfway house as a "specialized residential facility for
mentally ill patients." Wechsler surveyed nine transitional residences
for the mentally ill in 1961 and attempted to classify two types: the
halfway house model and the work camp model. However, his paper
simply amplified the degree of variation which existed between and
within the categories (Wechsler, 1961).

Huseth differentiated between types of facilities on the basis of

type of patient accepted in residence and distinguished between rehabilitative, preventive, and mixed halfway houses; short-term and
long-term facilities; and psychiatric halfway houses as distinguished
from houses for other special groups such as alcoholics, the mentally
retarded, and ex-convicts (Huseth, 1961). Goertzel (1965) estimated
that there were approximately one hundred psychiatric halfway houses
in the United States in 1964. Of the twelve he selected for survey,
eight were of the residential model and four of the "day center–social
recreational" variety. Rothwell and Doniger (1966) estimated there
were about fifty halfway houses by 1963. They pointed out that halfway houses were increasingly performing a variety of functions; persons who had never been hospitalized, but who had severe difficulties
which could conceivably lead to hospitalization, were being accepted
for admission. Additionally, nonresidential, social-vocational rehabilitation centers which provide post-hospital services were also being referred to as halfway houses. A differential definition of halfway houses
continues to be elusive. These programs continue to differ greatly in
orientation, emphasis, staffing, sponsorship, size, types of patients accepted, length of stay, and a multitude of other factors.

Perhaps one of the most significant differences is the extent to
which a house program is patterned around the medical model as contrasted to the sociological model. Houses that have a medical model
orientation provide more direct services, such as individual and group
psychotherapy, nursing, and medical supervision. These programs are
often closely affiliated with, or even sponsored by, psychiatric hospitals,
and some are located on hospital grounds. A multitude of services are
provided within the house rather than by community resources. The
rationale of the sociological model according to Gumrukcu (1966) is
that:

Relationships with other residents and volunteers is the key and
appropriate means of conditioning for community living. This rationale assumes patient leadership and responsibility of action within
the house setting, and emphasis on spontaneous rather than structured social activities, and on self-care and autonomy rather than
meals and room maintenance provided by staff. With patient-resi-
dent leadership there is needed a fairly wide continuum of health-
pathology, with the healthier ones serving as catalysts and leaders.
The house may include some non-patients to allow for the patient

population to identify with the normal community and reduce the stigmatization of the patient label. . . . Psychiatric and other professional personnel serve best as consultants or background help.

El Camino House is modeled along sociological lines as described above. The basic philosophy of El Camino House is that patients recovering from mental illness, who may not have adequate family or residential resources, can best be rehabilitated in a setting that is as free of hospital-type institutionality as possible and that provides an atmosphere and structure conducive to social recovery and self-care. The internal social system of the house is regarded as a vital force for creating a milieu that will maximize the individual's ability for performance in society and adjustment to social roles.

Important to the theoretical orientation of El Camino House is the acceptance of a conceptual and operational distinction between rehabilitation and treatment. While it may be said that both of these activities are provided for within the service simultaneously, and both are an integral part of the therapeutic process, the primary focus is on rehabilitation. We accept Rapoport's (1960) definition of rehabilitation as ". . . those measures that have as their immediate aim, the fitting of a particular personality to the demands of an ongoing social system." Treatment, defined as those attempts to enhance characterological or personality change, also occurs within our setting; however, efforts aimed toward such change are not of the consultation room variety, but rather emanate through the existence of a therapeutic milieu, informal encounters between residents, volunteers, and staff, and utilization of role models.

Our rationale for distinguishing between treatment and rehabilitation and emphasizing the latter is our belief that the halfway house should be as unlike the hospital and other treatment settings as possible in order to more closely emulate the community at large. The milieu of the halfway house must be sufficiently different so that the resident does not regard it simply as an extension of the hospital within the community, where he can continue maladaptive behavior patterns. Although therapeutic in its own right, the halfway house is part of a total treatment program which includes day treatment, vocational rehabilitation, and traditional modes of psychotherapy which residents receive outside of the halfway house.

The concept of self-determination is of prime importance to the El Camino House program. Residents are regarded as self-determining individuals with both the responsibilities and privileges of that status. A core element is the provision of opportunities for residents to take an active part in the affairs of the house. Residents have their own keys, and may come and go as they wish, as there are no curfews; they are responsible for their own personal hygiene, for the taking of prescribed medications, for the cooking of all meals, and for the housekeeping of the entire house. In essence, they are responsible for any and all activities which they will have to assume when they reenter the larger community.

Behavioral expectations are outlined to prospective residents at the time of intake and as needed throughout the resident's house tenure. In summary, expectations are: behavior which is acceptable in the community at large or in an ordinary family, that is, common courtesy and consideration of others. Any behavior that infringes upon the rights of other residents is unacceptable. In some respects it can be said of the halfway house that expectations exceed those of the general society. Attention paid to pathology is minimized, while the concept of residual strength and abilities is emphasized. A crucial, oft-repeated theme is that no matter how upset or depressed a resident might feel, he still has the capacity to function at some reasonable level, even if this means merely procuring a substitute for one of the jobs within the house to which he is assigned. In keeping with this philosophy, residents who do not plan to be at dinner or who do not feel well enough to be with the resident group at dinner must still call in or sign out as a courtesy to the resident cooking teams. Persons expecting to be away for a weekend or those who do not expect to return to the house from a date or for some other reason until the early morning hours are requested merely to inform a staff member of the hour they can be expected to return. One very stringent requirement, however, is that each resident must be involved in some structured daytime activity—job, school, day treatment center, vocational workshop, work experience placement, vocational training—between 9:00 A.M. and 4:00 P.M. weekdays. During my previous halfway house association at Harvey House in Palo Alto, California, I observed that those residents who were inactive or resistive to some structuring of daytime hours tended to deteriorate or were seldom successful in their attempts to achieve self-sufficiency. Where there was uncertainty or lack of clarity on the part of staff or residents as to the need for participation in a daily routine, residents would spend a great deal of time and energy manipulating and testing the staff on this issue. Hence, spending idle time at El Camino House during the day is not generally permitted. There are exceptions, of course, for physical illness or, for instance, when a resident must wait for a phone call from a prospective employer.

El Camino House accommodates nineteen men and women in a three-story, stucco, thirty-year-old apartment building located on the main thoroughfare in Belmont, California—the most central city in San Mateo County. The neighborhood is zoned commercial and is quite varied. The halfway house itself is sandwiched between a lapidary shop and a modern, small office building. To the north is a mixed array of businesses, including a motel, office building, and drive-in restaurants. Two blocks to the south are located the major intersection of Belmont and a small shopping area. Belmont is a suburban, residential city. A large proportion of the population commutes to places of employment in San Francisco. A major advantage of the location of the house is ease of access to both bus and train transportation. The automobile is the major source of transportation in the area, but the majority of halfway house residents do not own cars.

The San Mateo County Department of Public Health and Welfare is located only one and one-half miles away. Not only are psychiatric emergency (available day and night), outpatient, inpatient, and day hospital services of the Mental Health Services Division available, but also medical care, through County General Hospital. The vocational services center, providing vocational counseling and a sheltered workshop, is located three miles south of the house.

In addition to being oriented along sociological lines, El Camino House presents still another variation in mode of operation and emphasis: a performance-oriented system of work teams or crews. Our program fits the pattern of a high-expectation halfway house as distinguished from a low-expectation or "nurturing approach," as defined by one recent study (Wilder, Kessell, and Caulfield, 1968). This concept for our facility refers to the expectation that each resident live up to his potential, that he attempt to muster sufficient strength so that he may perform in full accord with his individual resources. No paid cook or housekeeper is employed at El Camino House. Once each week house residents sign up for work crews and prepare the following week's menu. A staff member may be present at this meeting, but it is conducted by a chairman selected from the resident group. At least two people sign up for each evening's cooking crew. In addition, there are crews for kitchen clean-up, dishwashing, stove and refrigerator care, maintenance of the living room, recreation room, hallways, and exterior sidewalks and gardens. Ordinarily, it is not necessary that each resident sign up for more than two crews each week. Efforts are made to encourage the rotation of assignments so that each resident has as broad an exposure as possible to all facets of cooperative living and individual responsibility. Moreover, residents are expected to maintain their own living units with a modicum of neatness. The crew system has proven to be an effective method of teaching responsibility and social skills and has provided a structure to which residents could easily relate. Once acclimated to the program, groups of residents begin voluntarily to adopt the system for their individual living units within the house. Chairmen are chosen, meetings initiated within groups to assign duties. Assignment lists for the cleaning of bathrooms, the vacuuming of floors, and similar jobs, appear on the walls of the apartments.

The entire house is inspected weekly by a committee of two residents and one staff member. Should it be found that an area of the house or an apartment has not been properly maintained, the person(s) responsible is contacted and informed of the committee's evaluation. If the area or job is not attended to within a reasonable period of time, the matter is brought before the group at the house meeting. Even residents who are initially resistant, whether actively or passively, find, once group pressure mobilizes their performance, that they have capacities and abilities of which they were previously unaware. We have observed that those residents who accept in principle the philosophy of the house and attempt to fulfill the expectations make a significantly better post-house adjustment. Nakajima and Ishii (1967), reporting on an evening hospital, have observed that the two prognostic signs by which they could evaluate a patient's capacity to be rehabilitated were the ability to keep personal belongings in order and the ability to handle money.

Resident Responsibility

In the first few months of house operation, the crew system for the most part worked well; however, there were residents who made no attempt to fulfill their in-house responsibilities, who manipulated themselves out of crew jobs, or involved themselves in house activities on a minimal basis. These residents simply continued the same pathological behavior patterns that had necessitated their referral to a rehabilitation program. Unless there was intervention in the form of social pressure from other residents and from the staff, these deviant members gained little from their house experience. An undesirable practice evolved: residents would complain about deviant members to the staff and request staff intervention; staff would suggest the matter be brought up in the house meeting and would encourage such confrontation, but this was seldom done. Thus, the residents saw their responsibilities to the community as limited to "tattling" to the parental figures, the house managers. The expectation was that staff would "take care of things" and this, of course, placed staff in a role contrary to house philosophy. Under the original work crew system, there were no means of enforcing expectations, few sanctions, other than pressure from staff, subtle and covert pressure from residents, or prolonged delay until a situation became so grievous that expulsion from the house might be necessary. Although house pride, the desire to be involved and succeed, and the desire to meet staff expectations motivated some members, it could not be relied upon as a motivating factor for all residents. It was seen that social pressure would have to be fostered and facilitated, that more structure was required to facilitate social pressure and provide sanctions. At the same time, this would have to be congruent with the house philosophy of minimal structure and institutionality.

In August, 1967, we began gradually to introduce our present program. We received consultation from George W. Fairweather and David H. Sanders, who had developed an intentional social system at the Palo Alto, California, Veterans Administration Hospital (Fairweather, 1964). Several aspects of that system were adapted to the particular needs, goals, and philosophy of the halfway house. A journal was instituted. In it staff record, on a day-to-day basis, their observations, impressions, and factual information relevant to the operation of the house and residents. Complaints from one resident about another are carefully recorded, including the name of the offending member and the name of the person complaining. Residents are advised that any communication to a staff member which is relevant to the other members of the group and the functioning of the house will be noted in the journal and later placed on the agenda for discussion at the house meeting. Once weekly, on the afternoon before the house meeting, the journal is scrutinized, and an agenda for that evening's meeting compiled. The agenda is divided into two parts: the information notes, comprising any information of general interest to the resident group, such as anticipated new admissions to the house, names of persons who have given notice that they will be leaving the house, names of new volunteers who are involved in the program, general announcements of, or comments on, any social events that are being planned by the residents, and reports on the progress of people who have left the house or who have been rehospitalized. Also included are commendations to residents who have functioned well or outstandingly on their crew jobs, prepared particularly good meals, or made positive changes in behavior. Every opportunity is taken in the informational notes and subsequent discussion to acknowledge the efforts of those who are doing well. This practice evolved directly from residents' requests for just such acknowledgment as a means of providing incentive for good performance and enhancing house morale.

The action notes comprise the second section of the agenda. These are a listing of any reports of infractions, listing both the person reporting the infractions and the violators. Any policy infractions or lack of consideration observed by staff members or residents are reported in the action notes. Also recorded are any expressions of concern about the behavior of residents which, though not an infraction of policies, may be relevant to the well-being of an individual or the house as a whole. Copies of the "house notes," as the informational notes and action notes are called, are posted on the bulletin board and distributed to house members before supper on the evening of the house meeting. An example of typical action notes:

*Action Notes:*

1. No resident signed up for morning kitchen clean-up during Tuesday's crew sign-up meeting.
2. Sally J. and Peggy D. have expressed concern because Alice D,

seems to be withdrawing and has little to do with her roommates
or other people in the house. They fear that she is upset about
something but has not been able to talk about it.

3. Ann H. and Patty C. have complained that Vera F. comes in
and out of the apartment at late hours at night, is frequently
noisy, and often wakes her roommates. They have expressed concern about her staying up many evenings until 2:00–3:00 A.M.
and then not being able to get to work on time. They are particularly concerned with the lack of consideration which they
feel she shows toward them.

4. Janice R. missed dinner and did not sign out on Tuesday.

5. John C. did not return from his weekend visit at home until
Tuesday and did not attend the day treatment center on Mon-
day and Tuesday.

6. Leslie H. and Denise R. did not sign up for any crew job for the
coming week.

7. It has been observed by staff that James M. is not taking his
medications as prescribed by his doctor.

When the house meeting convenes, the major responsibility of
the resident group is to consider carefully each action note and recommend a method for dealing with the member who breaks the rules or
fails to meet expectations of the program. On the premise that the
more information the group has, the better able it will be to make intelligent and meaningful decisions, the staff attempt to clarify any
questions with regard to the notes and offer as much additional information as necessary for the group to make its recommendations. When
the group has sufficient information the second phase of the meeting
begins. All staff leave the room and the resident group alone begins
their deliberations.* They choose a chairman who conducts their
meeting and after considering each of the action notes, call the staff
back into the meeting to report their recommendations. At this point
staff may ask questions for clarification, will discuss the degree to
which, in the staff's opinion, the proposed recommendations adequately dealt with the problem, and then in the presence of the resi-

---

* Lerner and Fairweather (1963) having shown the greater cohesiveness of chronic schizophrenic groups when they functioned without staff leaders,
it was decided the residents would operate autonomously during this portion of
the meeting.

dent group and by staff consensus, will either (1) agree with and accept the recommendations of the group; (2) disagree with some of the recommendations, stating reasons why, but still accept the group's recommendation; or (3) choose not to accept the recommendations and request reconsideration. Instances in which the staff disagree with but still accept the recommendations of the group are usually situations of little serious consequence. For example, the group may respond to the problem of John B.'s not doing an adequate job in cleaning the recreation room for two successive weeks by recommending: "No action. John promises to do his jobs next time and will clean the recreation room tonight." The staff might point out that this is a decision of immediacy, expressing the group's uncertainty as to what to do about John's several poor performances and implying that he and they can get off the hook if he takes care of the job that evening. Further, the staff may suggest that the group has been manipulated into accepting and perhaps approving repeated incidents of irresponsible behavior, that there were no assurances by the group or sanctions developed to insure that John really would try to improve, and consequently the infraction could be expected to be repeated, so the matter would be likely to come before the group again very soon. The rationale behind accepting recommendations which staff disagree with is that people cannot be expected to make good decisions all the time and that groups learn from past error, particularly if they have access to persons who can help them review past actions. When staff veto a group recommendation and request reconsideration, the group may reconsider and come up with a more acceptable solution or it may choose not to reconsider. In such cases the staff make a counter recommendation, which is, in effect, the decision.

No attempt is made to create the illusion that the system is democratic or self-governing. The system exists primarily to mobilize social pressure and at the same time to allow residents the maximum opportunity for developing decision-making skills. The group actions are carefully labeled as recommendations, not decisions. The resident group does not have the authority to abolish the crew system, or delete the requirement that residents have daytime activities. They may, however, make, and have made, major policy recommendations which have been accepted by the staff.

As Childers (1967) points out, the staff cannot help influencing, consciously or unconsciously, the residents' decisions, and the fact that staff retain final authority may make it difficult to communicate to the residents the real and meaningful responsibility we wish them to have. Maintaining the proper balance between staff and resident control requires constant awareness of the ways in which staff may tend to assume responsibilities which are the proper jurisdiction of the residents. Soon after initiating the system, we learned the absolute necssity of stating clearly what we expected and what we did not expect the group to handle. We had to specify that professional and medical decisions, such as the decision to rehospitalize, were the responsibility of the staff but that we would on occasion, where appropriate, ask for opinions from the resident group. The setting of discharge dates is, for instance, a responsibility shared by the staff and the resident's therapist. The group, however, is usually asked for its recommendations with reference to discharge dates. On the other hand, all problems which do not require professional action or an immediate staff decision are referred to the group. The group's recommendations are for the most part marked by fairness. Although there is occasionally a punitive quality to their approach, they will more often than not simply discuss a situation and issue a warning to an offender who does not habitually cause difficulty. For repeated offenses, the group has taken such action as "grounding" the offending member to the house during the evening hours, or recommending that a person does not visit his family as frequently when his behavior in the house seems related to a "difficult time at home." They have reorganized the work crew system to make it more effective. The assignment of extra crew jobs to an errant member is a frequent recommendation. On two occasions, the house voted to expel a resident, and in both instances the staff concurred that the recommendation was appropriate.

The program was well planned, and the flaws we encountered were primarily related to staff fears that the system would not work, that a group loaded as it was with chronic schizophrenics would not be able to organize themselves sufficiently to choose leadership and proceed with the problem-solving process. There was also concern that some of the patients with greater verbal facility and a tendency to manipulate would use the meeting to act out negative feelings toward other members and the staff. To be sure, this has occurred, but rarely. Under these circumstances the recommendations for the most part would be unacceptable, reconsideration would be requested, and this would give staff the opportunity to point out directly acquiescence to the manipulative or acting out behavior of a few.

Our observations corroborate those of Fairweather (1964) that leaders can emerge just as frequently from the most chronic psychotic groups as from the least chronic psychotic and neurotic groups. We also found, observationally, that the quality of group performance is in direct relationship to the quality of leadership.

When the system was first introduced, the response from the group was highly negative. They reflected the staff's view that it could not be done and expressed feelings of hostility, helplessness, and abandonment. Reviewing the rationale for the plan did not seem to ameliorate their anxieties. The major problem seemed concerned with group uncertainty about what sanctions they had at their disposal and the limits of their responsibility. Once these points were clarified, the group was able to come up with highly innovative and successful recommendations, and the negative feelings quickly diminished.

Like the community group meeting of a therapeutic community, the house meeting serves multiple purposes. In addition to its vital role in the house social system the meeting provides a forum for reenforcing and reorienting residents to the purposes, philosophy, and expectations of the house. An occasional reindoctrination is particularly necessary to carry on the house culture when there is a high degree of turnover. Another function of the meeting is to deal with feelings related to staff changes, anxieties generated by the rehospitalization of a member of the group, or the stresses produced by a catastrophic national occurrence such as the King and Kennedy assassinations. House morale may be enhanced within the meeting, through recognition of acceptable group performance and acknowledgment of the group's leaders. Finally, the house meeting may be used for announcements by both residents and staff and for the initiation of special social activities such as a holiday party.

### Staffing

The El Camino House staff consists of a full-time director, who is a psychiatric social worker, a part-time psychiatric consultant, two resident house managers, a coordinator of the apartment program, and an administrative secretary. We studiously avoid referring to the live-in staff as "house mothers." Although this term may add to the feeling that the house is an extension of the family, we feel it detracts from our objectives to assist people in their emanicipation from parental figures. To be sure, residents often see the male and female house managers as parental figures, regardless of what they are called; but the designation "house manager" seems better to define the role of the staff person as facilitating rather than nurturing, and therefore, indirectly influences his mode of functioning and the manner in which he is perceived by the residents. The house manager's primary role is to inculcate the high expectations culture. In addition, it is to be available in time of crisis, to teach, to coordinate, and to be supportive, as well as handling some of the more mundane aspects of house operation, such as seeing to it that maintenance and repair work is attended to. The managers alternate on-duty time.

The director has overall responsibility for the administration and operation of the facility. He is, of course, responsible to the board of directors. His duties include the hiring, training and supervision of staff, the screening and evaluation of applicants, coordination and liaison with agencies and therapists, public relations and fund-raising. El Camino House has developed excellent coordination with the key rehabilitation facilities in the county. The director regularly attends staff meetings at the county day hospital and vocational services center. Liaison personnel have been assigned to the house by the local welfare agency, Bureau of Social Work (a state-operated aftercare program), and the state hospital. This cooperation is of obvious benefit to the patient and additionally helps to lighten the burden of the director.

During the planning stages there was some question as to whether a full-time rather than a half-time director would be needed. The soundness of the decision to have a full-time director has since clearly been affirmed. A considerable expenditure of time and energy is necessary if a small agency is to be run effectively. Indeed, as Duval (1968) points out, the small rehabilitation agency has many problems as a result of its smallness. There are less staff to whom authority and detail work can be delegated. The struggle to obtain funds can consume a considerable portion of the administrator-director's time, and as a result, the quality of the program can suffer. Furthermore, the staff of small agencies must be deeply motivated for their work since they are called upon to work an irregular schedule, including evenings and weekends.

The psychiatrist operates primarily as a consultant to the staff in matters of psychiatric or medical import. He confers with the director once weekly and is also called upon to assist staff in dealing with emergency situations, difficult management problems or any other areas where it is deemed advisable to seek psychiatric opinion. He is a member of the admissions committee and assumes overall medical responsibility for the agency.

In order for a patient to become a resident of El Camino House, a written application must be submitted by the referring agency or therapist. The submission of a letter of application on behalf of the patient implies a certain commitment on the part of the referral source to the idea of halfway house residence and, therefore, frequently enhances communication and collaboration between house staff and therapist during the patient's stay. Following receipt of the application letter—which outlines briefly the patient's problem, diagnosis, history of antisocial acting out, problems which house staff could expect to encounter, the name of the therapist who will follow the patient throughout his residence, and the physician who will supervise his medications—an interview is conducted with the applicant for purposes of screening and orientation. Subsequent to the interview, telephone conferences between the house director and the referring professional are usually arranged in order to work out details. The admissions committee, composed of the consultant psychiatrist, house director, and a member of the Professional Advisory Board, meets weekly to determine each applicant's appropriateness for admission. The factors evaluated in considering each referral are course of hospitalization, current mental status, and the presence of rehabilitative rather than custodial goals.

Basic requirements of house residency are that the applicant will remain under the care of a therapist during his stay; that he will be involved in some regular daytime activity, that he has the ability, or at least the potential, to care for his own personal hygiene and take prescribed medication without house staff supervision. Persons with recent histories of antisocial behavior generally are not admitted; however, some alcoholics and persons with drug abuse problems may be admitted. Patients accepted may include: (1) patients at state and private hospitals who require a supportive residence during their initial post-hospital period; (2) patients discharged from hospitals but suffering exacerbation of symptomatology as the result of living in environments not conducive to social recovery; and (3) patients receiving outpatient treatment from private therapists or public and private outpatient agencies where the therapist believes that removal from an unsuitable environment will assist the patient's therapeutic program or prevent hospitalization.

Many of the patients accepted by El Camino House are severely limited in their ability to function, have a very limited experience in living independently, and are lacking in interpersonal skills. These patients are routinely accepted for admission. In addition, a research project, undertaken in cooperation with Agnews State Hospital, the county day treatment center, and the vocational services center, requires admission of all long-term hospitalized chronic patients referred to us under the project (Rehabilitation Services Administration grant RD-2847-P). The research group is comprised of patients who for the most part would not ordinarily be accepted, even under the existing liberal admission criteria, and may include patients who have had multiple hospitalizations over a long period of time, who have histories of acting out, or who have been lobotomized, as well as other high-risk patients not usually seen in a halfway house.

We had expected that many of these patients, who had experienced long periods of hospitalization and who initially appeared very difficult to deal with in an open setting, would not be able to adjust to the halfway house and community. Many have been able to do so and we attribute this in part to their preconditioning in the hospital to an acceptance of routine and regulations. Thus, ironically, the very fact of institutionalization renders these patients more amenable to fitting in than we would anticipate.

Originally the applicant's motivation for halfway house residence was considered an important factor in determining whether an individual would be accepted. We quickly observed that a significant number of prospective residents were either poorly motivated or markedly ambivalent about leaving the protective environment of the hospital upon which they had become extremely dependent. Some were being discharged from the hospital not entirely voluntarily but in accordance with administrative policies to move patients out as soon as possible. Furthermore, there were patients who used referral to the halfway house as a ticket for release from the hospital. These patients were able to perform within the institution adequately enough to warrant referral and discharge; however, they usually had little investment in the referral, and had poorly formulated goals for their reentry into society, or none at all. Although it was never intended to take only the best motivated patients, it was also recognized that, if services were to be provided to post-hospitalized patients and if we were to be of service to those who needed us the most, we would also have to accept the more poorly motivated. The orientation portion of the screening interview takes on a different character with these reluctant applicants. Attempts are made to motivate the patient to enter the house and efforts made to establish a contract which is mutually acceptable. Frequently more than one interview is necessary. Should the applicant decide to enter the halfway house, regardless of how reluctantly this decision is made, or how inappropriate his reasons might be, the contract stipulates that no less will be expected of him in the way of performance. It is further agreed that he may leave the house at any time by simply giving ten days notice and that he could also be asked to leave if his behavior is not acceptable. A contract of this kind often serves to enhance the patients' motivation to enter the facility. It also clearly differentiates the house from the hospital. Patients who prefer to remain and live at the hospital are often reassured by the possibility they can return and are more likely to risk what at first seems to them like a giant step toward independence.

### Symbiotic Relationships

Many referring professionals tend to use the halfway house to attempt to assist patients to extricate themselves from symbiotic family ties or as a means of dealing head on with the patient's excessive and incapacitating dependency on a friend or lover. The halfway house is, therefore, seen as a vehicle through which liberation from symbiotic relationships can be accomplished. The fact that it may be deemed beneficial by the therapist for such relationships to be broken, or at least diluted, is often a goal not shared by the patient and his counterpart even though one or both may pay lip service to the idea. A patient will frequently go along with the therapist's plan in order to please him.

Sometimes the referral really reflects the therapist's own unresolved dependence-independence conflicts that have become projected upon the patient and his family. In such instances, the patient has very little if any investment in breaking the symbiotic relationship, and both parties attempt to manipulate and undermine the "desired" separation. When these patients become residents in the halfway house, they are generally minimally involved in house activities or only superficially go through the motions of fulfilling expectations. Their tenure is marked by continual visits, telephone calls, and excursions with the family member or person with whom they are aligned.

The essential problem of assessing the patient's motivation and ego strength for separation is a vexing one. Patients often are intellectually aware that they should remove themselves from the union for their own benefit, but on the emotional level are simply not able or willing. These patients can be highly convincing, and the intake worker is easily seduced into believing that the house can, in fact, deal with the patient's interminable tie. Often patients will appear highly motivated to leave a mutually dependent counterpart whom they feel is overly protective and depriving them of their independence; but these patients are often unaware of their own corresponding dependency needs and the secondary gains of the relationship. If admitted to the house, they remain a very brief period. A pathological symbiotic relationship in many instances may be the main factor in keeping one or both parties from ego disintegration and hospitalization.

This is not to suggest that all of these patients are unable to achieve some degree of emancipation. The question remains, however, whether such referrals to the halfway house should be accepted since so few do achieve the goal of independence. The fact that some make it may be justification enough, but this hardly deals with the frustration of working with the many who do not. In an analysis of patterns of residence at Rutland Corner House in Boston, it was observed that of twenty residents who lived with parents prior to last hospitalization, sixteen ultimately returned to their parental homes (Landy and Greenblatt, 1965). While these residents who ultimately return to the unhealthy relationships from whence they came may appear to be halfway house failures, we have come to view such situations in a different light. We have observed that the experience of attempting to separate and not being able to do so may frequently bring into focus the intensity and nature of the mutual dependency and provide better perspective for the patient, his family, and the therapist. It is also conceivable that as a result of greater comprehension of the situation the patient and his family are better able to accommodate each other following the separation. What then ostensibly appears to be a failure to achieve goals may ultimately serve the patient well.

### Termination

The halfway house represents a home, a family, albeit temporary, but nonetheless a pleasant, comfortable social environment where the resident is treated with respect and understanding. He may therefore be expected to resist departing from such surroundings. Staff may also experience some reluctance to discharge the "good resident" who takes on responsibilities, assumes a leadership role in the house, and presents few problems. It may be even more difficult to terminate the resident whose destination is vague, whose plans are unclear and remain so despite staff intervention. The resident's ambivalence or resistance to leaving is often acted out through failure to concretize plans or simply by making no plans at all. Setting limits with such patients becomes tantamount to eviction and carries with it for staff, in particular, all the attending guilt. This pattern is familiar to hospital and outpatient clinic staff, who must often set specific dates for discharge or termination. The halfway house is no exception.

The usual period of residence in El Camino House varies from three to five months for patients with greater ego strength to a maximum of one year for those who are both chronically and more severely disturbed. In our experience, an extended period of residence beyond the initial three months has no correlation with ability to function in the community; in fact, the reverse may be true. All residents, however, are expected ultimately to leave the house and to find permanent quarters of their own. During the initial months of operation, staff were preoccupied with setting up administrative procedures, coordinating with other facilities, learning to work together, renovating the building, as well as other types of "nest-building." As a result, little attention was paid to discharge planning and to the resident's long-range plans. Many of the early residents, therefore, settled in for long stays. When this error was realized and the concept of discharge from the house began to be discussed with the residents, a barrage of acting out ensued, including suicidal gestures and attempts. Planning for the patient's discharge now begins at the time of intake and is both an integral part of the program and a real part of the resident-patient's expectations.

### Establishing a Halfway House

From the foregoing, the reader will have perceived the extent to which existing community service patterns and expectations influence the basic mission of the halfway house. In San Mateo County, for instance, the organizational groundwork was carried out by a voluntary organization; nevertheless, this organizing or sponsoring group early enlisted the interest, cooperation, and support of the local community mental health program operated by the county government. Subsequently, the halfway house staff has carefully developed viable liaison arrangements with the state hospital, the local welfare program, and many other private and voluntary services in the mental health orbit of the community.

It can be said without reservation that the form each house takes is the direct or indirect result of the particular history of the facility, the personalities of its leaders, the type of sponsorship within which it occurs (hospital-affiliated or privately sponsored), the attitudes of the community, the rehabilitative ideology of the staff, geographic location and nature of the physical plant. Residential halfway houses do, however, share numerous common goals, including providing residence, providing a protective base for transition from hospital to community, providing for socialization and resocialization experiences, and encouraging use of vocational and other rehabilitation services.

Establishing a halfway house can be a long and arduous task. Sound community organization is necessary to establish a transitional residence and insure its continued existence. The remainder of this section is devoted to discussing the steps we believe necessary for effective planning of a halfway house. We draw on our experience at El

Camino House as well as previous association at Harvey House in Palo Alto, California.

*Determining the need for the facility* is of course the logical first step. A fact-finding survey of the existing institutions for the mentally ill, especially private and public hospitals, but also including outpatient clinics and private practitioners, should be initiated. Attempts to learn something about the characteristics and diagnosis of the prospective residents, that is, whether chronic, acute, or mixed, should be included in the survey. Since many of the existing community agencies would be involved in the survey, an excellent and early opportunity is presented to bring agency personnel into the planning. This would enhance the future possibilities of coordination between house and agencies.

Second, once it is established that a facility is needed and the sources of referral and patient characteristics are known, a *general conception of program orientation and philosophy* is needed. This includes consideration of such factors as high expectations versus low, degree of emphasis on employment or vocational training, extent to which professional staff will be used and how, and the methods through which socialization will be achieved. Also necessary is the establishment of a minimum and maximum resident census, anticipated length of stay, intake procedures, selection criteria, and a decision as to whether the facility should include only one or both sexes. These considerations are best dealt with by professionals who have knowledge of or interest in halfway houses. During the planning of El Camino House, a professional advisory committee was formed, composed of the assistant superintendent of the state hospital, a psychiatrist with a local private hospital, a social worker representing a state aftercare program, the chief of the county psychiatric rehabilitation services, and the executive director of the Mental Health Association. This body drew up general guidelines with reference to many of the above factors.

Third, a *determination of the most effective administrative structure* should be made, that is, should the new service operate independently, as an extension of an existing agency, or in cooperative federation with a presently operating agency? Another question is, should the project be hospital sponsored, community sponsored—that is, initiated by private citizens—or some combination thereof? The administrative structure chosen will depend greatly on the history of the planning body, the source from which the idea and the implementation of the idea of a halfway house emanated. There are certainly advantages in terms of flexibility of community sponsorship; however, there may be financial advantages to being associated with a well-funded, existing structure, public or private.

Fourth, *establishment of community support and interest* involves seeking the assistance of service clubs, women's clubs, or perhaps the establishment of a volunteer auxiliary or women's guild for fund-raising, volunteer, and public relations purposes. A professional advisory committee should be considered. It is presumed that the new organization, if community sponsored, will organize a board of directors or similar governing body from interested and influential members of the community.

Fifth, *establishment of sources of financial support* (governmental, private foundations, donations, fees) is one of the most important of the variables. The fund-raising potential of the planning group must be objectively assessed, especially if it is a new organization. Future deficits should be anticipated and concrete plans made to deal with them. Total support from community contributions alone is unrealistic in most instances; a combination of support from local contributions, federal and state funds and fees is most practical. Halfway houses, like so many small voluntary agencies, tend to experience financial crisis after financial crisis as the result of an insufficiently broad base of funding. The need for sound business planning from the outset cannot be emphasized enough. Halfway houses for alcoholics seem especially prone to financial failure or continual crisis due to lack of funds. Perhaps this is because these houses often employ non-professionals, who double as live-in house manager and director, and whose primary duty is counseling and supervising residents. Consequently, little time, energy, and perhaps inclination, is left to deal with monetary problems. Although the rehabilitation of the patient is the most important consideration, it is foolhardy to think that good intentions are enough. It must be anticipated that a significant portion of the director's time will have to be spent in fund-raising activities such as gathering statistical data, preparing grant applications for presentation before philanthropic and governmental bodies, and working with his governing body in developing fund-raising contacts within the community.

Sixth, *determination of the initial costs and operational costs* involves drawing up one or more budgets. An important consideration is that of leasing as opposed to the buying of housing. Our organization chose to lease, simply because we did not have sufficient capital to buy. Financial estimates are likely to vary over the planning period more than any other factor. Although costs are contingent upon the size and location of the facility selected and the number of residents to be accommodated, they are most closely related to the staffing pattern.

Seventh, provision must also be made for the *establishment of basic guidelines for internal administrative procedure,* such areas as staff job descriptions, lines of authority and responsibility, and personnel practices. Too often the working out of such details as salary ranges, increments, health insurance and retirement benefits is left until employment of staff. This can make for complications in hiring or keeping staff.

Finally, familiarity with the *zoning regulations of the community* is essential. Organizations which are able to procure for use as a halfway house a building previously used as a boarding house or an apartment building which does not require structural renovation to adapt it for use are fortunate indeed. Harvey House, in Palo Alto, California, simply took over an existing boarding house, moved in the house staff and gradually replaced the occupants with previously hospitalized patients as they were referred. The process is not always so smooth. Often a building selected as ideal for a halfway house is located in an area which is not zoned for group living. To complicate matters further, zoning regulations seldom include the concept of the halfway house. The halfway house fits into no existing category: it is not just a boarding house, not a single family dwelling, not exactly a business, and not an ordinary apartment house. It fails to fit precisely into any zoning category, and therefore may be assigned to any of them or, depending upon the attitudes in the community, may not be allowed to fit into any category. Where the establishment of a halfway house depends upon approval by the local officials and, in essence, its prospective neighbors, a public controversy is assured. All manner of objections are declared, ranging from depreciation of property values, inadequate parking space, failure to meet building code requirements, to that of operating a hospital without a license and being Communist inspired. The citizenry acts on preexisting notions and is hard put to conceptualize a place that is said to rehabilitate patients but is not a hospital. Although zoning and building regulations are used as the legal mechanism of opposition, the evidence suggests that fear, prejudice, and bigotry are the base of the resistance. Community feeling may become highly emotional with calm and objective discussion rare.

Prejudicial opposition may be broken down into four categories: first, fear of the mental patient, who is seen as aggressive, dangerously out of control, bizarre and different; second, a decreased sense of distance from mental illness and the mentally ill, which renders one no longer able to ignore and defend against one's own real or imagined illness, for expample, fear of being "found out," "maybe they will see that I am really like them"; third, fear of sexuality, for example, "they will molest our children and accost women on the street"; and finally, distrust of psychiatry and social workers—"they will manipulate our minds and make us accept things we do not wish to accept."

In order to cope with such volatile antagonists, the petitioning organization must be sufficiently well-organized to provide for a well-formulated, documented presentation with legal opinion and precedent, massive community support of the project from all segments of the community possible, and have phenomenal good fortune.

In the case of El Camino House, planning was carried on under the auspices of the Mental Health Association of San Mateo County. The membership of that organization formed a committee which later became the nucleus of a separate non-profit corporation, which assumed the responsibility for establishment of the first halfway house for the mentally ill in the county. Since the new corporation had no paid staff, the executive director of the Mental Health Association served as a consultant and community organizer and did much of the research and required leg-work. Other interested members of the community were added to the board of the new organization and a professional advisory committee was formed.

The search for an appropriate physical plant consumed a large portion of the planning time. Many buildings which at first appeared adequate for the purpose ultimately had to be rejected as a result of high costs of renovation or improper zoning. Fortunately, the building

finally procured has proved to be ideal in almost all respects. It meets
the multiple criteria of being centrally located, close to transportation,
is able to accommodate both men and women and has adequate space
to make operations reasonably economical. In addition, there is ample
living room, recreational and storage space, and a private apartment
for one of the house managers.

Partial financial support for the administrative-professional
portions of the program was procured through a contract with the
County of San Mateo under the provisions of the California Short-
Doyle (Community Mental Health Services) Act. It was decided that
room, board, and a portion of the supervisory cost would be borne by
the residents. A minimum fee was established within the means of welfare recipients which still left them sufficient other funds for personal
and transportation expenses. A total of $9,000 was raised and donated
by one local volunteer women's organization, and $1,000 by another.
These funds were earmarked for use in necessary renovation of the selected site, furniture, and other initial expenses. A yearly deficit was
still anticipated since the Short-Doyle contract paid only up to 80 per
cent of the professional and administrative cost. It was planned that
future deficits would be met through continued support by local service organizations and donations by individuals and private foundations.
There were pledges of sufficient donations in kind to furnish the house,
including the office, almost completely. Present sources of financial
support are:

| | |
|---|---|
| Room and Board charges | 40.0 per cent |
| Short-Doyle (State and Local) | 41.0 " " |
| Satellite Apartment Program (Grant) | 8.0 " " |
| Donations | 4.2 " " |
| Fees | 3.6 " " |
| Miscellaneous | 3.2 " " |

Because of sound planning and excellent community support we have,
in a relatively brief period of time, been able to initiate new services
which extend our activities beyond the physical confines of the halfway house.

### Satellite Housing Program

The rapid establishment of halfway houses throughout the
United States attests to the belief that adequate and suitable living

accommodations are an essential part of the patient's readjustment. Today, however, transitional living accommodations must be employed on behalf of individuals whose impairments are much more severe, whose potential for fully independent living is much more limited than has formerly been true. As state hospitals continue to rapidly discharge patients who can be maintained in the community on drug therapy and with minimal supervision, halfway houses receive more referrals of the hard-core chronic patients and of patients who are difficult to manage in the community. Patients with limited ego strength and overwhelming dependency needs often require more than a transitional living experience. The severity of illness necessitates living arrangements which will not require a fully independent existence. Post-halfway house accommodations must be established which can provide an adequate physical and psychological milieu, the necessary sustaining supports, as well as geographical accessibility to such facilities as medical clinics, day treatment centers, sheltered workshops, ex-patient social clubs, and outpatient clinics.

During our short history, we have become acutely aware of the difficulties the halfway house resident faces when his time comes to terminate. Despite attempts, often successful, to decrease dependency and enhance feelings of self-sufficiency, the typical halfway house resident continues to exhibit strong residual dependency. We must also recognize that in addition to certain psychological problems, the patient may encounter some very real obstacles to hinder his transition from the halfway house to the community. The area served by El Camino House, for instance, has practically no residence clubs, an extremely small number of boarding houses, and even a paucity of residence hotels. The typical mode of living in this suburban community is either in houses or apartments, and the problem is even further complicated by the fact that apartment rentals are high in cost and there is a very low vacancy rate.

We felt it was important to help people leaving the halfway house find adequate accommodations which were typical of the community. We observed, however, that the difficulties in finding a vacant apartment, finding compatible roommates, procuring furniture and kitchen utensils, paying security and cleaning deposits in advance, and signing a complicated lease, were enough to make patients in good remission decide to return to an unsuitable home or to the hospital. We, therefore, instituted a program we hoped would help the patient cope with these problems while providing minimally supervised and largely independent living situations which could unobtrusively gratify needs for protection and dependence.

The use of apartments as transitional placements was originally conceived by Fountain House in New York City (Beard, Smith, and Sorokin, 1963; Beard et al., 1964). This type of program offers considerable advantages to the sponsoring organization as well as to the patient. The programs are relatively low in cost, as the occupants are usually able to assume the full cost of the rent and utilities. Expenditures for staffing and a reserve rental and deposit fund are minimal, since the project can be developed gradually as the need arises. This avoids large initial outlays of funds for physical facilities, furniture and equipment, and numerous staff.

Under our Satellite Housing Program, selected residents who will require continued supervision while in the community are discharged from the house to live in apartments, duplexes, or houses procured with the assistance of staff. Usually groups of two, three, or four residents who have lived together within the halfway house and appear compatible are discharged simultaneously. Efforts are made to locate apartments or other housing in areas reasonably close to transportation. No more than one apartment is used in an apartment building, thereby avoiding creation of another institution and offering the additional advantage that the placement is not easily identifiable as housing for a special group.

In order to qualify for placement in a satellite apartment the resident must demonstrate, during his halfway house occupancy, his ability to assume responsibility for various crew jobs, reasonable ability to cook for himself, to care for his personal hygiene, and to live compatibly with others. The housing program is only one of many alternatives for halfway house residents being discharged. The resident may shop for an apartment on his own, with or without staff assistance, may move in with friends or relatives, return to his family home, return to the hospital, or secure any other accommodations at his disposal. The satellite housing program, however, provides another positive alternative in addition to the traditional modes of leaving a halfway house. At the very core of the program is the mutuality of expectations and responsibilities, which are shared by the apartment occupant and El Camino House.

The halfway house resident who requests inclusion in the housing program and is accepted agrees to assume full responsibility for his share of the apartment rental and utilities. The organization assumes responsibility for furnishing the apartment, primarily through donations made to El Camino House. The organization also pays all initial costs necessary to secure the apartment, including security and cleaning deposits. The agency, in addition, assumes responsibility for full occupancy of the living unit. Should a tenant vacate an apartment for any reason, efforts are made to find another resident from the halfway house to occupy that space. In the event there is no one readily available and the apartment cannot be filled, the rental payment is assumed by the organization. If, however, the organization has someone deemed by staff to be compatible with the remaining members of the apartment, but who is rejected as a roommate by the other members of the dwelling, the remaining partners in the unit must share in payment of that portion of the rent until another roommate is secured and acceptable.

A contract, a clearly and simply written agreement between the agency and the satellite housing occupants, is executed. In addition to the above-mentioned mutual responsibilities, it also specified that the apartment occupant will remain in outpatient treatment until terminated by mutual agreement with his therapist. Of prime importance is the agreement to attend a meeting of satellite housing residents at least twice monthly, or more frequently, if necessary. Excepting stipulations of the contract, the occupants are free agents. They regard the apartment as their own and take responsibility for their own actions in regard to guests, drinking, sexual activity, and any other aspect of living. In most instances, the occupants themselves hold the lease and are, therefore, accountable to the landlord should care of the apartment or conduct of the occupants be questioned. Where El Camino House holds the lease and sublets, the occupants are accountable to us as landlord, in the same fashion.

The bimonthly meetings of satellite housing residents have become a key factor in the success of the program. In order to avoid establishing large and unwieldy groups, the apartments are divided into units, with the occupants of three apartments comprising one unit. Members of each unit meet together in a group with an agency staff member. Each apartment in the unit alternates in hosting meetings. Each of the units, therefore, comprises between nine and twelve individuals. This small size greatly facilitates interaction; perhaps partly for this reason the discussions take the character of reality-oriented group therapy. The content of the discussions revolves around here-and-now, real life problems—conflicts between roommates, structuring of housekeeping, resistances to taking medications and remaining in therapy, problems with employment, and the overall difficulties of adjusting to a more independent existence.

For the resident, the housing program as operated by El Camino House offers a nontransitional placement. Occupants may stay as long as they wish, thus affording the resident permanence in housing, allowing him to avoid still another termination together with the attending problems of adjustment to new situations. Individual tenants, however, are free to vacate the apartment at any time by simply giving two weeks notice of termination. Should all members of an apartment wish to break ties with the agency, they may do so by requesting cancellation of the contract and refunding the deposits advanced by the agency.

One criticism that has been made is that we do not really terminate some patients, that we are attempting to do too much for the patient, fostering dependency and not letting our patients go. The question of termination is fraught with controversy and double meanings when related to social psychiatry follow-up aftercare services. We liken the process to that of the diabetic patient who, although he is on his own and administers his own medication, still remains under a physician's care for the remainder of his life. If periodic health and dental check-ups are appropriate for the general populace, then availability of groups where the mentally disordered can check out their problems seems equally valid. Terminating a patient whose dependency and lack of ego strength are such that there is a continued need for therapeutic intervention is not appropriate. Much, of course, depends on the quality, frequency, and intensity of the contact provided. Terminating a patient when he truly no longer needs the service or refuses the service is quite appropriate.

**The Camino Club**

From the foregoing it is apparent that we believe follow-up services are as important as the halfway house itself. The satellite housing program provides a multiplicity of groups to which the former resident may relate. Besides being a member of the group in his own individual apartment, he is also a member of a unit of apartments and a member of the total satellite housing program, which meets as a group occasionally for social purposes. In addition, if he so chooses, he may attend the Camino Club. This is a combination open house and social club which convenes weekly at El Camino House, for residents, ex-residents, and any interested persons from the community. Its function is to facilitate social contact, to expose the patient to functioning members of the community, and bring the community into contact with the "mental patient."

Establishment of the Camino Club emanated from the needs of discharged residents to maintain contact with staff and friends at the house. Former residents had already been coming by on a haphazard basis. We felt it important, however, to designate a specific evening each week as a reunion evening for former residents who wished to return. We invited members of the community to attend in order to dilute continual patient-to-patient contact and expand the members' social spheres. Generally, however, the only outsiders who attend are students and friends of residents and staff. We believe that having a variety of groups with whom the patient can interact dilutes feelings of isolation and loneliness for those who have left the congenial, larger group living situation of the halfway house. The tie which exists between the ex-resident and the "mother institution" can diminish the anxiety and resistance related to separation and fear of independence.

In conclusion, El Camino House, the Satellite Housing Program, and the Camino Club are dynamic programs which attempt to provide an appropriate gratification of the dependency needs of the severely mentally ill coupled with maximum expectations for independence. Involvement with the patient in a wide range of ways, both psychological and practical, while providing structure for optimum performance, is essential if we wish to effectively assist patients to live in the community in a manner that will enrich their lives.

# CHAPTER 7

# The Role of Nursing

*Pauline Bowen, Lina S. Wygant and Don Heath,*
*Mildred L. Mouw and Clarice H. Haylett\**

ϟϟϟϟϟϟϟϟϟϟϟϟϟϟϟϟϟϟϟϟϟϟ

In community mental health, the nurse is faced with perplexing new challenges and demands, each of which arises from the special professional distinctions which nursing brings to the tasks of prevention, treatment, and rehabilitation. This chapter discloses the extent to which nurses in community mental health are learning to use themselves and their discipline as a creative, therapeutic social force, both within the hospital and day hospital treatment setting and in the community at large. In the first two sections, the emphasis is on San Mateo's experiences in the developing

---

\* This chapter has three sections, each by different authors. The first section, "The Day Hospital Nurse," is by Pauline Bowen; the second, "Working with Hospitalized Patients," is by Lina S. Wygant and Don Heath; the third, "The Public Health Nurse," is by Mildred L. Mouw and Clarice H. Haylett.

functions of nurses employed in community treatment programs—both part-day and full-time hospital settings. Building upon this clinical base, the chapter then turns to what we consider to be an extremely important area of community mental health: the role of the public health nurse.

## The Day Hospital Nurse (Bowen)

When the day hospital opened in 1961, there seems to have been a hazy and uncertain grasp of the functions that nursing might contribute. In the original planning for the day hospital, special emphasis was placed on hiring nurses trained in public health nursing as well as psychiatric nursing. The nurse, it was assumed, would be used extensively to evaluate the patient in his home environment. Indeed, early in the history of the day hospital, the nurse did make home visits to patients who telephoned complaining of ailments which prevented scheduled day hospital attendance. The nurse making the home visit usually found the absence was due more to resistance to the treatment program than to actual physical illness. During the home visit, this resistance to treatment was dealt with, and the home visit often proved instrumental in helping the patient return to treatment.

As the day hospital census increased, it became increasingly difficult for nurses to make home visits on anything like a routine basis or even to do so in those cases for which it was definitely and specifically indicated. The nurse had become more involved in the activities within the day hospital itself. Moreover, liaison between mental health services and the public health nursing program was improving. The day hospital staff began to recognize the vital contribution to be made by the public health nurse as a member of the day hospital treatment team. Consequently, the public health nurse was regarded as the logical person to make the home visit, especially if she already knew the patient and his family.

There are still instances when the day hospital nurse will make a home visit, either because the public health nurse is not available or because it is felt that the day hospital nurse's visit would be especially valuable. But such a home visit might also be made by another member of the treatment team—the psychiatrist, the social worker, or any combination of the three. The treatment team decides who will make the visit; the factor governing this decision is usually a determination of which of them has the most meaningful relationship with the patient.

In the early stages of the day hospital, separate nursing staff meetings were held. These were traditional nursing conferences to discuss medication, treatment goals, and the day's activities. Later, the occupational therapist joined the meeting because she felt left out of essential communication about patients and treatment plans. However, she was quiet and passive, more like a spectator than a participant. With the addition of the recreational therapist, it soon became apparent that all three disciplines were working toward the same goals for patients and in ways that were, in many respects, quite similar. All were involved in the crucial minute-to-minute contact with patients, and all were involved with the patient group throughout the day. The staff's participation in varying functions frequently overlapped. It was at this point that the staff discovered how a close working relationship between nursing, occupational therapy, and recreational therapy was an important ingredient in guaranteeing consistency, continuity, and effectiveness of the program and patient treatment.

To this end, the nurses, the occupational therapist, and the recreational therapist now meet together each day. The total time involved in such meetings is three and one-half hours per week. This group calls itself the activity staff (to distinguish it from the treatment team, consisting of nurse, psychiatrist, and social worker). The nursing staff never meets in the absence of the other two disciplines. The activity staff meetings emphasize the sharing of information about patients among all participants, as well as joint planning of the day hospital day.

"The nurse who understands the therapeutic benefits of activity therapy is a vital force in helping the patient to gain full benefit from them. Her support, interest, and cooperation are directly dependent on her understanding of and attitude toward these therapies and the kind of relationship existing between her and the activity therapist (Hofling and Leininger, 1960)." At the same time, availability of full-time specialists in occupational and recreational therapy, allows the nurse to relinquish some of her responsibilities in these spheres, devoting her energies more fully to the nursing functions—even while participating in the activities.

Understanding the nurse's role in the day hospital has been a most valuable ingredient in conceptualizing the day hospital treatment program itself, since nursing is an integral part of every aspect of that program. The treatment team, as the day hospital chapter explains, consists of a psychiatrist, a social worker, and a nurse. Each team is responsible for twelve or thirteen patients. The nurse is an extremely important member of this team. The nurse is with the patient group from 9:00 A.M. to 4:00 P.M. up to five days a week. Consequently, she can be aware of a particular patient's functioning under many different circumstances. Her observations of patients throughout the day are especially valuable, for example, in determining whether the patient is able to return home for the evening after the day hospital day. Communications between members of the treatment team are on-going throughout the day; the nurse will frequently report her observations to the team and may ask that the patient be seen by the psychiatrist or social worker, if she believes the patient to be especially upset or suicidal and in need of an increase in medications or of admission to the inpatient service in lieu of returning home.

As a participant in activity staff meetings, the nurse can pass along information about the patient's history, family contacts, and treatment decisions to the other nurses and the occupational and recreational therapists. This information contributes to a multidisciplinary conclusion as to whether a particular bit of patient behavior represents progress, or resistance, or a realistic limitation, or a reaction to a temporary stress. The activity staff is thus able to decide whether the behavior should be encouraged or discouraged or whether a particular patient should be included or excluded from an activity.

The nurse also functions as a co-therapist in small group psychotherapy as well as a participant in larger community meetings. In group therapy, she can be helpful because her contact with patients throughout the day is more comprehensive than that of other staff professionals who spend more time in individual and family contacts. As a result, she is more often aware of group anxieties and tensions than the doctor or social worker, especially if these are related to a problem within the treatment community.

Traditionally, the essence of the nursing role concerned direct patient care as an extension of the doctor's treatment plans. In our day hospital, treatment plans are usually prescribed by the treatment team including the nurse and are not solely the responsibility of the doctor, even though he is the administrator of the team.

On an inpatient service, a patient relates to numerous nurses on various shifts. In the day hospital setting, he relates primarily to one nurse, thus intensifying the relationship. Very often the nurse is introduced to the patient prior to the patient's actual admission day. The relationship, once established, can continue after discharge if the patient returns for aftercare. When readmissions occur, the patient usually will be assigned to the same treatment team (although often the resident psychiatrist may have changed). For this reason the patient often feels more comfortable in returning, since he can relate to staff whom he knew during his previous admission. If he feels ashamed or guilty about having to return, he frequently can express these feelings to the nurse. Furthermore, as one of the persons who has known the patient in the past, the nurse can be helpful in assessing differences in behavior between the past and present admissions.

The patient directs many questions to the nurse throughout the day. These may range from inquiries about medication to vocational services, to concerns about financial problems. The nurse is a resource person within the treatment social setting who listens and encourages the patient to select the course of action which will most benefit him at that particular time. This does not mean the nurse does things for the patient. Rather she evaluates the situation and tries to help the patient help himself. "Aiding patients to develop the competence essential for living with people in a democratic society is part of the day-to-day nursing service in a psychiatric setting (Peplau, 1967)." Sometimes the nurse does little more than listen while the patient thinks things through out loud. Or she may point out self-destructive tendencies and other pathological trends, perhaps reinforcing a therapeutic intervention made earlier in group or individual therapy. On other occasions, the patient may be far too disorganized to arrive at anything resembling a meaningful decision, even on relatively minor matters, and in such instances the nurse is much more actively involved, often to the point of acting as a bridge to reality for a psychotic person.

The nurse involves herself in the patient's therapy in a very practical way, applying and putting into action throughout the day her knowledge of the patient's psychodynamics. For example, one patient may repeatedly get himself into psychological difficulty because of his tendency to take on more responsibility than he can realistically handle. A nurse, noting frequent examples of this throughout the day, may point it out and encourage him to allow other patients to assume more of the responsibility. On the other hand, if a patient avoids responsibility, even when he is able to handle it, a nurse can interpret this behavior to him in a multitude of ways and encourage him to try to take on more responsibility. Seeing one patient distressed by inappropriate guilt, which stems from a hypertrophied superego, the nurse can on a day-to-day basis help reduce this guilt. Conversely, the nurse can attempt to reinforce and strengthen the superego in another patient where lack of a sense of responsibility and conscience interferes with his ability to function effectively in the community. This experiential learning provided throughout the day by the psychiatric nurse supplements, and in many instances is more effective than, clarification and interpretation of behavior patterns in a therapy hour.

New nurses coming into the day hospital often have difficulty adjusting to their new roles in the treatment team. They find it difficult to disagree with and question statements made by professionals from other disciplines, especially doctors. One new nurse described her reluctance to question the doctor as an "inbred anxiety" due to past nurse-doctor work relationships. We think it is important for the nurse to be an active treatment team member and not just sit idly by, passively taking and carrying out the doctor's orders. Furthermore, we attempt to avoid the doctor-nurse game (Stein, 1967) where everyone goes to great lengths to perpetuate a fantasy that all decisions have come from the doctor, even though many actually may have originated with the nurse. The nurse should feel free to express her observations and suggestions and the psychiatrist should be secure enough to listen and to act on the nurse's advice, if he concurs, without feeling any loss of face or status.

In our experience, individual supervision helps the new nurse gain enough self-confidence to express herself more freely and to disagree with those who possess different or higher badges of authority. For the nursing staff to function effectively, support is essential. Nurses need to be encouraged to speak.

By defining the nurse's role and by giving her an important and specific function in the treatment team, we have avoided some of the competitiveness between nurses and other disciplines sometimes en-

countered in other psychiatric settings. For instance, the struggle between the doctor and the nurse or between the social worker and the
nurse, as to who is to be the "one-to-one therapist," has not been an
issue here. The nurse is convinced she is fulfilling a vital role without
having to take the patient into an office to do "psychotherapy."

"Certain nursing skills and traditions lend distinctive features to
the nurse's position in the day hospital, particularly the nurturant role
implied in the term 'nurse.' Skilled in the management of large numbers
of patients, tutored in the art of looking after the patient's total well-
being, and trained to note and report discomfort, the psychiatric nurse
is also particularly able to exert skills in interpersonal relations as a
means of helping troubled patients (Kramer, 1962)."

The role of the nurse in the day hospital is many-sided. She
assumes responsibility for patients who would often be on a twenty-
four-hour service if the day hospital were not available. This requires
continual observation and reporting of behavior. Most nurses find this
work exciting and a constant challenge. Perhaps the most difficult task
is learning to work closely with other team members. A collaborative
effort between nursing and each of the other community mental health
disciplines is necessary if patients are to receive good nursing service
(Matte, 1967).

### Working with Hospitalized Patients (Wygant and Heath)

Psychiatric nursing on the inpatient ward is influenced by a
combination of many factors. For instance, changes in personnel bring
changes in the way inpatient service staff work. Many other incidental
circumstances have an influence: the problems presented by those admitted for treatment, the fact that nurses are on the staff of a general
hospital and that the ward is one element in a comprehensive mental
health center, as well as the fact that this service is part of a psychiatric
teaching program.

Our inpatient ward is described in detail in Chapter 4. The
pace is rapid and often hectic, for we receive over one hundred admissions to our thirty-one-bed facility each month. The average length
of stay is seven days, with a range from overnight to something less
than a month. Treatment that will help the patient return to the community must be available here, even though symptoms virtually run
the gamut of serious, acute psychiatric problems. To supply this treat-

ment in so short a time, we must selectively limit our attention to those aspects of the patient's problem that have made necessary the positive prescription of a full-time hospital ward. It is the mission of this ward to help the patient through his crisis and to support his active efforts to improve his functioning to the point at which his treatment can continue in another less inclusive and less costly program—a day treatment center or an outpatient clinic.

All of these circumstances, and others beyond the scope of this brief summary, can be considered a changing field of factors which regularly brings about changes in work and changes in the nurse's view of her work. The important point is that nurses do not have and do not try to impose rigid rules or preconceived ideas about the procedures or methods they expect people—either patients or staff—to follow. Flexibility is a basic stance for all staff.

Half of our twenty-two nurses are registered nurses; the others have training as licensed vocational nurses (broadly equivalent to the licensed practical nurse in other states) or as psychiatric aids. The relatively large complement of R.N.s is a luxury that allows us to put greater emphasis upon patient care and to participate in a team approach.

A newly admitted patient may need close support, perhaps even one-to-one nursing for the first few hours or for a day; but the nurse's task, as a member of a team, is to help the patient move quickly out of this dependence and to encourage him to achieve more independent functioning as soon as possible. We try to maintain a nursing pattern in which all nurses, including the L.V.N.s and the aides, feel comfortable in making frequent revisions in their patterns of service and degree of support for each patient, as he moves toward increased independence, often on an hour-to-hour basis. In this service, each nurse recognizes the fact that she will have changing patterns of work all day long.

Nurses participate with all other staff and all patients in the six-morning-a-week community group, as well as in the patient government groups, which meet twice weekly. Nurses and social workers are the co-leaders of the small groups, which meet three mornings a week, and of the joint patient-relatives group each Tuesday evening. In addition, nurses take part in case conferences, general staff meetings, and meetings in which planning for treatment and aftercare is discussed. In these activities, our nurses make an important contribution to assessment and evaluation of patients and planning and its implementation.

Inpatient service nurses are on the staff of the general hospital; technically, our nurses are under the administration of the director of nurses in the hospital. Although the nursing director assists in the recruiting of staff, she allows the service to interview and select its own staff. Practically speaking, the lines of authority run from the psychiatric nursing supervisor to both the chief psychiatrist and the director of nurses. If a conflict develops or there is need for bilateral decision-making, it is handled promptly by a conference. Thus, nurses feel no division of loyalty between the nursing office and the ward administration; they are given the latitude to blend their skills with those of the other mental health disciplines in the service and to accept the leadership of the chief psychiatrist, who is the ward administrator. It is our experience that an effective milieu treatment program depends upon good, stable work relationships and the development of a cohesive staff team. Therefore, nurses do not rotate regularly through other departments, although they may do so by request as a refresher. The same holds true for nurses from other departments spending time on our psychiatric ward to gain experience.

We do put much emphasis on the many significant relationships between our nurses and those in other parts of the hospital. Our supervising nurses routinely attend the weekly meetings of hospital nursing supervisors and head nurses and our nurses participate in interdisciplinary case presentations in the departments of internal medicine and surgery. These conferences bring together residents, medical social workers, personnel from psychiatry, and hospital nurses.

We expect the nurse in the therapeutic community to work toward the goal of accepting responsibilities as a staff member working with others from her own and other disciplines. Nurses whose formal psychiatric training emphasized one-to-one interpersonal techniques often find this broader collaborative team role difficult at first. A continuing learning attitude is essential.

Patients are persons who have been so overwhelmed by some crisis in their lives that they require twenty-four-hour hospitalization. But with varying capacities they can still assume real responsibilities. It is in this sense that we say the appeal in the therapeutic community is to the well, or potentially well, part of each patient. Our belief—constantly reaffirmed—is that, in addition to working toward assuming responsibilities for themselves, patients can and will grow to share in responsibilities to each other.

Our understanding of *permissiveness* and its application to our work is evidently not the same as the implication the word has come to convey in the United States. One of the authors (L. S. W.), who worked for a time in Maxwell Jones' therapeutic community in England, found the British connotation of the word implies "permission to take part in." In this country, *permissiveness* is widely taken to mean "anything goes." Consequently, Americans often misunderstand Jones' idea and find themselves in conflict when they attempt to apply it. Here in San Mateo we mean by it that we do not take responsibility *from*—we allow people to function in those ways that are appropriate. In all respects, it is the same as we encounter it in life—except that more support is given to people in this situation. The subtleties surrounding our interpretation of permissiveness, democracy, and the egalitarian trends in the therapeutic community are discussed in more detail in Chapter 3.

*Support* is the key word to describe the nurse's work, but it is used in the sense of calling upon people to develop their individual patterns of appropriate functioning. The term *guide,* if it is understood to imply a combination of teacher and companion, might serve reasonably well to indicate the nursing role. We think of the nursing "presence," instead of using images that suggest taking care of people. It is a supportive thing rather than a limiting thing. People are encouraged to do things for themselves. Nurses try to show people a way to move toward more functional behavior, but they ask the patient to find his own way—the way that has real meaning for him. In supplying her presence to the patient, the nurse is seeking to elicit increased coping powers on the part of the patient, helping him acquire new dimensions of social problem-solving versatility. Hopefully, these will contribute in a meaningful way to his life after discharge from the hospital.

It is not imperative that the nurse perform some highly technical skill. The nurse finds that her presence with another person has meaning. She learns it is the kind of feeling she communicates, the messages she transmits by word, deed, and mood that are often crucial determinants of the patient's ability to use the program effectively. Patients realize that they are not going to be mistreated. They do not have to go through the experience alone. Nobody can do it for them, but they are not alone.

These feelings of isolation constitute a tremendous problem, common to the vast majority of our patients. This is why the nurse is such an important person in the early hours of hospitalization. Our patients are admitted in the emergency room of the hospital. In the early minutes of the patient's contact with the psychiatrist in the emergency room, the seeds of trust begin to take root. When the physician has succeeded in establishing a preliminary and perhaps inchoate understanding with the patient, when the patient has found it possible to impose tentative controls over his own impulses and fears, he is ready to come to the psychiatric ward. The usual practice is to have a nurse from the ward go to the emergency room to meet the new patient and work with the doctor. The nurse and patient (and family members, when present) walk to the ward together.

Cumming and Cumming (1962) observe that "The success of military psychiatry in swiftly returning patients with cases of battle fatigue, or acute ego disorganization, to their duties has demonstrated the crucial importance of the early hours in the hospital." They proceed to recall a comment they attribute to Edward Stainbrook that "One hour in the first day in the hospital is worth five in the second week. In other words, for many acutely ill people the admission process is a major part of therapy." We have found that a large part of the effective early work with a patient consists of a very simple achievement: giving the patient the assurance that he knows one person. The nurse who admitted him will spend whatever time may be necessary to help him begin to feel comfortable on the ward and to feel a certain familiarity with these surroundings. Afterward, she may not be as much involved with him as other nurses. Nevertheless, nurses can recall individuals whom they have admitted coming to them a week later—although in the intervening period they had not been working directly with them—to talk about an upsetting telephone call from home. It then becomes clear again that the admitting nurse's presence each day has been a source of support to a particular patient, because of their initial work together, even though other staff and patients have been much more actively involved with him.

Next to other patients, nurses spend more time with patients and are more actively involved with them than anyone else. What the nurse does between the admission and discharge of a patient is individualized—both for the patient and for the group of which the patient is a participant. Her interventions are usually at a very basic level. She must use her judgment in deciding on individualized decisions: should this patient be encouraged to get up in the morning? Or should he be allowed to remain in bed? Should she (or someone) sit with him? We like to encourage people to participate actively in the program; but the nurse often has to decide whether a patient should be helped to get to the table for his meals, given a tray in his room or, in fact, whether it is desirable at a particular stage to avoid making an issue about food. It is up to her to notice symptoms which indicate the need to withhold or otherwise modify medication, and to call this to the attention of the patient's doctor for verification. She must consider whether to encourage a person to join activities or to encourage less active stimulation for him. She must feel free to depart from ward routine when special circumstances demand it.

A fourteen-year-old boy, who was very disturbed, was having difficulty staying on the ward. He was six feet tall and probably could not have been handled by the staff, if our handling were based upon a contest of physical strength. He was actively hallucinating. When he came into the conference room as the nurses gathered for morning report, it was decided to let him stay. It seemed evident he would leave the ward otherwise, and he appeared to be less frightened when he was with the staff. When the night nurse got to him in the report, she talked with him about the troubled night he had had. Several times during the report, he stood up, saying the voices were telling him to leave, but he would sit down again, when asked. During this meeting, he also accepted the liquid medication he had earlier refused. The staff considered this a very rewarding experience, because they could see this youngster was trying very hard, and they felt the message got across to him that they were trying too.

When the nurse makes a decision, she assumes the responsibility for stating her decision and for explaining its basis, rather than couching this action in the terminology of a thinly-disguised rationalization or excuse. An example: a patient has been given permission by his doctor to go on an outing; the nurse (or occupational therapist) does not feel comfortable in escorting that patient off the ward. The staff member is not required to take the patient, but she must explain to the patient the basis for this decision in such a way as to permit the patient to take a look with her at the elements of his behavior that have caused the staff member to believe it inadvisable for him to join the outing. Later, the staff member is expected to go over this decision with the patient's doctor, also.

There are few rules to go by. The staff work more from a philosophy than within the rigidity of rules. Naturally, this creates intermittent problems and dilemmas. We still hear a nurse say, "We can't have any visitors at mealtime." But, the truth is, there are times when the family is invited to stay for a meal. A wife had to spend two hours on a bus to get in to see her husband. It seemed absurd to ask her to leave at mealtime, which came shortly after she arrived. She had a four-hour trip to visit her husband. When she was invited to remain for the meal, the staff were telling her that they cared about her, as well as about her husband. It clearly meant a great deal to both of them—and, in any case, it would not have been right to send her away; the principle is very simple and basic: you just do not treat people that way.

It should not be supposed this pattern of interpersonal involvement and responsibility-sharing is a "sugar-coated" method. It demands much of patients, as well as of staff. Sometimes we ask too much. Not all of our patients go back to the community, by any means. Approximately 20 per cent are unable, in the brief time we can keep them with us, to achieve the functioning level that would permit them to remain in the community with the support that is available; these patients move into our regionalized state hospital wards, where the program is not quite so fast-moving and people have more time to develop their sources of strength.

A newly-admitted patient complained, during a community meeting, that he was not being taken care of—he said no one had told him how to do certain things. The discussion developed the question of how much responsibility each person has for taking the initiative in meeting the demands of daily living on the ward. A second person—having been on the ward for three days—observed that people did need to be dependent at first, saying too much had happened to you at once, so you need to have someone who can guide you. Staff members spoke of the importance of expecting people to function independently and to accept responsibility. It was at this point that a third patient summarized for all of us, saying he thought the new patient was right about dependence and the staff was right about taking responsibility. But this patient's actual words contained an interesting revelation for all of us. Addressing his comment to the staff, he said "You are about 50 per cent right." Then, quickly revising, he added, "I mean, it's fifty-fifty." Without doubt, the demands we make on patients often prove to be very heavy burdens.

From this brief discussion, it can perhaps be understood that we expect our nurses to be somewhat unusual people. The nurse we try to recruit blends the hospital nurse and the mental health worker, with plenty of scope for her own personality. There are no carbon copies.

### The Public Health Nurse (Mouw and Haylett)

San Mateo's challenging community mental health adventure has been shared by public health nurses since enactment of the California Short-Doyle Community Mental Health Act in 1957. Although they are not actually psychiatric personnel, these nurses were recognized as caregiving professionals who were concerned with the mental health aspects of their work, and they were considered an appropriate instrumentality for the further extension of mental health into the community.

Public health nurses function in many areas where mental health principles can be practiced: prenatal clinics, schools, child health conferences, and in the family itself. They have entrée to many individuals and families who need help to adjust to the problems of physical illness and emotional stress. In their daily work, they encounter a wide variety of emotional reactions and can refer, for further study and treatment, persons for whom their own counseling and guidance may seem insufficient.

As these nurses engage in casefinding and in assisting those who are in need of rehabilitation, they must have a working knowledge of the various mental health facilities in the community. To initiate their acquaintance with community mental health services, a one-and-one-half day orientation visit to the psychiatric inpatient ward and the day hospital is scheduled for all newly-employed nurses. In addition to learning something about the philosophy, function, and purposes of these services, the nurses are told that further contacts are welcomed; they are encouraged to discuss patients with physicians, social workers, and staff nurses, to visit patients on the ward and in the day hospital, when appropriate, and to attend case conferences. In particular, the multiphasic staffing conference offers the opportunity for professionals from different disciplines to collaborate, a reciprocal process which may occasion an expansion of each caregiver's understanding of the patient and his family, as well as an increased appreciation of each other's roles.

In a public health nursing service, nurses have a multitude of opportunities for interventions that may promote and maintain mental health, as well as for activities that expedite recovery and rehabilitation. Guidance and counseling about emotional as well as physical health matters are now a familiar part of the public health nurse's daily work. The nurse's roles as an early identifier of mental disorder and referral-expediter to appropriate community resources also are well established. However, in our community, the public health nurse's role in the management and treatment of diagnosed mentally ill persons was not well defined initially.

As nurses were requested to undertake expanded responsibilities in the aftercare of mental patients, many questions of role and function were raised. Physicians from public hospitals and clinics and some in private practice began to ask nurses to make home visits to recently discharged patients. Sometimes the charge was vague: "See how things are going and be supportive." Nurses who had limited experience in psychiatric settings requested both inservice training in the subject area of major mental illnesses and mental health consultation. They needed to know in considerably more detail what was expected of them and what they could do. In the course of the consultative relationship, three roles came to be identified: observer, expediter, and auxiliary therapist.

In the role of observer, the nurse has the responsibility of assessing the patient's adjustment to the home situation. She is especially aware of the quality of his interaction with the family and other important persons in the home. She notes his attitudes toward his drug therapy and his motivation to follow through with aftercare plans. The nurse is also in a key position to determine the family's receptivity to the patient. She considers their understanding of the illness and the aftercare plans as well as their needs for support and counseling. In addition, the nurse is concerned about the general health status of the entire family.

As expediter, she assists the patient or family to follow through on aftercare recommendations. This might involve getting the patient to clinic appointments or expediting referrals to other programs, such as those provided by vocational rehabilitation or social welfare.

The role of auxiliary therapist initially caused the greatest uncertainty and resultant anxiety. Several nurses were concerned that "just visiting and talking" was somehow not as real a service as those nursing arts where there was "laying on of hands." As these nurses came to understand how their interaction with patients could be therapeutic as well as important, however, many began to enjoy the challenge and stimulation of this new dimension in the professional use of self.

In mental illness, as in physical infirmity, the nurse serves as a mothering person who aims to alleviate discomfort, and as a vehicle for the physician's healing instructions. The nurse who comes to the patient's home is, symbolically, one who cares. She becomes available as a model for identification. She may clarify issues, give advice, or suggest environmental changes. Many of these activities are used in supportive psychotherapy. Shared, too, is the professional use of self in an interpersonal transaction.

Nurses have been given administrative sanction to use the nursing hour in an imaginative and creative way. The format of a nursing visit to the home of a recently hospitalized housewife illustrates the nontraditional pattern of interaction that may be necessary when the assignment calls for socializing and facilitation of increased social functions. The housewife was having difficulty in mobilizing her energy to buy the food for the family. The nurse and mother studied the grocery ads in the newspaper and made a shopping list. Together they went to the market. When they returned, the mother asked, "Now what do I do the rest of the day?" Together they worked out a step-by-step plan for the remainder of the day. Included were the all-important, albeit prosaic, details involved in cooking the evening meal.

In another instance, a nurse who had been visiting a chronically ill woman for several months arrived one day moments after the patient's husband had died. The nurse assisted the patient in calling her physician and went with her to the hospital where the husband was pronounced dead. Later the nurse accompanied the patient to the funeral home where she gave support while the necessary arrangements were being made.

Patterns of visiting are based on patient and family needs. Visits may vary from as often as once a day or several times a week to once a month. A nurse visited a depressed patient who had been discharged from the state hospital. She found him in his night clothes at two o'clock in the afternoon. The shades were drawn and the atmosphere was one of gloom and despair. He told her he saw no need for her visits. She stated simply that the doctor was concerned and wanted her to come. She indicated that she, too, was concerned and that she would sit with him quietly for a time and would return in two days. The visits continued. Ultimately, the nurse arrived to find the patient dressed and the shades up. One day the nurse accompanied this patient to a neighborhood recreation center. In each of these instances the nurse used her professional self in a series of interpersonal transactions which were rewarding and satisfying to both patient and nurse.

The nurse's psychotherapeutic role technically differs from more formal psychotherapy in several respects. The primary intent and setting are different. The depth of discussion is generally limited to the conscious and current without probing or encouraging free association. Furthermore, as in other home nursing activities, the nurse's self-identification is clearly that of a team member working with medical direction.

As a team member, the nurse is encouraged to assess the nursing needs of patients based on her observations and then to formulate a plan of action. This plan frequently means that the nurse can use her own creativity and ingenuity. As she becomes more secure with that which is nursing, her relationship with the physician becomes more collaborative and reciprocal.

Communication between nurses and doctors is imperative. An interagency referral form has been worked out for use between physicians, hospitals, and service personnel. All orders for public health nursing visits to patients must be renewed every two months. This means that nurses must review and evaluate their services to patients and request renewal of orders from the medical source. Physicians, too, must assess the patient's needs for nursing care, medications, and treatment at these regular intervals. There are times when patients or their families decline to seek the needed medical supervision, despite nurses' attempts to motivate this necessary step. In those instances, nurses must then discontinue service.

That the public health nurse can function comfortably and effectively in the aftercare of patients who have been sick enough to need hospitalization is well documented (Collard, 1966; Donnelly et al., 1962; New Haven V.N.A., 1966; Zolik, Lantz, and Sommers, 1968). She is often able to reach and establish contact with a poorly motivated segment of the population. Because she goes to the patient and has a generally helpful approach, she may be seen as less professionally demanding and more personally caring than others. Furthermore, the public health nurse is frequently viewed by the patient and his family as the least stigmatizing of all public representatives. Not only is she likely to be accorded the easy entrée of a trusted family friend, but, unlike the social visitor, she brings a rich professional armamentarium.

She is a trained observer who sees and hears much but knows the ethics of confidentiality. She knows her community and can help her patient establish new contacts when these are indicated. Increasingly, she individualizes her professional approach, supplementing her intuition with considered interventions. Finally, she knows the importance of keeping communication flowing between herself, her supervisor, and the responsible physician.

It soon became apparent to public health nursing administration that if public health nurses were to contribute to the early detection of mental and emotional disorders as well as to improve their services to patients with diagnoses of mental illness, and their families, a specialist in the field was needed. A request for a mental health nurse consultant was made to the Consultation, Education and Information Service of the Mental Health Services Division in 1961. This request was granted in the division's 1963–64 budget. A mental health nurse consultant, who was intimately acquainted with the system of public health and public health nursing and who had training in the techniques of mental health consultation, was employed and assigned to work primarily with public health nurses.

Goals of the mental health nurse consultant and the consultee group were initially lacking in precision, and methods of working most productively with administration and staff needed to be explored. As nurses were requested to expand their responsibilities in the aftercare of mental patients, roles and functions needed to be identified and clarified. In addition, as the nurse consultant became familiar with the mental health services within the San Mateo County Department of Public Health and Welfare and the state hospital system, it became more clear that a liaison function between these services and public health nursing would serve a useful purpose. Thus, the nurse consultant moved in all of these directions, attempting to improve liaison and to bring greater clarity and structure into consultation transactions.

A great deal has been written about nursing services to the mentally ill person and his family during the hospital interlude and after the patient's return to the community. Such a service has been given various labels: *aftercare, follow-up care,* or *continuity of care.* Perhaps the last term best conveys the idea of the succession and connection of care that presumably will contribute much to the patient's welfare.

Mental health services in San Mateo County are highly complex, and it is difficult to know how or where to "plug in" to this complexity in order to give nursing service to those who might profit from it most. The mental health nurse consultant soon learned that patients moved in a wide variety of ways between services. For example, a patient receiving therapy at the adult psychiatric clinic might be referred to the day hospital or a patient presenting himself at the emergency room might be referred to the inpatient service or to the state hospital. It soon became apparent that by assuming the role of liaison between the mental health units and public health nursing, the nurse consultant could serve to interpret and clarify roles and functions of both.

First, communication between the mental health nurse consultant and the supervising nurses on the inpatient service and the day hospital was established. With administrative sanction, a plan was worked out in which public health nurses are notified daily about new admissions to each of these services. Upon receipt of such notification, the nursing files are checked to learn if this patient is, or was, known to the public health nurse. If he is known, a summary is written and sent to the mental health professionals who are caring for him. Case conferences, telephone conversations, joint conferences bringing together the patient, the public health nurse, and ward personnel, and requests for visits with the family and patient are examples of patterns of service that have resulted from such communication. When a patient has not been known to the public health nursing service, a referral to this service can be initiated by the inpatient or day hospital personnel. Communication has been further facilitated by the planned conferences between the nurse consultant and the supervising nurses on the inpatient service and in the day hospital. The latter two nurses have assisted greatly in the interpretation of public health nursing services to psychiatrists (including residents who may soon be practicing in this or in other communities) and social workers who heretofore were not acquainted with their services.

A modified but similar system of communication has been worked out with the other units of the Mental Health Services Division. These include the adult psychiatric clinic, child guidance clinic, and the regional North County Mental Health Center.

The mental health nurse consultant also serves as liaison between public health nursing and the San Mateo County patients in the regionalized state hospital wards. Regular weekly visits with the state hospital ward personnel are scheduled to discuss discharge plans for patients. Public health nursing aftercare has been extremely helpful for the woman who will be assuming the role of wife, mother, and household manager upon returning home; for the patient who needs encouragement to maintain his drug regime and his appointments at the psychiatric clinic; for the family who refuses to accept the patient as ill and in need of care; or for the patient who needs support to resume his place in the family, in the labor market, or in the community.

The supportive role that the nurse can play by seeing the patient and his family at home is recognized by many psychiatrists, social workers, and psychologists as adding a valuable ingredient, different from those supplied by the traditional clinical disciplines working within clinics or hospitals. Public health nurses are talking with these workers with increasing self-confidence and ease.

As a result of direct channels of communication between nurses and the professional staff at Agnews State Hospital, an understanding of roles and responsibilities has evolved to such a degree that far more comprehensive services are provided to patients and families in the home as well as to patients in the hospital. The public health nurse has frequently enabled the hospital to get better cooperation from family members, thereby contributing to the hospitalized patient's welfare. The assessment and evaluation of the home situation often has led to a more realistic aftercare plan for the patient. Similarly, the public health nurse has been able to formulate her plans with the patient and family more realistically as the result of the assessment and evaluation of the patient in the hospital. Thus, on the part of all workers there is a growing respect for each other and each other's competence.

Another example of mutually helpful cooperation can be found in the relationship with the regional North County Mental Health Center, where each of three team psychiatrists visits the district public health nursing office once a month. At these meetings, the psychiatrists, the supervising nurse, and the staff nurse discuss patients active in both services, with a view to optimum caregiving collaboration.

The numbers of persons with a diagnosis of mental illness referred to public health nurses have increased from 88 in 1962 to 183 in 1968. The number of nursing visits have jumped from 717 in 1962 to 2,105 in 1968. These numbers compare favorably with the statistics from other disease categories such as cardiovascular disease, cerebralvascular accidents, and cancer. However, when compared with the large numbers of patients discharged from the acute psychiatric ward of the county hospital and Agnews State Hospital, the numbers referred to public health nursing for aftercare are very small indeed. Large numbers of emotionally ill persons present themselves at the emergency room and many are sent back home. Many of these patients could benefit from nursing surveillance to see if they respond to the medications prescribed, to see what further medical or nursing service is indicated, or to give support and guidance to family members as they attempt to cope with the sick person. It is obvious that new methods of closing these gaps of service to people in need are yet to be created.

As experience was gained and shared by consultants from several disciplines, working with many different consultee groups, consultation goals of the mental health nurse consultant became more precise. In general, consultation is now seen as having three aims: (1)

helping the visiting nurse with specific work problems, (2) educating the visiting nurse to be more effective in the mental health aspects of her professional role, and (3) educating the mental health nurse consultant, not only in regard to the epidemiology of mental illness, but also in awareness of how she may be more effective in her consulting role.

The public health nurse consultant has proceeded on the premise that a long-term, working relationship with the public health nursing service is a desirable goal. This has provided a variety of indirect services in response to changing interests and needs. In addition to regularly scheduled individual and group consultation, the nurse consultant has been used for emergency consultation, for inservice training, and for collaboration with public health nursing colleagues. As a result of continuing work together, the nurse consultant has been used flexibly and creatively at various levels within the nursing system for consultation about specific cases, administrative policy, and even some aspects of program planning.

Goals for nurse consultees have also become better defined. Our impression is that there have been modifications in performance that we could now consider goals, even though these were not formulated as such in advance. Nurses have become increasingly sensitive to the emotional aspects of their work. Many nurses now consciously listen for "the question behind the question" and systematically consider possible determinants or perplexing behavior. They now tend to individualize each patient in each family, thus lessening the use of stereotypes.

There has been greater acceptance among the nurses of their own strengths and abilities and more tolerance of limitations, both personal and professional. Professional role refinement has occurred, leading to a clearer definition of the nurses' particular contributions to the treatment and rehabilitation of mentally ill patients. This has helped to allay the needless anxiety and guilt that they cannot be all things to all people, and to increase their satisfaction and self-confidence in working with the mentally ill.

In addition to "sanction at all administrative levels," orienting new staff members in detail to the purposes, methods, and process of consultation is especially desirable. In their academic preparation, many nurses have had little exposure to mental health consultants or to the nature of this type of a helping relationship. Thus, careful preparation and structuring of early consultation experience is necessary if both unrealistic expectations and unnecessary fears are to be minimized.

Orientation meetings are now planned with the consultant on a regular basis. A group of newly employed nurses has an opportunity to be a part of a session in which a typical nursing situation is presented and all enter into the problem-solving. Through this demonstration it is hoped that nurses have a beginning understanding of consultation—its values and limitations.

From the outset, the mental health consultants have worked with district office supervisors and nurses as a group. The supervisor generally assumes responsibility for chairing the meeting and for deciding which patients or situations will be discussed. Thus, the consultant is free to interact as a clearly nonadministrative, resource person. Usually, one nurse presents a case or situation of current concern and the group participates in clarifying issues and suggesting ways to understand and deal with problems.

The consultant, as well as the supervisor, may facilitate the group process. At the same time, she may make some independent hypotheses about the nature of the problem. She may raise questions that lead to a different conceptualization of the problem or invite group members to share their perceptions and experience with similar cases. In thinking through a problem with her colleagues, the presenting nurse frequently sees its nature in a different context and feels free to proceed with renewed conviction and self-confidence.

Sometimes, the consultant supplements the group's knowledge of child development, personality dynamics, or mental illness. Most often, however, the consultation is a process of shared thinking, which gains strength from the professional relationship with the consultant and from the group interaction.

In addition to regularly scheduled group sessions, individual consultation time is available to district offices. Staff nurses sign up for scheduled time as needed. The supervisor may reserve part of the time to review the problems and concerns she has in developing the potential of staff nurses or to discuss program issues. When early attention is needed, a telephone discussion may suffice or additional consultation time is arranged. It is highly desirable that the consultant have enough flexibility in her schedule to be available for occasional emergency contacts.

Although separating the impact of mental health consultation from many other experiential variables is not possible, shifts in the relationship between the consultant and consultee are noted and are reflected in their communication. In time, a nurse consultee tends to shift her emphasis from what patients say to what she herself says and does, and finally to include how she herself feels about it. Our impression is that a parallel change takes place in many nurse-patient relationships. As the nurse progresses from an intellectual acceptance to an emotional acceptance of a patient's behavior, a more comfortable, warm, individualized transactional pattern results.

Since the initiation of our mental health consultation program, psychiatrists, psychologists, psychiatric social workers, and a mental health nurse have all consulted with the nursing division. Our experience suggests that consultants from various professional disciplines are useful, as each has a special body of knowledge and experience to offer. In practice, however, most of the consultation has been with a psychiatrist or the mental health nurse or both. When both have been simultaneously available to the nursing division, the advantages have been qualitative as well as quantitive. The different disciplines seem to potentiate each other. Each has special assets.

A mental health nurse consultant, for example, already knows nursing as a profession. Although a new nurse consultant must become acquainted with the unique aspects of a particular nursing program, she need not learn a new language or professional philosophy. Her identity is as a nurse. She is not likely, inadvertently, to encourage a nurse consultee toward inappropriate roles. Furthermore, where the nurse consultant can have an office in proximity to the nursing division, she is available for a variety of informal as well as formal consultative activities. On the other hand, a consultant from the same discipline as the consultee does not bring a markedly different knowledge base or perspective. Nor is the potential for interdisciplinary stimulation the same. Although the nurse consultant may not have the advantages or disadvantages of any traditional, interprofessional status differential, staff usually come to associate her with their own supervisory and administrative echelon.

In the San Mateo program, one of the mental health nurse

consultant's major contributions has been to bring greater clarity and structure into consultation transactions. She has helped to define roles and functions for supervisors, consultants, and consultee nurses. She also has helped to conceptualize public health nursing roles in mental health.

CHAPTER **8**

# Vocational Rehabilitation Services

*H. Richard Lamb, Cecile Mackota*

⁍⁍⁍⁍⁍⁍⁍⁍⁍⁍⁍⁍⁍⁍⁍⁍⁍⁍⁍⁍⁍⁍⁍⁍

With the evolution of society, and especially in the Western democracies, achievement has become more and more important as a factor in establishing one's identity. Self-esteem and one's self-image depend in large measure on what one does occupationally and how successful one is in doing it. No longer, as in earlier societies, is one classified primarily by birth, family, and station. For these reasons any attempt at treatment of the mentally ill and emotionally troubled must, in some way, deal with the issues of occupational choice and vocational satisfaction.

Most persons find it difficult to feel themselves a part of society if they are not in the working community. In general, our society disapproves of those who do not work. Most people, consciously or unconsciously, accept society's view and suffer a lowered self-esteem if they do not meet the standards of society. Conversely, the ability to work and to be productive heightens one's self-esteem. The feeling that one is conforming to the norms of society is very much bound up in one's sense of well-being. The contribution of a sense of occupational failure to many cases of depression illustrates this point.

With the establishment of comprehensive community mental health services in San Mateo County, there gradually emerged a recognition of our lack of more extensive and sophisticated vocational services. As will be described, we have resolved this by developing within our own program vocational services specifically geared to the needs of psychiatric patients.

These needs fall within a wide range. For instance, with the more chronically disabled patients from the state hospital or our own day hospital, inpatient, or outpatient services, we realized that in many cases we were dealing with people who were in need of a whole new vocational structure. It was not just a question of planning and direction in a counseling relationship, but a necessity for working with people's basic attitudes toward work and helping them form work habits such as learning how to get to a job on time, remaining the full day, and understanding and adjusting to the need for authority from supervisors on the job. These basic lacks in such an important area of life made even more apparent the inadequacy of trying to treat chronic schizophrenics with only psychotherapy and drugs. Lindner and Landy (1958) have stressed the need for vocational rehabilitation services for "those whose illness occurred so early that they never established a vocation." With these very sick people we are dealing with persons who have never resolved one of the major tasks of adolescence, namely, choice of a vocation, and in many cases choice between entering the world of work or the world of dependency on institutions and agencies.

But the gap in services was not limited to this group. For instance, in outpatient treatment with more healthy patients, we became aware that vocational matters were being discussed in the artificial atmosphere of the consultation room which, while providing an ideal setting for psychotherapy as such, did not necessarily provide sufficient reality for meaningful discussion of vocational problems. Much can be meaningfully discussed and worked through in psychotherapy, as in such areas as interpersonal problems which interfere with vocational adjustment, but lacking are the hard facts of an objective appraisal of a patient's skills, aptitudes, work habits, and other aspects of functioning in a job situation. Furthermore, we saw that providing this service required the separate and distinct skills of vocational counselors. These are skills which all therapists do not have and probably should not be expected to have.

### Pitfalls in Counseling

"The counselor of the emotionally disturbed must be prepared to deal with a higher rate of failure than he might find in working with other disability groups," warns Hediger (1967), and adds that counselors will often select "good risks" as feasible for counseling, sometimes because of the policy or regulations of the agency, and sometimes for reasons connected with lack of interest or comfort in dealing with the mentally ill. Furthermore, the emotionally disturbed often need a great deal more time for the rehabilitation process than do other forms of disability (Burling, 1950). Our experience has confirmed these observations.

Information about patients' work performance while in the hospital is frequently available. Ethridge (1968) has shown that this information, if properly collected and evaluated, can be significantly related to successful vocational placement. However, systematic data collection and analysis is not done in most hospital industrial therapy departments. This probably accounts for Walker and McCourt's findings (1965) that hospital work performance of patients is not a reliable indicator of what a patient can and will accomplish in the community. We, too, have found that it is necessary to do a thorough vocational evaluation from the beginning in the community rather than placing heavy reliance upon the vocational evaluation done in the hospital.

We have come to appreciate the need for counselors who understand psychodynamics. Important examples are the concepts of ego strength and dependence-independence conflicts, and the effects of these factors on a patient's capabilities. Trying to evaluate a patient's vocational and intellectual capacity apart from his emotional strengths and weaknesses provides only a very incomplete picture of what a patient can do vocationally. This seems almost self-evident and yet, in our experience with our own and other agencies, we have found that failure to take into account a patient's emotional capacity has been a leading cause of unsuccessful vocational plans. A patient may be fully qualified in an occupation but be overwhelmed by the prospect of returning to it. To do so may represent a major step toward independence or a major increase in pressure for which he is not ready. The counselor must be able to recognize when more time and support are needed or when perhaps goals must be scaled down to the individual's emotional strength. For instance, a paranoid schizophrenic graduate engineer may need a period of time in a sheltered workshop and, for that matter, perhaps a permanent lowering of goals.

Vocational goals must be seen in their proper context, that is, as part of the overall treatment goals for a patient. Those goals should all lead to helping him have a life satisfying in all respects, including a lifelong work experience that will be satisfying and contribute to overall mental health. Just an immediate job placement, we have learned, is not enough.

Thus we recognized that vocational services must meet the varying needs of psychiatric patients, ranging from people who need only counseling to the very sick people who need to begin at the beginning insofar as vocational choice and vocational services are concerned. Services were required in which vocational counselors understood mental illness and its effects on work and felt comfortable in working with psychiatric patients—and with the mental health professional. We found that we had to be able to allow considerable periods of time for vocational rehabilitation without an expectation of the agency or the counselor himself, or both, of quick success.

The existing agencies were unable to provide what we wanted and we therefore found it necessary to set up our own services. In addition to meeting our particular needs, several other advantages emerged. We have been able to tailor our services specifically to the needs of psychiatric patients with all the advantages of specialization in any field. Further, by having these services administratively together with the mental health center, we eliminated the administrative difficulties in having to deal with another agency. Vocational referrals became intramural.

## Problems in Defining Roles

Some of the most difficult problems we encountered involved defining staff roles. We want to mention such problems and others in succeeding sections which might well be expected in any community mental health center that includes vocational services.

Initially, many mental health professionals were not clear as to where the role of the therapist ended and that of the vocational counselor began. Some psychotherapists found it difficult to give up their former roles in the vocational area to admit their lack of competence and skill to do vocational counseling. For instance, a patient might be referred to a vocational counselor with a vocational plan already formulated by the therapist. Further, the usual training of most mental health professionals does not provide an understanding in depth of the nature and philosophy of vocational services. This, too, often made it more difficult for the therapist to properly prepare his patients for the vocational referral.

Defining their own roles also presented problems for the vocational services people. Just as it was difficult at times for the therapist to see where the job as therapist ended and that of vocational counselor began, so was it difficult for the counselors to draw this line and not become seduced into the role of therapist, sometimes through the manipulation of the patient, sometimes through their own inexperience.

The initial definition of roles was crucial for all concerned. As roles gradually became better defined, staff, both in and out of vocational services, felt more comfortable and worked more effectively. In-service training, both formal and informal, was directed toward helping both therapists and vocational counselors better understand the role of vocational services.

As we conceptualize it, the counselor's role is to face the patient with the reality of his functioning, in terms of skills performance and relations to other people on the job. All of these things, of course, reflect his interpersonal problems and strengths and style of living in general. In this sense vocational counseling cannot be seen as totally different from psychotherapy. In fact, some aspects of vocational services and psychotherapy are very similar and overlap. However, the vocational counselor hopefully limits his discussion with the patient to these things only insofar as they relate to work. The vocational counselor frequently finds himself saying, "That would be better discussed with your therapist. Let us concentrate on your vocational problems."

The goal of vocational services is work, but vocational goals must be recognized as only part of the total therapeutic goals. The vocational counselor is part of a team that treats mental illness. Thus, although the vocational counselor has a very specific role, he sees himself as working toward the total therapeutic goals rather than working only toward the limited area of vocational goals. The vocational counselor brings to the total treatment picture the reality of the real world —the here-and-now workaday world. The counselor is not involved as a psychotherapist per se, or involved in dealing with fantasy material or irrational thinking or the working through of unconscious conflict. Rather, he uses various reality-oriented techniques to modify working behavior.

The vocational counselor sees himself not as trying to eliminate symptoms, but rather as trying to help the patient contain them so that they do not interfere with the patient's work performance. A graphic example of this would be advising a patient not to talk about or respond to his hallucinations while at work. The patient learns acceptable behavior, which then gradually becomes part of his personality pattern. The gratification of achieving acceptable behavior adds to his self-esteem and confidence and enables him to gather strength to attack further problems both in and outside of work.

It has been important to emphasize that vocational services involve a collaborative effort between the therapist and the vocational counselor. This means that cases cannot be closed when referred for vocational services and that the therapist needs to remain involved throughout the period of vocational services. Vocational services are an adjunct to therapy but not a substitute for it nor a dumping ground for unwanted cases. Occasionally a therapist has tended to see a patient who is difficult to treat or with whom he has reached an impasse as being suddenly and solely a vocational problem, in order to find a way out of a therapeutic stalemate. Having a patient in vocational counseling or in the vocational workshop is only rarely a complete solution to his problems without other treatment and support.

As pointed out by Olshansky and Unterberger (1963), "The work experience of nonprofessional workers is apparently an unknown area for many psychiatrists whose contact occupationally and socially is with the professional worker." With their knowledge of the work world, counselors not only can help patients to view and respond to work in a different way but also can open up for them the whole spectrum of occupational possibilities. This provides a range of choices unavailable to most patients through their own limited experience. Further, the counselor, unlike most psychotherapists, is by skill and training equipped to make two kinds of appraisal: first, an evaluation of the patient to determine his particular aptitudes, interests, and temperament; second, an appraisal of the skills and aptitudes required and the stresses and difficulties encountered in different occupations. Thus, the counselor, in addition to matching up patient and job in terms of skill and aptitudes, also is able to observe, evaluate and help a patient to see how he is reacting to the particular stresses of a job and how his particular personality and life style fits in with his chosen occupation. With this knowledge the counselor can become engaged in a process which increases the patient's self-knowledge with regard to work and helps the patient use what is learned to make a choice that enhances the possibilities of his achieving success and enriching his life. Even with vocational counselors, we should add, it has frequently been necessary to stress the importance of knowing the specifics of occupations rather than just the techniques of effective counseling.

## Other Problem Areas

In working with the more severely ill patients in particular, we have found it necessary for mental health professionals to accept the responsibility to help, and in many cases push patients toward higher levels of social participation and work performance. As Freeman and Simmons (1963) have said, "It is crucial that we maintain as high expectations of social participation and work performance as is realistic, because low expectations simply support the socially deviant performance and reinforce the patient's failure to perform in ways defined by the role expectations of the larger society." However, some therapists criticize that philosophy as being synonymous with an attempt to indoctrinate patients with "middle-class morality." Perhaps professionals, themselves middle-class, are burdened by guilt, a strong sense of responsibility and emphasis on achievement; they are therefore loath to see themselves as maintaining high expectations of their patients, who have already failed to meet so many of society's demands. Perhaps sometimes the professional derives vicarious pleasure from seeing patients dependent and regressed. Yet for many patients, high staff expectations are a crying need if we hope to motivate them and help them improve their life patterns.

Although most of the therapists considered vocational counseling a valuable adjunct to therapy, some felt that the sheltered workshop was demeaning to patients and bespoke the failure of therapeutic efforts. They seemed to feel that including a sheltered workshop in our program meant that therapy would become less sophisticated, less like "therapy." That feeling was especially strong in day hospital, where because of the chronicity and severity of both illness and vocational problems, most patients needed the workshop experience before, and in many cases long before, they could consider competitive employment. Some professionals whose identities were those of practitioners of intensive psychotherapy and casework felt they were being asked to abandon their skills and assume a role "that anyone could do." Frequently referrals to the sheltered workshop also involved lowering of goals, at least initially, for patients, but to some staff it also seemed as if the standards of therapy were being lowered. It was almost as if some professionals feared that their treatment facility would hark back to a bygone age and become like a poorhouse where people would be made to work in a manner which was demeaning to both themselves and to the therapist.

One goal of treatment may sometimes be to help a patient discard his striving toward unrealistic levels on which he cannot function, because of his emotional or intellectual limitations. But the necessity of lowering vocational goals was often difficult for staff and patients to accept. Sometimes, for instance, a staff member would overidentify with a patient and set vocational goals for him that would have been more appropriate for his own son. Or a patient would identify with a staff member and decide to become a psychiatric technician, even though his emotional limitations made such a goal impossible. He had not yet developed the capacity, required by such a job, to take care of needy, disturbed people. There was a need for both vocational and mental health staff to see that the concept of limited goals and lowering goals, which at first may seem discouraging, can often result in the restoration of a disabled and dependent patient to the role of a functioning member of society, even though at a humble level, if this is the extent of his total social and vocational capabilities.

A seemingly opposite but oftentimes related problem is a lack of therapeutic optimism on the part of some mental health professionals. In the words of Benney and Waltzer (1958), "This optimism needs to be based on the conviction that people have some drive toward health, however weak this may appear; that the psychotic symptoms are defenses; and that energy can be mobilized and channeled providing the professional and environmental resources are available." In some cases, a judicious lowering of goals can make the prospect of rehabilitation much brighter. In other instances an objective appraisal by the vocational counselor who is not intimately involved with the patient—as is the therapist—can add a whole new perspective to the case and contribute to the formulation of more optimistic vocational goals.

These observations have helped lead us to our conviction that the referral form should be extremely brief. For one thing this makes referral easy. Moreover the vocational counselor then does not have a preconceived idea of the patient's vocational potential. The presentation of some cases by the therapist may paint a gloomy picture indeed, even to the most optimistic vocational counselor. It is after the initial contact with the patient that the counselor may collect more complete psychiatric and social information. We have found that the counselor is freer to evaluate and plan with the patient if he sees him initially as an employer would. For example, one woman had been attending our psychiatric clinic and admitted to our inpatient service intermittently for ten years. Her inch-thick record reflected a chaotic and disturbed life and family pattern. After counseling and testing she elected to train as a nurse's aide. Her record in training was excellent and when she graduated she was hired by the training institution. After being on welfare for many years, she is now self-supporting and seems content in her work. If the counselor had read her case record prior to seeing her, we doubt that he would have been optimistic enough about her chances of success to have planned with her as he did.

Our vocational services program handles appointments directly with the client; appointments are not made for the client by his therapist. Referrals can be made not only from county mental health services, but from any psychiatric or social agency or private therapist, as long as the patient is in treatment.

Patients referred to us range from employed professionals to teenagers who have never worked. We have tried to develop a comprehensive service that will provide help at whatever level the individual needs it. Sometimes only counseling is involved, either one-to-one or group. Here, types of problems handled include: selection of an appropriate and satisfying occupation, being able to look for work more effectively, interpersonal problems on the job, learning acceptable work behavior, and control of symptoms while working.

In our work experience program, we place clients with particular skills or skill potential in various county departments. This is not "made work"; the people so placed function as regular employees and are required to conform to all of the rules and regulations of the job. Through this method we are able to provide a real operating work environment for those not quite ready to meet the pressures of a competitive job. Here they can brush up on their skills, learn new operations, and gain the confidence they need. We have found that these need be only relatively short-term placements and are very effective preparation for regular work. We have used the engineers' office for draftsmen, the hospital lab for lab technicians and lab helpers, the typing pool for typists, and so on. In setting up and operating this program, we found that some supervisors of departments were fearful of mental health patients and needed much help and support. Some were oversolicitous and found it difficult to treat those referred as they would any other employee, and to set limits on inappropriate behavior. This attitude made the placement of little value. Gradually, however, as department heads have had more experience with our clients, they have come to accept and treat them as workers and have become enthusiastic about the program. Many have wanted the patients placed with them as permanent employees and have encouraged the civil service office to hire them. One key factor in the success of our work experience program has been the availability of the counselor to the supervisor as needed.

With those people who have selected an appropriate occupation and are ready, the counselor works to obtain proper training. This may be in public or private schools, training facilities or government programs. Some of our patients are able to finance their own training but have not, before this, been able to focus on any specific occupation. More often, at this point, the State Department of Vocational Rehabilitation is the source for finding and financing a training program. Our patients are frequently more acceptable to that agency following a period of therapy and vocational counseling.

Approximately 20 per cent of patients referred to our vocational services need and can use a sheltered workshop experience. This 20 per cent, however, constitutes a group that poses major psychiatric, social, and vocational problems in our society. We have found that if we are to reach this group it is essential to have a vocational workshop as part of comprehensive vocational services in a mental health setting.

Black (1965) feels that there must be industrial therapeutic services outside of the hospital and closer to normal work settings in the community, and this is very much in keeping with our own experience. Originally, we shared a sheltered workshop with the welfare division of the department. This was unsatisfactory, not only because of the differing focus of the welfare division and the mental health services, but also because the workshop was located within the physical plant of the county general hospital. It was very difficult for our patients to regard the workshop as being in any sense a realistic and meaningful work setting. They continued to see themselves primarily as patients, not as trainees or workers. It was with these ideas in mind that our own sheltered workshop was set up several miles from the hospital and in the midst of a bustling industrial park surrounded by busy factories and electronic plants.

We would like to emphasize that the role of the sheltered workshop is not simply to provide a baby-sitting service for chronic schizophrenics. We use it to help each individual identify himself as a worker rather than a patient and to change his self-image so that he perceives himself as someone who can function productively and be paid for his contribution. As a matter of fact, our clinical impression is that when in fact the patient truly sees himself as being a worker, he is ready to move on from the protected setting of the sheltered workshop. The workshop is also a means of measuring actual behavior, providing both the vocational counselor and the therapist with a concrete test of reality in terms of a patient's work readiness and his ability to function under stress. Here a former patient can work out problems and conflicts with fellow workers and supervisors; the workshop staff can help him solve some of these interpersonal problems in the sheltered setting, instead of leaving him to experience them again in a competitive job and risk being fired and thus another failure.

There are few persons available who have both of the two general categories of skills and experience needed by a vocational workshop floor supervisor: the ability to work with psychiatric patients and a solid background of industrial experience. The latter is essential and something in which it is difficult for us to provide training. We have, therefore, hired persons with industrial experience and little or no experience in working with psychiatric patients. We do, however, look for a potential in our workshop floor supervisors for working with and understanding the emotionally disturbed with the intention of our providing in-service training in this area.

This ongoing in-service training requires working with a variety of problems presented by the new workshop supervisor. For instance, they may be too permissive or conversely too demanding and rigid. A workshop floor supervisor may be too "motherly" toward patients and not expect enough of them. Sometimes overidentification with patients is part of the problem. Other floor supervisors present the opposite extreme of being too rigid and making too strict demands on patients without taking into consideration the psychiatric and rehabilitation problems involved. These difficulties have been resolved by both individual supervision of the workshop floor supervisors and by in-service training. New referrals to the workshop are discussed by the total vocational service staff. Here the purpose, expectations, and goals of the vocational placement are presented and clarified. Furthermore, sharing of problems between both the counselor and supervisor is helpful. All of this enables the supervisor, in addition to the counselor, to understand the rationale and plans for the patient so that the supervisor in the very minute-to-minute relationship with the client in the workshop is able to understand and reinforce vocational goals.

Role definition is fully as important in the workshop as anywhere else in the vocational services. Just as the therapist's role differs from that of a vocational counselor, so does the counselor's role differ from that of the workshop floor supervisor. The workshop floor supervisor must see that his role out on the floor directing and helping and observing the client is an important one, but a different one from taking the patient into the office and discussing vocational goals and interests as does the vocational counselor. At the same time, it is important for the vocational counselor to allow the vocational floor supervisor to run the workshop and not to attempt to take over this role. Again, staff discussions have been useful, as has been the vocational counselors' making themselves readily available to answer questions from the vocational workshop floor supervisors when they arise.

We have found the monthly evaluation invaluable in telling a patient how he is doing and indicating whether or not he is measuring up to our expectations of how he will use the workshop. In some cases we have suspended patients from the workshop for poor performance or inappropriate behavior as reflected in their evaluations; this has served as a powerful motivating force for some patients. For those patients who are suspended or discharged, and whose performance did not improve, we found that rather than denying services to people who could benefit from it, we were eliminating people for whom we had been making no positive contribution and were making room for other people who could benefit from our services.

We should add that we have found that it is extremely important to have our expectations realistic and to not move too fast with patients, especially those in the severely and chronically ill group. These patients may be well motivated to make good use of the workshop but require periods of time in the workshop up to two years.

Occasionally, there is a tendency for the workshop staff to be overpermissive. Many of our patients are people whom we get to know and to like, and who, furthermore, are able to evoke guilt in staff. It is sometimes difficult to maintain our policy of not allowing patients to remain in the workshop unless they are gaining some benefit from it and are showing some improvement. But when we do not set limits on inappropriate behavior or if we retain patients who are not making good use of the service, the morale of the whole workshop is impaired. Such staff inconsistencies give the patients a double message:

on the one hand, we say that we expect them to strive toward realizing their potential; and on the other hand, we permit them to do just the opposite. In the same vein, it is important to maintain a policy that the patients must, on any given day, work or leave. An example of this was patients complaining of feeling ill and asking to be able to lie down in a little room off the workshop containing a bed for emergencies. Allowing this quickly increased the number of such requests to lie down. This has been handled by telling patients they should go home if they are ill, and if they are to stay in the shop, then they must stay and work. This has resulted in the number of these requests being greatly reduced. Moreover, the number of patients going home because of illness has not appreciably increased.

Although the workshop operates as a small business and must operate as such to provide the proper setting, it is primarily a tool for rehabilitation of patients. Often good "profit practice" must be sacrificed to serve its main goal. Black (1965) points out that, "In the United States there is still much of the fiction at large that industrial therapy can be profit-making or at least break even." Recognition of this from the literature and from other agencies has helped us to keep from setting financial goals that are not attainable in a truly therapeutic agency. If profit is the goal, clients will be kept too long and there will be the danger of focusing on productivity and the business end of the operation at the expense of rehabilitation. It is important for administration organizing a sheltered workshop in this setting to be prepared to subsidize it, and especially to subsidize costs of vocational counseling, evaluation, and other costs specifically related to rehabilitation rather than production.

On the other hand, in accepting subcontracts from industry, it is necessary to compete with other small businesses and not expect to pass on to our customers costs related solely to rehabilitation. For example, there probably will be a larger amount of substandard work from some clients that must be corrected or redone. This cost must be borne by the workshop rather than passed on to industry in increased costs. In order to continue to be able to supply real work to our patients, we need to bid for jobs on the basis of quality and quantity as they would be in a "normal" business. If it takes three patients to do the job of one "normal" worker, we can bid only on the basis of what the "normal" worker would produce. We must meet delivery schedules and production standards so that private business can continue to use workshops, thereby benefiting us and themselves.

There has been question in the literature as to the validity and usefulness of vocational testing for psychiatric patients—that the symptoms of illness may interfere with the test results, or that the fluctuations of illness will make for fluctuating results (Gladis and Hale, 1965; Hediger, 1967). On the contrary, we have found vocational testing extremely valuable for our patients. Our psychologist administers a battery of aptitude, interest, performance, and personality tests. The counselors use these tests as one of the tools in the evaluation and planning process and find them extremely useful in determining the level on which the patient is functioning *now*. We carefully prepare our patients for testing, and we wait until an acute psychiatric episode has gone into at least partial remission and the patient's illness has stabilized. Under these circumstances, we find that testing gives us a reliable and meaningful idea of a patient's abilities, aptitudes, and interests. We feel also that it is important to recognize that tests are only one part of a vocational evaluation which supplements the clinical impression of the counselor and observation of the patient in a work-like situation.

In the area of job placement, we have found that our most effective activity is to provide clients with information about the labor market and the needs of industry in our area, and explain to them how and where to apply for jobs. We make direct placement only as a last resort. We have learned that once a person is really ready for work he does not have too much difficulty in finding a job. More important, we have found he shows a markedly different response to a job "I found myself" rather than one which we obtained for him. His self-esteem is greatly increased, and that helps carry him through the first difficult weeks of adjustment. Moreover, if we do find him a job, we are giving him another mixed message: we have told him he is ready to take his place as an independent productive citizen, yet we have taken him by the hand and done it for him again.

To realize the full potential of vocational services, we must be constantly alert to the need for new programs where gaps in service occur. For example, seeing one of our clients about to leave for a job interview poorly groomed (despite counseling in this area) sparked the idea for what we will call a "job clinic."

The job clinic will attempt to reproduce as closely as possible the whole application-interview procedure the client will face in industry. It will be a full dress-rehearsal of the actual performance for those persons ready to begin the hunt for a job. A client will be given an appointment to apply for one of a number of specific "job openings" which will be listed with our unit receptionist. He will approach her as he would apply at the front desk of any business or industry. She will give him an application form to complete, after which she will arrange for him to be interviewed by a counselor other than his own counselor. The receptionist will complete a rating form on details of appearance, manner, punctuality and the time it took to fill out the application form.

The vocational counselor will complete a rating form after the interview, covering such factors as personal hygiene, grooming, posture, facial expression, speech habits, manner, preparation for interview, appropriateness for the particular job classification, and whether or not the applicant would be hired. Immediate testing will be done for those skills which industry measures by testing, such as typing and finger dexterity. Following these procedures, there will be a group meeting to review the rating sheets and for interaction between applicants and counselors about what occurred. The following day, applicants will go out on regular job interview, returning for another group meeting for assessment of their experiences. There will possibly be other group meetings as needed.

We are also initiating a research program, the purpose of which is twofold: first, we are looking for an *objective* assessment of the actual results of our providing vocational services to our patients; second, we are attempting to define what specific factors contribute to successful vocational adjustment. For example, from the personal bias of counselors we believe that an increase in the patient's ability to socialize predicts success on a job. We hope to be able to establish whether or not this is so and what other factors contribute to achievement of realistic and satisfying job experiences.

An IBM card will be prepared at intake, covering such identifying data as age, sex, marital status, education, history of hospitalization, employment history, social class, and occupational level. At closing, vocational services provided, results of vocational testing, and vocational achievements will be coded. In addition, both an overall rating assessing mitigation of vocational problems and specific ratings of improvement on a number of factors will be made. These factors will include: socialization, ability to concentrate on work, reduction of inappropriate behavior and others. By these means we hope to improve the evaluation of our services and facilitate research in an area where objective data are sorely lacking.

We want to reemphasize the importance of specialization in the vocational rehabilitation of persons in psychiatric treatment. This specific area is exceedingly complex and in itself requires a broad range of knowledge, skill, and experience that differ from other areas of rehabilitation. Thus, it is a specialty both in mental health services and in vocational rehabilitation. It offers services to psychiatric patients which cannot be as effectively given by other mental health professionals or by traditional vocational rehabilitation agencies.

Freud felt that the criteria of a healthy personality were the ability to love and to work, and in these two areas in large part he measured the success or failure of psychoanalysis. Certainly in our society today it is taken for granted that part of health and recovery is taking one's rightful place in the working world. Any attempt at treating the mentally ill and emotionally troubled must in some way deal with the issues of occupational achievement and vocational satisfaction.

# CHAPTER 9

# Adult Outpatient Services

*Isadore Kamin and Bernice Birchess,*
*H. Richard Lamb and John Odenheimer* *

ᔑᔑᔑᔑᔑᔑᔑᔑᔑᔑᔑᔑᔑᔑᔑᔑᔑᔑᔑᔑᔑ

Can the new community mental health centers function in harmony with psychodynamic psychiatry? Or do they represent mutually exclusive doctrines?†

## Evolution of a Clinic (Kamin and Birchess)

Trying to keep pace with a society in the throes of rapid change, the psychiatrist has emerged from the isolation of his shel-

---

* This chapter has two sections, each by different authors. The first section, "Evolution of a Clinic," is by Isadore Kamin and Bernice Birchess; the second, "The Brief Service Clinic," is by H. Richard Lamb and John Odenheimer.

† For discussion of this issue see Rosenbaum and Zwerling, 1962; Sutherland, 1966; Wallerstein, 1968.

217

tered office and has plunged into "the community." From an absorption with one-to-one psychotherapy, he has become involved with entire organizations, agencies, and even rolled up his sleeves to confront huge social forces, the nature and boundaries of which he is only dimly aware.

Out of his feeling of responsibility and commitment to perform herculean tasks, there comes an awareness that he will have to dash in many directions. He will need to keep up with his familiar role as psychotherapist and also with innovations in his techniques. He will become a consultant to agencies—schools, public welfare, family service—and to key help-giving personnel—police, ministers, probation officers, and many others. Mindful of preventive services, he is concerned about home visits, maintaining continuity with those of his patients who are in the inpatient service or in the day hospital, "crisis intervention" whenever indicated, and even social action.

It is small wonder that the psychiatrist (or psychologist or social worker) feels he cannot afford to spend his time on lengthy individual psychotherapy, no matter how useful it might be. Preoccupation with digging back into the childhood of adult patients, working through involved transference reactions, is passé. The here and now assumes increasing attractiveness as an area of focus, and the new philosophy which underlines the socioenvironmental forces crowds out concern with intrapsychic factors. There are those who, aware of these trends, wish to reemphasize that "the [community] psychiatrist is clinically concerned with intrapsychic experiences as much as with the social situational factors" (Group for the Advancement of Psychiatry, 1967). Instead of a balance between the two, a rift is appearing, forcing polarization. Factionalism is being created instead of the needed mutual support and cooperation.

Our aim is to offer an individually tailored approach to fit the needs and capacities of each patient. Thus, we are committed to the fullest range of treatment techniques compatible with the skills of our staff and the use of the widest variety of resources within the limits of what is available in our county. Approximately one-fourth of the patients in the clinic are treated by group therapy and three-fourths are in individual therapy. Half of our applicants terminate therapy by the end of the fifth interview. This last statistic is typical of what most clinics report. This is not planned brief therapy. These are abbreviated contacts, because the patients unilaterally decide not to return.

Now that roles such as consultant, administrator, community organizer, in addition to that of psychotherapist, are in vogue, it is possible for staff members to assume various combinations of activities. Some will attempt to be "generalists" undertaking a wide spectrum of services, while others will prefer to restrict themselves to one specialty. We have concern about those specialists who are no longer treating any patients. "Prolonged and intimate exposure to the struggles of the individual patient is the *sine qua non* of the student's evolution toward human and clinical maturity (Kubie, 1968)." To a lesser degree this is pertinent beyond the student stage. Thus if one ceases to do psychotherapy we believe it detracts from one's ability to consult about patients, to do research about patients, and even to be the administrator who plans programs for patients. Therefore, every professional in our clinic treats patients, in addition to any other special tasks he may have.

When a program chief arrived in 1958, he found an active outpatient service which had considerable autonomy. In fact, the clinic enjoyed a unique situation. There was a group of about twenty-five professionals, who were volunteers, but who had an important role in the operation. They collaborated to set policy, to hire new personnel, to discharge personnel, to set rules and regulations. There was also a central core of paid staff. This association was appreciated by all and developed into a tightly-linked group with high morale.

With the inauguration of a central administration called the program office, the various units of the county's mental health service were to become linked together in a new fashion. The autonomy enjoyed by all units was bound to be reduced. For example, the volunteer staff in the clinic would have to relinquish their prerogative to hire and fire personnel and to set policy without interference from an overall program chief. As a consequence most of them decided to leave. Henceforth the clinic was operated by a paid full-time staff, aided by the two or three volunteer psychiatrists and psychologists who did remain.

This is a psychoanalytically oriented clinic, by which is meant that psychoanalytic principles are applied in order to create flexible programs for the patients. Our aim is to create a treatment plan to fit the patient. If the chief psychiatrist knows one therapy technique particularly well he may be tempted to cast the entire clinic in that mold. But no single modality can help all patients. Therefore we resisted any tendency to convert our entire operation into brief therapy or long-term therapy exclusively. Similarly, we do not focus our efforts entirely into group therapy nor into individual therapy. Elements of all these techniques are employed. The choice is based on the needs and capacities of the patient as well as the training and skill of the therapist. Ideally, these components match.

A most distressing issue was the long waiting list, the bane of most psychiatric clinics. It grew to the point where over one hundred patients were on it, and it took up to six or eight months to offer treatment in some cases. We knew that it was imperative to free many hours of staff time, in order that more patients could be treated by the same number of professionals. (It was then impossible to hire more staff.) Could we change any of our procedures without detracting from the quality of the service?

One of the first areas that received our attention was the intake process. Hitherto it had been the custom for patients to be seen from one to six visits in order to study in depth each applicant. The accumulated material was presented to a conference where up to twenty-five professionals deliberated in order to decide on diagnosis, disposition, and other pertinent factors. This was an extravagant use of time. The diagnosis did not seem to be of such importance that it warranted so much deliberation. Further, the treatment recommendation did not vary greatly from case to case. For most, the disposition was either individual therapy or group therapy. Since we had an experienced staff of social workers and psychiatrists, it was decided to reduce intake to one visit, during which one professional, either a psychiatrist or a social worker, would see the patient and make decisions about the treatment plan. When necessary, either the social worker or the psychiatrist could call on the other as a consultant, in order to finalize any program. Sometimes the social worker called in the psychiatrist on an issue of hospitalization or to confirm that outpatient treatment would make sense, in spite of the risk of suicide. In other cases it was for prescriptions of drugs. At other times the psychiatrist called in the social worker for consideration of other community resources.

This change in procedure dispensed with the presentations to a group, released much professional time, and maximized the number of patients who could be seen for intake. We felt that since ours was a community clinic, we should never close intake no matter what the demand on our services. This did create other problems for us, because we were not always able to begin treatment with those patients who had been seen for intake and for whom a treatment plan had been devised. The waiting list continued to grow, even after we had released much time by simplifying the intake process.

When the waiting list still remained very long, and the many months' delay was so preposterous, we made another important innovation: we began what we called a post-intake group. The post-intake group must be distinguished from what is frequently called an intake group. In our method, patients were first seen individually for intake as described above. When the recommendation was individual therapy but there was no treatment time available, the patient was offered the alternative of coming into a group immediately rather than going on the waiting list. If the patient refused, he still had the choice of going on the waiting list for individual therapy. Some patients, indeed, insisted that the latter was their preference, but the majority did accept immediate assignment to the post-intake group, with the assurance from us that if the group was not to their liking, they could still go back to the waiting list for an individual assignment.

The staff did not immediately take warmly to this concept. In fact, many had difficulty for months in understanding the choice patients had. They interpreted this innovation to mean that all patients would be assigned to groups and would have no choice. In various ways, they communicated these attitudes to their patients when they offered to them what they considered a rather questionable gift of the post-intake group. Consequently their patients turned down the opportunity of beginning treatment in a group. In time, the entire clinic was won over to the usefulness and practicality of this post-intake group. The staff now presents this group clearly and positively to each patient. As a result, more patients understand the real choice that is open to them.

The chief psychiatrist, chief social worker, and one of the psychologists formed a troika to run this group. Usually our therapy groups have one or two professionals in them, but we could foresee that this group would have heavy traffic in and out, extensive record keeping, and would easily keep three of us quite busy. Because there was a guaranteed heavy flow of patients into this group, we had to devise an egress that would be equally free. Our original plans have had to be altered only slightly. Some of the exits we devised should be mentioned briefly. For some patients a few sessions in the post-intake group were sufficient, due to such amelioration of their problems that we and they no longer felt the need for further therapy. In these cases termination was reached by mutual agreement between patient and group therapists. For many more patients the group was a test of their ability to use more conventional group therapy; if this appraisal was in the affirmative, these patients were transferred from the post-intake group to other groups in the clinic where there were openings for them. Sometimes two or more patients were transferred into the same group to make easier their entrance into a new situation. This meant that the existing, conventional groups in the clinic had a guaranteed steady inflow to replace those members who either dropped out or who graduated. Several new groups were created, in order to keep abreast of the demand for group therapy which emanated from the post-intake group.

One important discovery which cannot be minimized is that an appreciable number of patients dropped out of group therapy, either because they disliked it or because they found it not useful. Some told us so; others by their abrupt termination implied this. A few of these disappointed patients did go back to the waiting list for individual therapy. Others were disillusioned with the clinic and would no longer accept the waiting list.

The total effect of the post-intake group on the waiting list was dramatic. It was evident this was an important addition to our program; in fact, the waiting list was reduced, for a while, to zero. This created a state of euphoria in the clinic. We did, in fact, believe this was going to continue indefinitely and that we were now able to eliminate the waiting list with this post-intake group. However, the waiting list did grow. We could not keep pace with the demand for services. New programs were starting in the community and with increased acceptance of the county's psychiatric program many more people came to our doors than had hitherto been willing to come. Thus, with continued success in creating a positive public image for mental health services, we perpetuated our old nemesis, the waiting list. It would not be fair, however, to leave the impression that the waiting list is as bad as ever. It is now of modest proportions and has never grown to the immense size it was before the advent of the post-intake group.

The clinical operation of this group was a difficult one. We made no effort to screen out anyone. There were psychotic patients, neurotic patients, and those with character disorders. We reasoned that if we attempted to do any screening, we would create confusion both for staff and for patients. The rejection of patients might do even more harm than any possible benefits we had in mind. Also, we were not sure that we had the clinical wisdom and foresight on which to base any accurate or precise screening. We felt that if any patient was grossly unsuited, we could spot this quickly in the group session and remove him after one visit. This never turned out to be necessary. On the other hand, some patients probably screened themselves out when they felt extreme disharmony with other members of the group.

Patients were seen for varying lengths of time; there was no predetermined length of treatment. They stayed in the group until we, the therapists, could estimate what kind of treatment was indicated and what their capacities were to follow through with it. Thus, with some patients the length of stay was one visit, and for others it ran as high as ten, and in one case went up to eighteen visits.

There are disadvantages in transferring patients from one group to another. We have, in fact, a built-in disruption of the treatment program. In some cases patients have objected to being transferred because they felt we were demoting or penalizing them for not participating well. This highlighted how quickly camaraderie and group cohesion could develop, even though there were new faces almost weekly. This did not seem to bother the patients as much as it did the therapists. There were exceptions, of course, and those patients who were troubled by the constantly changing population were moved out quickly to groups where the patient membership was stable.

In order to keep the post-intake group as effective as possible, we rarely closed its doors; that is, we strived to keep it open for new additions. On rare occasions when its size was so large that additions were prohibitive, we did have to decline for one week to add any new members. Its maximum size did reach fourteen members. Clearly, it was inappropriate to add anybody else, if we sincerely intended that every member have a chance to participate actively.

This group is now a regular feature of our clinic. No eyebrows are raised, and no challenges come up with regard to its therapeutic value. New staff who join the clinic feel it has always been part of our program. If we had sufficient personnel, we would start an evening group of this nature, to accommodate those patients who have to decline membership because they are unable to get time off from work or, for other reasons, cannot come to a daytime group.

Because of a constant feeling of need for better treatment methods, we have encouraged innovations on the part of any staff member. When a psychiatrist and social worker wished to team up to try group intake, they discussed this at one of our staff conferences. The majority of the staff were skeptical, but, nevertheless, these two were given a green light to try out their plan. The idea was to institute a time-limited group lasting ten sessions, the first session of which would be the first actual contact these patients would have in the clinic with any professionals. After the experiment was over this team reported back to the staff about their experiences. In essence, they felt the ten interviews were worthwhile; however, if they had to do it again, they said they would make one change. They would have preferred to have each patient seen in an individual session for intake, thereafter placing him in a time-limited group. They believed this would result in better screening, in a better identification of the problems for which the patient was coming to the clinic, and in enhancing the efficacy of the ten sessions of group therapy.

Our general experience has dictated against any arbitrary number of visits set in advance. Consequently, brief therapy in the form of a design proposed at the beginning, is not undertaken to any great extent in the clinic. As stated previously, half of our patients terminate after a few sessions, but this is "accidental" brief therapy, not planned. It is usually decided unilaterally by the patient and rarely by mutual agreement of patient and therapist. Our research project described in Chapter 15 is an attempt to discover the differences between these patients and those who stay to become long-term patients. Better understanding of these differences will, we hope, lead to modifications in therapeutic approaches.

Our concern is about indiscriminate use of brief therapy. For certain categories of problems it is particularly unsuited. Many of our patients who have depressive constellations or have been sent to us after attempted suicide are particularly vulnerable. We must guard against precipitating the kind of trauma that has sent them to us in the first place; namely, the loss of an important person. Others require prolonged maintenance and support of damaged egos due to chronic schizophrenic life patterns.

There are those whose main complaint (impotence, homosexuality, alcoholism) does not lend itself readily to resolution in a few visits, and for some patients this predetermined end of therapy may come at a bad time. One patient had received ten interviews as part of a plan, set in advance, by one of our psychiatrists. His tenth visit, and the termination of his treatment, came right after his wife had left him. These two rejections in tandem precipitated a crisis in this patient. He handled this in a pattern which was characteristic for him. He lashed out in an orgy of violence. Dishes and furniture were the targets of his anger at first, but later he turned on himself and, following his attempted suicide, the neighbors called the police, who took him to the county hospital, whence he was shipped to the state hospital. There are many other details of the case, but relevant here is the ill-timed termination which was invoked because of a predetermined commitment by the therapist to a set number of visits.

Equally cogent examples could be cited to illustrate other kinds of treatment used inappropriately. Long-term therapy may be used aimlessly or in a manner that aggravates chronic dependency problems. Then it is to be decried just as vigorously. We have concentrated on the subject of brief therapy perhaps because of bias, but also because the pressures of "expediency" are pushing us in that direction. Thus we see it as a particular problem at this time.

We are constantly seeking to improve our methods, because psychotherapy, as it now exists, cannot allow any practitioner to be smug. There is so much more that needs to be done. We encourage our staff to be innovative and to present new concepts for discussion. In California currently there are many new kinds of groups being presented to the public. Sensitivity groups, marathon groups, groups in which bodies touch are proliferating. We hope that eventually we will be able to sort out which of the new borders represents a truly creative frontier; to reject prematurely runs the risk of discarding promising improvements. We need more time for proper assessment.

Occasionally an innovator insists that others must become converts. Although privileged to use brief therapy whenever his professional judgment dictated its use, one of our clinicians was dissatisfied. It was probably because of his disappointment that so few were adopting the technique, and then were using it too rarely, that he needed some reassurance that he was making impact on others. If the chief psychiatrist introduces, or has special enthusiasm about, a new procedure, this has greater impact on other staff members than when one of the staff holds forth. But no one, not even the chief, can really make anyone work differently than is his custom. Nor can the chief be effective, if he pretends to like something about which he really has reservations. Moreover, the therapeutic style of any therapist is a composite of many factors, including his personality and his training. Because of these many factors, there are many different kinds of therapists, each one favoring different modes of intervention. We feel that we ought to take more advantage of this diversity among our therapists.

The case load of active patients in the clinic varies between five and six hundred, with from eighty to 120 new applications per month. The staff consists of three psychiatrists, six full-time and one half-time social workers, and one psychologist. There are varying numbers of trainees, including social work students who are in their second year of postgraduate field placement and second-year psychiatric residents.

A clinic with only one psychologist reflects a concept from the past with regard to how psychologists should be used. Formerly their main contribution was considered to be diagnostic testing. Although testing is still done, it is not routine and is asked for when it is deemed essential to the treatment of the patient. Research is now the primary responsibility of the psychologist. This reflects the thinking of both the chief psychiatrist and psychologist. For the past two years, our psychologist has been principally involved in the research project described in Chapter 15, along with doing psychotherapy and testing. This meant that other potential projects had to be set aside or postponed. In the future, we hope to have more psychologists, which will permit more research to be done and would enable a more comprehensive evaluation of our clinical services, suggest further changes and innovations in our programs, and provide added stimulation to the entire staff.

The role of the social workers in the adult psychiatric clinic, alluded to in various ways heretofore in this account, deserves more detailed discussion. They are impressive in number and also by function and responsibility. Out of a total of twelve professional staff members, seven are social workers. They are given administrative approval to work as independently and self-reliantly as possible in the intake process and in individual and group psychotherapy. We try to eliminate ritualistic supervisory hours which are for the purpose of maintaining a status hierarchy. Our social workers also participate in training of student social workers and psychiatric residents and in program planning.

The professional satisfaction that individual staff members gain from their jobs enhances the quality of work they are doing. We have strived, therefore, to give high priority to this factor. For example, anyone who has a second area of interest, for example, child psychiatry or consultation, has an option to work in another service for half a day per week. This policy reduces the amount of work done in our clinic; but more important is what it accomplishes for the professional staff. They are permitted to conduct private practices as long as they put in forty hours a week on their clinic job. Some have been candidates in the Analytic Institute and have had to shift their schedules around to make up for the hours that they have had to be away from the clinic. As much as possible, therapists are permitted to choose what patients they wish to take on in treatment. Obviously there are some patients for whom no one expresses a preference. All clinic staff are asked to take their proper share of responsibility for these hard core, difficult, provocative patients.

Of all our patients, two-thirds are female; 20–25 per cent are psychotic; but all categories are represented, including alcoholics, character disorders, even the mentally retarded. As long as they have a willingness to come, and for that matter even when they are unwilling to come, but do show up, they are seen, and a plan is formulated. We start seeing patients at age eighteen, and no one is excluded because of old age. It is true, nevertheless, that very few in their seventies have come here, but those who do arrive are seen and have, for the most part, responded rather quickly and favorably in treatment.

We have made extensive use of vocational services. For many of our patients the work plan is just as important as psychotherapy, and for some it is even more important (see Chapter 8). Collaboration with public health nurses has added an important dimension to our treatment of patients (see Chapter 7).

Emphasis on the use of groups has been increased owing to the special group therapy interest of the chief psychiatrist. We have a dozen groups. Some of these are run by one therapist and some by co-therapists. The latter practice is recommended especially for new staff members who come to the clinic with limited group therapy experience. Aside from this, many therapists feel it is advantageous to have a partner; group sessions do not have to be canceled because of illness of one therapist, and staff vacations are staggered so the groups can continue uninterrupted during the summer. This is especially valuable for those sick patients to whom a missed session represents trauma and rejection.

Our groups are categorized as either psychotic or neurotic. These are not ironclad compartments. The borderline patient might be in either kind of grouping. Because of the preponderance of women in the clinic, we have some groups that are entirely women, and a few with both men and women. No groups are all male. The composition of the groups is as heterogeneous as we can make them, except for level of illness. We do not wish to confront very fragile patients with probing therapy nor, by the same token, to be too supportive of patients who have the capacity for more insight seeking processes.

The clinic is part of a hub of services and must dovetail with other clinical and nonclinical units in a spectrum of activities in the community mental health center. The relationship of the clinic to the psychiatric ward is of special interest. Patients may be hospitalized while they are in treatment in the outpatient clinic. The clinic therapist may or may not follow the patient in treatment sessions on the ward, according to his own wishes. Similarly, when patients are discharged from the ward, a frequent recommendation is for the patient to follow up with outpatient treatment in the clinic. We ran into many difficulties in the past when patients were designated for hospitalization by their clinic therapists and then were turned down in the emergency room by the hospital staff. Some patients had been arduously and painstakingly convinced to accept hospitalization by the therapist, only to be denied admission by the admitting psychiatrist, who had opportunity for only a brief encounter with the patient. To avoid such dilemmas and such disasters in the relationship between patient, therapist, and hospital, an agreement was worked out which represents current policy. The hospital staff agreed to accept every patient for whom hospitalization was recommended by one of the outpatient psychiatrists. As a reciprocal aspect of the agreement, any patient who is considered a candidate for outpatient treatment upon discharge from the hospital is offered treatment by the outpatient staff. This agreement has worked to the advantage of both staffs—outpatient and inpatient —and I am quite sure the patients who have been involved have also benefited greatly.

This seems to be a simple and obvious plan; yet, until it was established, there were many headaches in what should have been a smooth transition of patients from one unit to another. The autonomy which each unit enjoyed was apparently considered primary, until it was demonstrated to be an obstacle to good psychiatric practice.

A special service which we call the Friday morning clinic was created by the chief social worker, in order to facilitate referral of patients who were about to be discharged from the psychiatric ward. We knew that some patients, after leaving the hospital, and for whom outpatient services had been recommended, did not follow through. To bridge this gap and make it more likely that patients would return, those who were discharged from the inpatient service were referred to the chief social worker before actually leaving the hospital premises. When a patient was to be discharged, he would be asked to go to the clinic on that Friday which was closest to the day of his discharge. On that occasion, he met individually with the chief social worker, who clarified such items as financial eligibility and explained the procedures. Orientation of the patient, warm acceptance of him, and assurance that he could count on seeing her again when he returned for his first official visit as a patient, all made the path of the patient smoother. The Friday morning clinic thus has functioned as "red carpet" treatment and is bestowed on the patient *before* he has gone home. It makes possible very specialized attention to those patients who have already had a treatment process initiated in the hospital and who are ambivalent or resistant to any continuation once they are discharged from the hospital. This same service is offered to patients discharged from Agnews State Hospital. They too are assured that they will see the person who is designated by their therapist at Agnews. They, too, are accommodated on Friday morning. This makes for a rather busy session for the chief social worker, but she is convinced of its usefulness. She has not requested any other staff members to help her; it would certainly no longer be the same plan if there were several workers involved. The simplicity of it at our end enables the staff members from both Agnews and county general hospital to know, by name and personality, the one person with whom they are required to deal. This has greatly facilitated the referral process.

Collaboration with the child guidance clinic is much better now than it has ever been. The relationships we enjoy are most friendly and cordial, and yet the arrangements are not ideal. The main obstacle has to do with administrative structure. Both clinics are autonomous. Frequently families will be split up between the two clinics; one or both parents may have started treatment in the adult clinic, and later, if their children need help, they are evaluated and offered treatment in the child guidance clinic. At this point the number of therapists involved with the parents multiplies. There is need for child guidance staff to have conferences with the parents, and these parents may be placed by them in groups. There is need to confer with the entire family about the progress of the child. At the same time, the therapists in the adult clinic wish to continue with the parents the psychotherapy which predates the treatment of the children. On the other hand, the family may first enter into the child guidance clinic via the child patient, and later, when the problems of the parents seem to be extensive and to warrant referral to the adult clinic, we get once more into a proliferation of therapists, conferences, and collaborations. Treatment ideas may differ between the two staffs; therefore, sometimes we are going in different directions with the family. Perhaps this latter point is not the main issue, since it comes up infrequently; a greater problem is that there are too many people involved in two different clinics. To have one administration is desirable, and yet, having started as two separate clinics, their amalgamation is difficult to arrange.

In the relationship of the clinic to the community there have been some serious deficiencies. For example, in spite of the option offered to our staff to have one-half day a week on the consultation service, this option is selected rarely. We are so busy dealing with our patients, and get so swept up in the volume and the intense demands made on us, that for most of the staff, most of the time, it is the clinic exclusively that preoccupies us. Since we have an unusual consultation service with staff assigned full-time, it has been made easier for our treatment staff not to get involved at all in consultation work. This means ministers, teachers, school administrators, even physicians in the community are in contact with mental health consultants who are *not* involved with the clinic. The clinic staff has a buffer between itself and the community, but this buffer is not a useful one. It is a barrier to better understanding, particularly between the nonpsychiatric physicians in the community and the treatment staff of the clinic.

Aside from treatment, the clinic receives requests to do psychiatric evaluations for various purposes. One request that causes considerable concern is for us to recommend to the court whether or not a mother should retain custody of her children. These are frequently divorce cases where the father initiates the action. The psychiatrist is called into court by a subpoena and is asked to make comments that he feels will be traumatic to his patient who is present in court. In addition to the crucial issue of confidentiality, the therapist becomes embroiled in the adversary system of the court in a way which is often inappropriate. It is a situation in need of major revamping.

The psychiatric clinic has been involved in a variety of conflicts due to ideological differences, but the most intriguing issue has been the role of the clinic in therapeutic abortions. Formerly, California had a law which permitted therapeutic abortions only when the life of the mother was in danger, and psychiatrists played a relatively quiet and minor role. Abortions could be approved only when suicide was considered a probability or a strong likelihood. Pregnant women who were considered candidates for a therapeutic abortion were referred to the adult clinic from the obstetrics clinic of the county hospital.

Our involvement began when the new California law went into effect, November 8, 1967. It permitted a recommendation for therapeutic abortion when "continuance of the pregnancy would gravely impair the physical or mental health of the mother . . . the term *mental health* means mental illness to the extent that the woman is dangerous to herself or to the person or property of others or is in need of supervision or restraint." Now the referrals come in greater numbers.

Since the hospitals in this area required that two psychiatrists had to approve a therapeutic abortion before it could be recommended, we soon discovered that doctors have different attitudes and opinions on the same case. Because judgment is involved and because criteria are interpreted in varying fashion by different clinicians, we found ourselves in the midst of a complex controversy. Ethical, moral, and religious principles were stirred up whenever the issue of abortion was presented to the clinic for disposition. Abortion raises many grim issues: social class discrimination, the power of professionals to grant or deny a decision which has enormous significance for the individual patient, and beyond the psychological and social consequences that ensued, there always lurked the shadowy specter of criminal abortion whenever a woman was denied.

Therapeutic abortion evaluations throw into relief the difference in the way the rich and the poor are handled. We have here an outstanding opportunity to ameliorate gross social injustice. Those who can afford it shop for a private psychiatrist until they get two who will recommend a therapeutic abortion. The poor who know enough to come to the clinic are obstructed by a variety of screening devices. The resident obstetrician in the obstetrics-gynecology clinic, the medical social worker, and the psychiatric clinic staff psychiatrists are all usually involved. As she is referred from one to the other, the patient may drop out because of a feeling she is getting a runaround. She sometimes does not know how to run the maze properly. Those who do finally get to the clinic are almost always Caucasian. The mystery of what happens to the blacks I have not yet solved. They may be treated differently, or they may not be applying for help. The latter may be due to a lack of knowledge that such help exists. It is also possible that most of them choose to remain pregnant.

Among the clinic staff, there were practically no differences of opinion on specific recommendations. We tended to be liberal in our recommendation. But this very fact produced some unfortunate results. To some degree the chief of obstetrics began to doubt that we gave any serious consideration to the cases at all, so consistent was our agreement about them. And the psychiatrists began to be known around the community as "abortion doctors," encouraging referrals and voluntary requests from many other sources. We have since attempted to spread these evaluations around among all the psychiatrists involved in the entire mental health service, rather than limiting it to those originally involved from our own clinic. Although we have formal administrative approval for this plan, there remains considerable resistance to it.

"In some ways commitment to the protection and defense of the values of individual integrity has become the humanistic movement of our times, calling for many kinds of dedication as exemplified by the Civil Rights Movement and the Poverty Programs. Recent major changes in psychiatric programs, [such as] the community mental health center movement, reflect a similar concern with human dignity. Thus psychiatrists participate with their medical colleagues and members of other professions in responding to a sense of important historic change as they grow toward redefinitions of traditional psychiatric roles (Group for the Advancement of Psychiatry, 1967)."

In the light of our experience with therapeutic abortions it is more difficult than we have realized to change our roles. No doubt a decision to end a pregnancy stirs up very special conflicts. But going out into the ghetto will not be an easy task, either. The treatment for alcoholics is another chapter, which, if written, would resemble in many ways what I have discussed with regard to therapeutic abortions. "In the case of alcoholism past practices of most general hospitals and of the medical profession at large have reflected prejudice towards the victim of a disease (Straus, 1968)." Too often we psychiatrists deny this prejudice and resort to rationalization. Our standard of psychiatric practice must be that every individual has the right to the best treatment. The poor must have the same quality of care as those who can pay.

The future promises to be a very exciting one in the field of psychiatry generally and in San Mateo County specifically. But as we plan to develop regional centers throughout the county, the problems involved will increase, as the demands of time-consuming psychotherapy conflict with the need for the same personnel to perform other tasks related to the community. These problems involve not only issues of the specific skills and roles of the psychiatrist, but also their views on broad social policy. As Halleck (1968) observes, "the overwhelming needs of a mass society and the moral demands created by the emergence of community psychiatry are forcing [the psychiatrist] to take a position on issues which have political implications, issues which involve power, social conflict, and social change."

But our new identity as community mental health professionals has not yet solidified. We still lack courage to speak out on controversial subjects. We must find ways to decide what our views on these social issues are and learn how to make those views felt by the broader community. For example, "the psychiatrist stands in the eye of the hurricane of controversy around abortion. He knows the problem at the practice level but has done little to translate this knowledge into enlightened public policy (Brown, 1968)." Can we rise above such difficulties, above the forces in the community itself which resist change, the community of which we are a part? "While it is blatantly grandiose to presume that psychiatry will make the poor rich, the bad good, and intoxicated sober, the unhappy happy, it is fair to ask what we can contribute to these compelling human hopes . . . it is not only mental illness that concerns us, not even the amorphous matter of mental health, but an evanescent and evolutionary concept that encompasses both illness and health—the quality of life (Brown, 1968)."

## The Brief Service Clinic (Lamb and Odenheimer)

As a beginning step toward regionalization of our mental health services on a geographic basis, "walk-in" services were offered to a catchment area in the central part of the county. The major arm of these services, the brief service clinic, focuses on crisis intervention and has an upper limit of six individual interviews. In large measure the clinic draws from the philosophy and experience of the Benjamin Rush Clinic in Los Angeles (Jacobson et al., 1965; Paul, 1966).

We want to emphasize that the brief service clinic is but part of a complex of outpatient services available to the population of this catchment area in one multifaceted clinic. The need of community mental health to utilize its limited manpower to best meet the needs of a total population must be taken into account. Thus, group and activity therapies, brief individual contact with medication and home visits by public health nurses are offered to most patients needing more than six treatment visits. For many persons this is not simply a matter of expediency, but the treatment of choice (see description of the aftercare program in Chapter 5). Longer-term individual therapy is offered to a few patients. This is not only because of specific therapeutic indications, but also, as pointed out in the first section of this chapter, because experienced staff and trainees alike need some intensive one-to-one experience with patients as part of their ongoing training and development.

Crisis theory has received a growing amount of attention in the literature since the initial classic works (Lindemann, 1944; Klein and Lindemann, 1961; Caplan, 1961). It has been observed that crisis intervention, in addition to resolving the acute problem, may also lead to new ways of problem-solving that often persist and enhance the patient's coping powers after the current crisis has passed. All too frequently these are patients who would not be amenable to therapeutic work at other times.

Our experience, like that of the Rush Clinic, is that some acute personal crisis accompanied by identifiable precipitating events, often superimposed on chronic problems, is found in about three-fourths of the patients applying for outpatient services. Further, regardless of how they conceptualize or verbalize their reasons for seeking treatment, most patients basically are seeking alleviation of symptoms or help with a current life situation. This holds true not just for public clinics. For instance, a prominent senior psychoanalyst in private practice in San Francisco describes a similar experience. He estimates that only about 10 per cent of patients coming to him are really seeking personality change and the resolution of unconscious conflict (personal communication).

We cannot stress enough the importance of easy availability of treatment. Without it, a number of persons desiring help will not or cannot get help, and important therapeutic and preventive opportunities are lost for a large segment of the population. For our treatment to be effective, we cannot attempt in a few interviews what is attempted in much longer periods in intensive psychotherapy. Thus, the aim is not personality reconstruction, but resolution of crisis situations and symptom alleviation—goals which are appropriate and specific to the time allotted. For that matter, in our brief service clinic both patient and therapist frequently decide that termination is appropriate after three to four visits. Patients are also advised that they are welcome to return should another crisis arise.

The time-limited relationship is often helpful to patients whose reluctance to enter into treatment is due in part to their ambivalence about becoming dependent on the therapist. The short-term nature of the relationship discourages dependency by stressing the patient's ability to draw upon his own resources to resolve his current problems.

Flexibility in the screening process is crucial. After filling out a questionnaire, each patient is seen by an experienced social worker or nurse for twenty to twenty-five minutes. If it appears that hospitalization or day hospitalization is indicated (for instance, if the patient appears suicidal or acutely psychotic), a psychiatrist is called to evaluate the patient. An assessment is also made as to whether the patient is appropriate for time-limited, brief therapy. If such is the case (and roughly 80 per cent of our intakes are so assigned), the patient is told about the six interview limit and given an appointment. If it appears that the problem is urgent, the patient has his first therapeutic interview that day, usually with a psychiatric social worker. (Staff schedules are so arranged that time is left open daily for this purpose.) Otherwise the patient is scheduled within the next few days and never longer than one week from the time he walked into the clinic. In any case, we believe that further diagnostic assessment should not be separated from treatment—that treatment can and should begin in this first interview.

Though the brief service clinic is an important part of our outpatient services, it is known to referring sources that we also offer a wide range of outpatient treatment. Thus, our clinic receives a cross-section of all patients who normally come to a community mental health center for outpatient therapy. Part of the initial interview involves a determination of a need for long-term services; approximately 10 per cent of our intakes are referred immediately to longer-term supportive treatment. We should add here that the important question is not the degree of psychopathology but the level of functioning. Chronic poor functioning—which may result in intermittent hospitalization, withdrawal, or generally in the patient's being a chronic burden to the community—calls for ongoing care. However, many patients who are obviously psychotic, both acutely and chronically, may be candidates for crisis intervention and not long-term supportive care, if their level of functioning is satisfactory to them and to the community.

As noted above, therapy begins in the first hour. The therapist also in this first hour tentatively formulates the psychodynamics, a working diagnosis and a treatment plan. Jacobson et al. (1965) state that the initial step of the treatment process is to "actively explore the current situation in order to identify the precipitating event in the instances where it is not obvious. Ask: What is the most recent threat, challenge or loss that has caused present disequilibrium? What is new in the patient's ongoing situation? When did he begin to feel worse or become acutely upset? Who is the significant person or persons involved in the crisis? What is the immediate problem, as differentiated from the basic problem?"

Losses are the most readily identifiable cause of crisis and are usually present. The loss may be that of a loved one, loss of one's sexual power and attractiveness, loss as experienced in divorce, loss of a job or a change in job status. Some losses are less obvious, such as the first offender who is jailed for a brief period and then placed on probation; he may feel very keenly the loss of freedom and decision-making (however much he may also want these controls). In this category too is the parent who is slowly becoming aware of the loss of maturing children, or is confronted with evidence of loss of parental control when faced with destructive acting-out of teenage children; this feeling of helplessness, anger, and guilt in being unable to control his children may contribute to a loss of self-esteem and depression.

The therapist attempts to learn how the patient handled similar situations in the past as a possible key to how he may handle his present predicament. The therapist then describes the problem to the patient concisely, in language free of jargon and in terms that the patient can comprehend. Deep, underlying dynamics are avoided. For example, the therapist might say "All of the increased pressures on your job that you have just told me about are making you nervous," or "Your children growing up and leaving home are a great loss to you and leave you without a feeling of being needed." The patient needs to experience or re-experience current feelings which he has warded off. These might include feelings of mourning or, for teenagers, fear of separation from their parents. Incompletely realized dependency problems are brought to the patient's awareness. At this point a teenager contemplating leaving his parents or a person contemplating divorce, but who is very dependent on the marital partner, is in a position to make a decision as to what to do—to go back to the dependent situation, which is frequently the solution, or to find further support elsewhere and other means of coping with the separation.

Alleviating feelings of helplessness, such an integral part of most depressions (Bibring, 1953), can be accomplished by helping the patient see ways that he himself can deal with his problems. Thus, he gains a sense of mastery which heightens his self-esteem and eases his depression. Another powerful therapeutic tool is that of reducing inappropriate and self-destructive guilt. To varying degrees the therapist represents authority to patients. If the therapist "takes sides" against the superego and in effect says, "Do not feel guilty," guilt can often be reduced to a level that the patient can manage. Efforts are often made to restore ego defenses such as rationalization, denial, repression, and intellectualization to assist the patient's return to his formal level of coping.

Prolonged discussion of chronic problems is avoided at all times; this prevents furthering regression which undermines the crisis approach and can produce sticky dependency problems at termination. Our experience has also been that providing medications makes termination more difficult. However, we do give medications to patients who truly need this help to tide them through their crisis periods.

Though crisis intervention requires considerable diagnostic and therapeutic skills, they can readily be taught to competent mental health professionals. Further, many tasks, such as mobilizing and coordinating various community resources (welfare, child care, housing) as an adjunct to crisis intervention can and should be handled by subprofessionals, such as case aides. Community mental health outpatient services utilizing limited manpower can, in our view, best approach serving the needs of a total population by offering time-limited treatment focusing on crisis intervention, and group and activity therapies for most patients requiring longer-term treatment.

# CHAPTER 10

# Services for Children

### *David J. Schwartz, Lois Wynn,*
### *H. Richard Lamb*

$\int_{\ast}^{\ast}\int_{\ast}^{\ast}\int_{\ast}^{\ast}\int_{\ast}^{\ast}\int_{\ast}^{\ast}\int_{\ast}^{\ast}\int_{\ast}^{\ast}\int_{\ast}^{\ast}\int_{\ast}^{\ast}\int_{\ast}^{\ast}\int_{\ast}^{\ast}\int_{\ast}^{\ast}\int_{\ast}^{\ast}\int_{\ast}^{\ast}\int$

In 1964 the American Psychiatric Association estimated that there were 2.5 to 4.5 million children nationwide in need of psychiatric attention. How can the limited number of child guidance personnel in community mental health programs hope to scratch the surface of a problem of this magnitude with one-to-one therapy? Out of necessity, one-to-one long-term treatment, though it has a place in the treatment of selected cases, cannot be the main focus in such a setting.

What then should be the roles of child guidance personnel and what services should be offered for children in a community mental health setting? Some of us in San Mateo would answer: (1) consultation services to non-mental health personnel and agencies who have a major influence in the lives of children, such as schools, the juvenile probation department, and children's welfare services; (2) streamlined evaluation, which need not routinely include a psychiatrist; (3) brief treatment and crisis intervention; and (4) group and activity therapies. Such a philosophy seems almost self-evident in the light of recent developments in the theory and techniques of consultation and preventive services, crisis intervention, and the recognition that many sophisticated mental health services need not be performed by psychiatrists. Yet it has taken San Mateo many years to reach the philosophy outlined above. Even today, some staff disagree or are at best ambivalent. We anticipate that many other community mental health programs will experience similar difficulty. Why? We believe that a primary factor is the tendency to apply in community settings a model of practice developed for training in academic centers. The problem in large measure results from the fact that this is the training that most of us received.

### New Trends

Freud's (1909) treatment of "Little Hans," a child whose psychiatric problems were approached through the intermediation of parent conferences, stands as a beacon for indirect treatment of the emotional problems of children. Further successes of this kind ultimately shaped the subspecialty of child psychiatry, whose refined techniques for dealing with the mental disabilities of children focused to a certain extent upon those who most importantly shaped the child's environment—his parents, his teacher, and others. Also influential from the beginning were psychiatric teachers and clinicians like Adolf Meyer, who insisted upon responding to the crucial interaction of social and environmental as well as the intrapsychic components of illness (Lief, 1948).

In the evolution of child psychiatry and child guidance, one trend, among others, has been a clear and relatively uninterrupted development and further refinement of indirect intervention as a definitive mode of treatment. As this trend toward indirect intervention was pursued, child guidance clinics increasingly experimented with other patterns of service which seemed to offer some hope of broadening the scope of their service. To date, most guidance clinics still fall far short of the community mental health commitment to serve the total mental illness and health needs of the entire child population within their service regions. Nevertheless many conscientious efforts have been made in the past fifteen years to shape new therapeutic services which would extend and enlarge the service reach of these clinics. It is beyond the scope of this chapter to review the extensive literature, but, in passing, mention should be made of the Wellesley Human Relations Project under Klein and Lindemann (1961), where situational crisis intervention was subjected to empirical field testing. In this project, the focus of concern was upon the individual enmeshed in a social network rather than upon the individual alone. While these workers recognized the need to make a careful assessment of the intrapsychic structure and dynamics of personality, they extended the assessment to an equally and sometimes more important appraisal of the individual's social role and of the significant role relationships in which he is involved. They stressed the importance of crisis intervention and pointed out that in working with a crisis a maximum of change may be possible with a minimum of effort, as compared with intervention in a non-crisis situation. But this pattern, followed experimentally at Wellesley, profitable as it has proved for both adult and child psychiatry in the present community mental health era, was really no more revolutionary than the so-called "common-sense psychiatry" advocated and pioneered by Adolf Meyer during his forty-year tenure at the Phipps Clinic.

Mental health in general has been extensively enriched by a new format in which many of the theoretical riches of the behavioral and social sciences have been effectively intertwined. An outstanding example of the new union of sociocultural and psychodynamic concerns is that of Erikson (1950), whose crucial concepts of identity take into account not only the intrapsychic but the demands and effects of the larger society in which the individual must interact.

In the same vein, Shaw (1966) points out that a "characteristic of psychotherapy with children, and one which distinguishes it from treatment of adults, is that the child is usually living in the environment which contributed to his disorder. Thus one does not often deal with the patient's recollections. Rather, emphasis is on the present, on current problems and relationships, on what happened today or yesterday at home and in school, what his father did to him last night rather than five years ago. Moreover, because his present environment is most significant, a major function of therapy is to deal directly with the environment, and to manipulate it effectively."

Despite all these trends, the ultimate goal of most child therapist and child guidance clinics has usually been to supply individual play therapy to younger children with emotional problems, or more verbal, individual psychotherapy for adolescents. Even though most child guidance clinics routinely see parents of children receiving therapy, the prestige hour is the direct time spent with the child.

San Mateo is perhaps representative of a large class of communities in which local mental health services had their first expression in a successful campaign to establish a child guidance clinic. Such communities almost uniformly experienced early disappointment, the clinic having quickly become clogged with long-term treatment cases, its staff increasingly preoccupied with direct treatment demands and ever-growing waiting lists. The demand for children's services of all sorts is great in our child-oriented society, but individual psychiatric treatment presents special problems because such treatment is slow, frequently taking many hours of professional time for one child for many months. The time required can easily be doubled if the usual parent conferences are added.

The pattern is remarkably similar even in such localities as Boston, which may be more richly endowed with child guidance clinics than any other city. In essence, what is known, perhaps erroneously, as "conventional" child guidance clinic operational patterns have almost universally prevented such clinics from dealing with chronic waiting list dilemmas and from reaching very large segments of the population at risk in their catchment areas. Only those clinics which have arbitrarily deployed staff time into new spheres of operation have partially succeeded in meeting the basic community mental health mandate.

San Mateo's child guidance clinic, from its inception in 1947, can report a constant chronicle of frustration concerning the waiting list problem. There were repeated experiments with rearrangement of intake and other clinic procedures. Because these were attempts to modify but still use a model based on routine extensive evaluation and individual psychotherapy, the clinic was never able to meet the expressed demands for direct service. Our clinic, however, has increasingly moved out of the traditional clinical patterns, improvising collaborative services with other agencies—schools and juvenile probation, in particular. Thus, our child guidance clinic is in transition. Traditional individual psychotherapy with children, with associated collaborative conferences with their parents, is being offered less and less and the emphasis is on creating new treatment services geared more to the needs of the community.

It should be emphasized that this has been and continues to be a difficult process in San Mateo. Most child guidance personnel have, at best, mixed feelings about turning away from the model in which they were trained. Some, being unable or unwilling to make such a transition, leave the agency; others have responded by taking innovative approaches to the problem.

The child guidance clinic in San Mateo County is the only accredited children's service in the county. The staff of the clinic (including the mental health unit at the juvenile division of the probation department) consists of two full-time and two part-time child psychiatrists, two full-time and one half-time clinical psychologists, seven full-time and one half-time psychiatric social workers and several psychiatrists and psychologists in the community who serve as consultants to the staff. In addition, the clinic has been complemented in the San Mateo mental health program by a very active and effective consultation service (originally formed in 1958 from a core staff of four child guidance personnel) which from the beginning has placed child-serving systems—schools, public health nursing, family and children's welfare services, in particular—on the top of its consultee priority list. (See Chapter 12.)

## Juvenile Probation

A special mental health unit of the child guidance clinic was set up in 1958 to work exclusively with juvenile probation. It is housed on the grounds of that department in a building which includes the offices of the juvenile probation officers, the juvenile hall (detention facilities) and the juvenile court. The staff now consists of a part-time child psychiatrist, one full-time clinical psychologist, and two part-time psychiatric social workers.

The early development of this program was spurred by the realization that there were chronically disturbed families with "traditions" and family patterns of delinquency and impulsive antisocial behavior. These families and their children require social structure, legal limits, and control in order to function even marginally in society today. For these families and children, traditional child guidance out-patient treatment is neither appropriate nor effective. The youngsters often require residential placement, day-center programs, halfway houses, or group foster homes. Programs utilizing group psychotherapy are frequently required. Structured settings and group therapy appear to be the most effective therapeutic model in meeting their psychological needs.

That these extremely dependent, impulsive, and infantile persons are a tremendous psychosocial problem to the community is self-evident. A mental health unit working with them must be able to evaluate these families and then support the agency which has the legal and financial means and the philosophical orientation necessary to implement a structured program for these youngsters. Further, what has evolved has been a realization that much or even most of the responsibility for their treatment must rest with the probation department with the help of consultation from the mental health unit in dealing with these families and their children. This, of course, required an aggressive definition of mental health's role as one of an indirect consultative service to the probation department rather than simply assuming the direct treatment responsibility for these children and their families.

But these conclusions were not reached overnight. When the mental health unit was first established, it was thought that consultation services would be the most useful and appropriate to develop. But in the initial years the focus was instead upon diagnostic evaluations, often of chronic, long-term offenders for whom all felt that psychological types of help were already too late. The mental health unit used whatever time was left over for treatment. Both the mental health unit staff and the juvenile court judge became dissatisfied with these practices and the large number of clients who were not receiving, but clearly needed, service. It was at this point that we were able to confront both ourselves and the probation department with the need to develop indirect services more fully and the need for the probation department to assume responsibility for treatment. This was not only because of our limited staff time available but also because of the nature of the clients being served. An initial step was the requirement that diagnostic evaluation would be done by the mental health unit only after consultation of the probation officer with his mental health consultant and mutual agreement that the case could not be handled by consultation alone without the mental health consultant actually seeing the probationer.

The primary focus of the mental health unit's functioning is now considered to be its consultation services. Each of its staff members is assigned to consult on a regular basis with specific subunits of the juvenile probation division and also the staff of the juvenile detention facility, the chief probation officer, the juvenile court judge and the court referee, the staff of the medical unit at the detention facility, the staff of the girls' day center, and the staff of the boys' rehabilitation camp. Thus, each probation department staff member has one mental health consultant to whom he can turn and with whom he can establish an ongoing working relationship. Much of the consultation is case oriented, but consultee-oriented consultation is an equally important service function.

The usual procedure for case-oriented consultation occurs when the probation officer requests a consultation session with the consultant assigned to his unit. We feel that the probation officers generally have become quite comfortable in presenting to their consultants not only information about their cases, but also their feelings about the particular youngster. Only following this type of consultation session is a decision made by the consultant as to whether a diagnostic evaluation of the youngster should be undertaken.

Because of our limited staff time and the extremely large referral source (more than one hundred probation officers) certain criteria for a diagnostic evaluation by the mental health unit have been established. First, the probation officer must be conversant with the case history and have some idea of the nature of the problem and, above all, have a fairly specific request in mind that both he and his consultant feel the mental health unit can meet. This usually falls into the realm of clarification of the dynamics of the case so that the probation officer can work with the youngster more effectively. Sometimes a psychiatric evaluation and diagnosis is needed for obviously disturbed youngsters to determine whether hospitalization, rather than detention, is more appropriate. The mental health unit has been very helpful in advising the probation department in making the necessary decision when the youngster falls into the obvious category of being both mentally ill and antisocial, incorrigible, or delinquent. Most youngsters who are in trouble with the law have emotional problems; we hope to identitfy those cases where certain problem areas are best handled by more sophisticated psychological techniques, available to mental health professionals and not to the probation officer. This might involve accepting a youngster for brief crisis-oriented outpatient psychotherapy while he is still on probation, or recommending an appropriate form of residential treatment for the youngster. Determinations of the degree of organicity or psychosis contributing to his present behavior problem are significant diagnostic questions. Again, we would emphasize that in only about one in four cases brought to the mental health consultant by the probation officer is there a decision made to do a diagnostic evaluation.

Following the original case consultation and the decision to do a diagnostic evaluation, a social worker spends about two to two and one-half hours with the family; a psychiatrist interviews the child for about one to one and one-half hours; and there may be psychological testing. Then a conference is held with the probation officer, at which time our findings and recommendations are communicated directly to him. Following this conference, a family conference with the parents is usually held, with the probation officer frequently present, to discuss these recommendations with the parents, recognizing, of course, that the probation department has ultimate decision-making responsibility. If psychotherapy is agreed upon, a team approach is used, with the probation officer as part of the team. The parents are often involved either separately or in what amounts to brief family therapy. We refer to this as "focal therapy" since these brief therapeutic efforts are usually directed at a focal neurotic conflict or interaction within the family. The youngsters and their families are seen in the offices of the mental health unit at juvenile probation. The duration of treatment varies, but the upper limit is usually five visits beyond the family conference. Since we are usually dealing with families in crisis, our treatment in many cases could be described as crisis intervention.

During the calendar year of 1967, 140 psychiatric evaluations were done by the juvenile courts and corrections unit. Psychological testing was performed in forty-one of these cases. Parent conferences and follow-up limited to five visits with the families occurred in 120 cases. Thirty-four families were seen in more extensive treatment. However, consultation services reached over six hundred families in that same year. In these cases detailed information, clarification, and even recommendations were made to the probation officer directly. Occasional brief, informal "corridor conferences" between probation officers and mental health unit staff were held because of our geographic proximity. Thus, more troubled families gained some access to some mental health services. In all these ways, a small expenditure of professional time reaches out to a large number of disturbed and troubled children and adolescents and has a tremendous impact on a program with many non-mental health professionals who have potential to be effective mental health caregivers. Further, we hope that in our work with some of these hard core maladaptive families, treatment and parent counseling will affect indirectly other children in the family at high risk of becoming delinquent but not yet identified as such. Thus we see a preventive aspect in our efforts with these families who would rarely seek out help elsewhere. In addition to those services which can be counted and measured to some extent, the mental health unit has many other indications of its influence being felt with the probation department. Various probation units have developed therapeutic intervention of their own, some with and some without consultation from the mental health unit. For instance, on their own initiative one unit developed activity groups and group psychotherapy, using consultation from the mental health unit. Other unique treatment programs include the development of a girls' activity group in which a probation officer takes the girls on various outings and trips to help develop their social skills. Another probation officer leads a karate class for boys on probation who have particular problems with authority, feelings of inadequacy, and poor masculine identification. The karate lesson itself lasts half an hour and is followed by a discussion of these youngsters' feelings about their bodies and masculinity. Karate is a formalized way of strengthening controls. The total experience gives the boys a greater sense of strength, masculine identity, and control of aggressive impulses. Further we have observed these boys get into fewer fights because they now have less of a need to prove their masculinity. Extremely significant has been the probation department's development of a day treatment program for delinquent adolescent girls. All these programs help further the hope of preventing some of the otherwise inevitable psychological and social problems this group will present.

The population dealt with at this facility is a high-risk group for various kinds of psychiatric and social disability in the future as well as the present. Robins (1966) did a study of 524 children diagnosed as socially deviant in a child guidance clinic. His study was a follow-up of these children thirty years later. He stated that, "we had expected that children referred for antisocial behavior would provide a high rate of antisocial adults, but we had not anticipated finding differences invading so many areas of their lives. Not only were antisocial children arrested and imprisoned as adults, as expected, but they were more mobile geographically, had more marital difficulties, poorer occupational and economic histories, impoverished social and organizational relationships, poor armed services records, excessive use of alcohol, and, to some extent, even poor physical health."

Because of the high risks in this group, it is an area ripe for preventive services as well as evaluation and direct services. In addition to the need for service at juvenile probation itself, the staff of the mental health unit also feel they could perform essential service by going into the schools to serve as consultants in behavior management, as, for instance, in helping school personnel understand delinquent and antisocial behavior in terms of the psychodynamics of the family. Upon this understanding can often be based more rational and effective management.

### The Screening Process

As staff time in the main child guidance clinic became increasingly committed to long-term, one-to-one treatment cases and extensive and prolonged diagnostic evaluations, the waiting list for both treatment and evaluation lengthened. Concern about the possible effects of the delay between the family's application for treatment and the time they were first seen led to a study which showed that the longer the delay, the higher the family's dropout rate before reaching the first appointment of their evaluation (see Chapter 15). Though some rationalized this as a screening process which weeded out the poorly motivated and left only the well-motivated families, there was sufficient concern that a number of different revisions of the screening process were tried. All had two things in common: first, none attacked the basic problem—the need for a sweeping reexamination of the functions of the clinic and its responsibility to the total community; second, they all failed to serve more children and decrease the dropout rate. A description of one of these attempts will illustrate this point.

About five years ago, a group intake program was initiated in an attempt to streamline the screening process. Parents' orientation meetings, as they were called, were scheduled twice a week, once in the morning and once in the afternoon for a two-hour period. All families applying at the clinic were scheduled for one of these meetings within a week of their first inquiry. Conducted by the clinical director and chief social worker, the parents' orientation meetings explained the clinic's purpose, fee schedules, and procedures, and then hopefully provided an opportunity to review each family's problems. Referrals to other agencies were made when appropriate. Those interested in help from our clinic made application. However, the complete diagnostic then proceeded in the usual way with the same wait as before—two weeks to two months for the first appointment. Moreover, the dropout rate, instead of decreasing, sharply increased. Perhaps an early appointment seemed to hold promise of equally quick help, a promise that was not kept. For many parents the problem that brought them to the clinic seemed to be, or in fact was, a crisis, for which they wanted early intervention. It was also thought that many parents felt too threatened to reveal their family problems before a group so early in their contact with mental health professionals. In any event, many families withdrew from the clinic at this point.

In the fall of 1967, a new approach was initiated. All of the social workers participated in brief screening of families shortly after their application to the clinic. The purpose was to give immediate individual attention. The social workers met with the parents and sometimes the child, if of adolescent age, and either directly helped the family assess and resolve the problem, or referred the family to other resources, or scheduled a "telescoped" diagnostic evaluation. In the latter instance, the whole family came in and met with the clinical team. The social worker saw the parents for about forty-five minutes while the psychiatrist met with the child. Usually school and medical reports were available to the team, with the parents having signed releases of information at the initial screening interview.

After seeing the family, the team conferred and came up with recommendations which were then discussed with the family that same day. If further evaluation seemed indicated, psychological testing and neurological evaluation were scheduled. If treatment seemed appropriate, then modes of treatment were discussed, and a treatment contract made with the family. Sometimes an extended evaluation to explore and clarify the family's interaction and dynamics seemed necessary, and another appointment was made. Yet, the diagnostic evaluation usually could be completed in two and one-half to three hours in one day rather than over a period of months.

Gradually, as the teams became more skillful, another innovation was instituted, namely, differentiated evaluations. With a shortage of psychiatric time (only three psychiatrists, of whom one was part-time), long waiting periods for psychiatric evaluation appointments developed. The experienced social workers who saw families initially for screening, continued with them and did the evaluation of both parent and child. An evaluation with a child psychiatrist could be scheduled, of course, if the child seemed seriously disturbed, or had medical or neurological complications. If the pathology seemed clear, however, the social worker saw the child and family and then staffed them at a weekly intake team staff meeting which served to give the social workers consultation and confirm their impressions and treatment plan. If short-term therapy or extended evaluation was indicated, the same social worker continued with the family.

Since many social workers initially felt inadequate to do screening evaluations of children, the staff psychiatrists conducted an in-service training program which enabled the social workers to be more definitive in their ability to formulate the psychodynamics of their cases and make recommendations and treatment plans. This streamlining of evaluations doubled the number of families seen in a three-month period in the spring of 1968 and made possible quicker and more efficient service based on the needs of families rather than ritualistic adherence to a standard procedure. It is recognized that new or inexperienced staff will not immediately be able to assume the sophisticated functions described above. However, we are pleased with the results of these differentiated evaluations and will be continuing the program.

### Evaluation as Treatment

The mental health evaluation is the total service provided to about one third of the families seen. They receive some clarification as to "what is wrong" and recommendations are made. Thus, the evaluation also becomes a brief treatment service and is sometimes extended to several extra parent conferences which may include the child. Two examples will illustrate how an evaluation ending with a prescriptive family conference can meet the needs of many families.

*Example A:* A six-year-old boy was brought to the clinic following episodes of fire setting. His parents practiced an inappropriate overpermissiveness for the purpose of allowing the child "to express himself." This philosophy seemed to stem from the parents' inability to deal with their own aggression both toward the child and, in the past, toward their parents. At the final family conference the parents were strongly urged to take active steps to stop the boy's pathological behavior and to physically restrain him if need be at such times. This was effective in stopping the fire setting and generally improving the child's adjustment. Moreover, the parents reported that shortly after their setting some limits on their child that the boy spontaneously said to them, "I didn't realize that you really loved me." We are not implying that the deepest emotional problems of children can be resolved in some miraculous short-term contact. Instead, we are suggesting that many significant benefits can be achieved through brief intervention and the use of adjunctive resources.

*Example B:* The prescription may be that the parents be more authoritarian or less. It may be pointed out to the parents how the child picks up inconsistencies in parental attitude involving management of the children and uses this to play one parent against another. The parents may be shown how the child is used by the parents to fight their battles for them; for example, two authoritarian parents brought their nine-year-old boy to the clinic because of marked over-aggressive and disruptive behavior which was at times overtly sadistic toward other children. It quickly became clear that this was an identification with the father's sadistic treatment of the child. The social worker saw the mother and the father individually and in a third interview, saw the parents together. The mother appeared frigid; the father felt that the only way that he could "get a rise" out of his wife was to harshly treat the child so that the mother would become upset and come to the rescue of the child. This was the only way that father could feel that he had any power over mother—the only way he could feel like a man. The parents became gradually more aware of this pattern in the diagnostic and it was made more explicit in the final family conference where the parents saw more clearly how their own interpersonal difficulties were affecting their child. At the same time the parents were supported so that they were not overwhelmed by guilt and given a feeling that they had permanently damaged their child. The mother was referred to a gynecologist for birth control pills and sex information which were badly needed, and the parents were now able to openly discuss their problems with each other and involve the boy less. Their handling of their child changed and the child's aggressive and disruptive behavior subsided.

A formal treatment contract need not be made. We believe more service can be given by not trying to involve people in long-term treatment who may not want it or be able to benefit from it. Many families can function better by being supported and directed at times of crisis and being allowed to return if another crisis occurs. The frequency of canceled and failed appointments is considerably lower and professional staff can more efficiently utilize their time. Community resources are often called upon, such as the public health nurses, who can make home visits and maintain contact with multiproblem families who are too poorly motivated to reach the clinic except under great stress.

Lest we have overstated our point of view, we want to add that we recognize the importance of keeping a place for some long-term conventional psychotherapy and casework, even in an overcrowded and understaffed clinic. "The importance of long-term psychotherapy depends, first of all, on the fact that some patients can be helped by nothing else. Furthermore, it is only through a thorough understanding of personality, achieved by conducting long-term psychotherapy, that staff members can become sufficiently skilled to use shorter, more active, and more experimental methods (Newman, 1966)."

Many community recreational facilities, such as the YMCA,

YWCA, and city and county recreation department programs, can be interested in helping children with emotional problems if alerted to their special needs. Thus a troubled child can be offered daily therapeutic activity, if necessary. The local big brothers are an example of another valuable community resource. This well-known organization provides dedicated men to assume responsibility for helping boys in the community who need a positive male relationship to facilitate the formation of a healthy male identification.

For children under five, nursery schools or preschool summer programs with the proper degree of structure, or lack of it, appropriate to the needs of the individual child can be recommended. If overinvolvement with mother and child is the problem, a nursery school with little parent involvement is recommended. Some mothers who need to learn about mothering can be referred to a cooperative nursery school where they learn from observation of interaction between other mothers and nursery school staff and the children.

It often takes ingenuity and creativeness to find or develop ways of meeting a child's needs, other than adding him to one's own treatment case load. However, if the clinical orientation encourages staff to utilize all available resources, then greater flexibility and innovation becomes possible.

Our activity groups have proven of great benefit to many latency-aged youngsters. Here, for one hour each week, a group of children play out their problems with other children in activities such as basketball, billiards, and other games. Sometimes these groups resemble psychodrama. After the activities the children sit around drinking Kool-Aid, eating cookies, and talking about what has happened. We have had groups for the seven- and eight-year-olds, nine- and ten-year-olds, and ten- and eleven-year-olds. We are planning to expand this group program and form groups which will continue for two years in addition to our current groups, which last for one school year.

Groups for older children gradually move from an activity focus to a verbal one. Junior-high-aged children meet in the activity center and many play pool for half of the session and then have food and sit around a table for discussion the rest of the meeting. The high school groups of both boys and girls meet in the conference rooms of the clinic with a still more verbal approach to the expression and resolution of their problems. Sometimes, soft drinks are provided for the high-school groups, too, if a particular group seems to have special needs to be fed.

### Skills in the Community

The lack of male staff co-therapists for boys' therapy groups was a real problem. Many felt it essential for latency-age boys, many of whom came from fatherless homes, or homes with inadequate or disinterested fathers, to have male therapists. We discovered that male staff from the juvenile probation department and the school counseling offices were interested in increasing their therapeutic skills. For the past two years, therefore, men from each of these sources have participated in our group program, each as co-therapist with a group therapist from our clinic, in a boys' therapy group. This provides more and better service to our youngsters as well as training for other community professionals who can then utilize these skills in their own settings. These men also participated in weekly group seminars which focused on group therapy techniques and group dynamics such as destructiveness or scapegoating; examples from their own groups made these seminars come alive.

The schools have long complained that the clinic did not meet their needs. The traditional evaluation of a child was helpful but did not seem to be enough to a frustrated teacher or an angry principal who wanted the youngster "cured" or at least wanted to be told "what to do with him!" Although the number of school conferences between school and clinic staff were increased, both school and clinic felt there was too little service, excessively long waiting lists, too infrequent contacts with teachers who saw the child daily, and too little reaching out to those families who needed our services the most.

A new approach was needed. In one of the more creative school districts, the psychologists and counselors who handle problem children began meeting with clinic staff to extend direct mental health services to the school. This took the form of the clinic providing staff to be co-therapists with the school counselors and psychologists for classroom group therapy in the special classes. Consultation was made available to teachers of special classes with the principal and psychologist often sitting in.

Gradually the program has expanded over a three-year period.

It has been shaped to meet the individual needs of this particular school's personnel and to make maximum use of the school's resources. The program is being extended to other school districts. Since school districts in this community vary greatly, we find that the first year is spent getting acquainted with and establishing meaningful communication with school personnel. Emphasis is placed on working in the areas where the school feels the greatest need and discomfort. This may change in the second year with the schools acquiring a better understanding of psychiatric services and more reasonable expectations of what can be accomplished. We try to incorporate school personnel into direct service whenever possible, as co-therapists for children's and parents' groups; or by means of training seminars to help them to carry on programs started by staff from our clinic. Our role then changes to that of consultant, and more time can be given to the next school district.

Stickney (1968) feels that schools can be helped to become, in effect, mental health centers. The first stage of this process is promptly responding to crisis referrals and providing practical assistance. In this way the mental health consultant becomes initiated into the school's complex subculture. Our experience likewise bears out the importance of beginning with a situation in which the school is hurting. Helping in these crisis situations varies from working directly with some of the most disturbed children in classroom discussion groups to talking with their parents who perhaps had been referred to the clinic earlier but had been too resistant to come. Permission is received from the parents allowing the youngsters to participate in group therapy within the school structure. Sometimes a group is bussed to the clinic for an activity group if the school lacks facilities or appears to be too inhibiting an environment for such a group or is unable or unwilling to cope with the acting out and anger often released by the children in these groups. Parents have been very cooperative in permitting their children to come to the clinic through the school program, even in cases where they have refused to come on their own initiative. Similarly, parents who were too frightened or otherwise resistant to coming to the clinic have been willing to participate in evening groups at the school.

A summer activity program has been instituted which provides therapeutic group experiences for emotionally disturbed youngsters in the form of a two-day-a-week day camp. Children attending the program are either already in treatment or on the treatment waiting list. The goals are therapy for the child and providing the clinic staff with more knowledge about the child through direct observation of his present functioning, interactions, and needs. Four clinic staff members, two student social workers and twelve volunteers gave part of their time to this program. The volunteers included high school and college students as well as arts and crafts specialists from the community. Clinic staff provided orientation and training sessions for the volunteer staff. Last year forty children participated, meeting twice weekly for six weeks from 10:00 A.M. to 3:00 P.M. The program included such activities as swimming, active games, crafts, story times, music, and special events like treasure hunts and track meets. Special emphasis was placed on individual needs. Significant gains in emotional maturity, peer relationships, and heightened self-esteem and self-confidence were made by a majority of the children. A relatively small amount of professional staff time created quite an impact on a large number of children. Two examples will illustrate the value of this program.

*Example A:* Bryan, a very disturbed, frightened, twelve-year-old boy with problems of isolation, was too fearful to go into the swimming pool the first two days. His parents had tried unsuccessfully the previous three summers to get him into the water. With much coaxing he stood in the shallow end of the pool, holding hands with a volunteer on the third day, and gradually began entering into the water games and participating in the group play. He became more involved in other activities following the many comments on his success in the swimming pool. His therapist further noted that the group achievements had been more ego-enhancing for this youngster than individual therapy had been and recommended further group programs for this boy.

*Example B:* The program proved to be of diagnostic value for Scott, a nine-year-old boy evaluated earlier as being mildly disturbed, and at the time of camp still on the treatment waiting list. After several days of group interaction, Scott's manipulative behavior with adults and younger children revealed a highly complex defensive structure which would have taken many months of individual therapy to unravel and understand.

Most of the volunteers indicated that this summer activity project had been a growth experience for them and indicated further interest in working with children in the mental health field. The program thus had a mental health education function. Further, a parents' group for neurologically handicapped children contributed funds for crafts and special events for the program. They were impressed by its effectiveness and set up their own program with local recreational centers to provide more summer activities for children with neurological handicaps. The child guidance clinic provided consultation for these activities too.

The next summer activity program for child guidance clinic patients is being planned in conjunction with our local junior college as a special laboratory class for students majoring in sociology and psychology. Child guidance clinic staff will provide supervision and consultation. Again in addition to providing treatment and diagnostic evaluation for our children, we hope to interest some of these students in coming into the field.

Last spring a companionship project (Goodman, 1969) was initiated with the local junior college as a one-credit course in psychology. The students were recruited from psychology classes and individually interviewed for the project; five female and three male students were selected. The students were matched with eight children who had been evaluated in the clinic and who were felt to need a big brother or a big sister experience. One child had elderly parents and no siblings at home and was felt to be quite inhibited and adversely affected by an overprotective, restrictive environment. The child would probably have benefited from individual psychotherapy, but was referred, to the project instead, where she had eight outings with the college student, seeing many new places in the community and receiving the special attention of a young adult who was obviously very much interested in her. Gradually her self-confidence grew, and she made a friend in her own neighborhood. She asked if she could write to her new college friend after the project ended.

The project was helpful for both students and children. A clinic staff member provided consultation through a series of hourly seminars with the students. The students were also asked to fill out observation sheets on each outing, describing their activity, the interaction with the child and their feelings about it. These reports were duplicated and given to the child's therapist, and reviewed by the clinical consultant and college program advisor.

The one criticism of the program was its brevity, and plans are now being made to expand to twelve outings or sessions between student and child and to enlarge the program to serve twelve children each semester. Currently arrangements are being made for graduate students in education to do a field placement at the clinic with children with learning handicaps. This therapeutic tutor program has been tried at the University of Washington (Goodman, in press) and elsewhere (Prentice and Sperry, 1965; Templeton, Sperry, and Prentice, 1967), successfully meeting both the emotional and tutorial needs of disturbed youngsters with learning problems. The clinic expects to provide consultation to the students and will work with the families of the children involved as well as the children's teachers.

### Other Resources

We feel, as does Newman (1966), it is important to emphasize that the child guidance clinic is not the only source of help within the community for children with emotional problems. In the family service, Jewish family service, and Catholic social service agencies and within the group of private practitioners, we find social workers, psychologists, psychiatrists, and pediatricians with knowledge about and skills in dealing with the emotional problems of children. Schools offer special classes for the mentally retarded, emotionally handicapped, and neurologically handicapped. Schools are staffed with psychologists, social workers, and counselors who help identify children with problems and offer continuing help when they can and refer elsewhere cases requiring more comprehensive diagnostic procedures or therapeutic skills. Several recreational centers in the community have extensive activity programs and work well with our child guidance clinic and give special attention to children with emotional problems.

Public health nurses work closely with the clinic. They are an important casefinding resource and refer special problems which they encounter to the clinic; in turn they make home visits to families serviced by the clinic at the clinic's request. For instance, in one multiproblem family, the child was able to come to the clinic on his own and did so, but the mother was disorganized and neither able nor motivated to come for help for herself or to accompany her child. In this case a Public Health Nurse made regular visits to give support to the mother and to help with organizing the household. This was helpful not only to the identified patient but to others in the home.

Medications are also being more and more freely used in our clinic, especially with neurologically handicapped and severely disturbed children. If appropriate drugs are chosen, they can control symptoms that do not respond readily to other measures. Drug therapy combined with supportive psychotherapy is frequently the treatment regimen used in our clinic to stabilize the child and relieve the current stress in the family. The mothers are seen at least biweekly to report the child's behavior and attitude and any side effects of the medication.

Johnny, a hyperactive nine-year-old, was placed in a special class for emotionally handicapped children who were functioning below grade level, but seen as having an average intellectual potential. He was referred to the clinic with complaints of unmanageability, rebelliousness to authority, difficulty with peers, and temper tantrums. The diagnostic evaluation revealed neurological handicap and a long history of inconsistency of parental discipline by the parents. Both psychotherapy and medication were recommended, and the teachers noted an immediate improvement with better physical control in Johnny, and subsequent attitudinal changes.

There is a growing recognition in the literature of the effectiveness of drugs for many target symptoms and in a variety of treatment patterns, including counseling and psychotherapy with less disturbed children (Fish, 1968; Kraft, 1968). Used properly, drugs can actually facilitate the educational and psychotherapeutic aspects of treatment (Fish, 1960). But "a fundamental and crucial factor is the attitude of the psychiatrist. If he considers drug therapy to be a lower order procedure, the child's mother or, in the case of an adolescent, the patient himself, will sense it (Kraft, 1968)."

As noted elsewhere, the San Mateo mental health services are being regionalized; each of four geographic regions of approximately equal population will be served by a community mental health center (see Chapters 17, 18, and 19 on regionalization). We plan to have a child psychiatrist, psychologist, and one or two social workers in each regional center. They will provide the full range of direct treatment and diagnostic evaluation services along the lines described earlier in this chapter. These children's specialists within each region will also consult with agencies in the region who work directly with children or whose work affects children. The major thrust in this area will be with the schools and children's welfare agencies. We will thus be able to expand these services, heretofore in large part handled by the separate county-wide mental health consultation service. We also plan to stress community organization and utilize and further develop local resources for children. For example, several of the churches are interested in developing teenage programs to reach delinquent and fringe group adolescents. With mental health guidance, they would be willing to undertake teen-club projects. Civic groups, looking for activities to sponsor, will collaborate with staff to meet local needs of children for such services as recreation, special education classes and part-time jobs.

A central child guidance office will continue to function. It will provide in-service training programs for staff in the regions, and supervise the training in evaluation and treatment of children of social work students, psychiatric residents, and psychology interns. It will also continue to supervise programs such as the juvenile probation mental health unit, the summer activity program and the companionship project, and develop new services such as a day treatment service for adolescents and a children's inpatient service. Neurological and EEG testing as well as speech evaluations will also be handled by this central office.

Thus has our child guidance clinic, through numerous struggles and problems, metamorphosed into a service oriented to meet most effectively the mental health needs of most children in the community. It has not been an easy transition. It has meant a willingness to adopt a new model rather than attempt to patch and renovate and yet still cling to the old. The essential ingredients of this new model are consultation services, streamlined evaluation, brief treatment and crisis intervention, group and activity therapies and maximum utilization of community resources.

CHAPTER **11**

# Mental Retardation

*George Hexter*

"Mrs. Jones, I'm very sorry to have to inform you," said the pediatrician, "that your son has Down's syndrome—it's the kind of difficulty that in times gone by was referred to as mongolism. I want you to understand . . ." Mrs. Jones never heard the rest of that comment. As literally as if she had been involved in a major automobile accident in which she herself was not physically injured, she underwent the physiological reactions of shock. A kind of numbness overcame her. Words of all sorts seemed distant . . . voices small and thin . . . their meanings seemed to float through her rather than to register in some useful fashion. Mechanically she responded to the doctor's query, "Yes, doctor, I understand." But, of course, she did not understand in any real emotional sense, and her intellectual powers were disorganized by the enormity of her loss and grief.

261

What has just been described is the opening incident in a long series of actions and reactions comprising the lengthy scenario sometimes called the parent's coping reaction. Later this initial stage of shock gives way to succeeding stages of denial, guilt, hostility, intellectualization, involvement, and (ideally) resolution.

This chapter discusses this longitudinal coping reaction in more detail as a way of (1) putting into better perspective the reactions of the parents of retarded children, and (2) extending this schema to understand the reactions of groups of these parents and their spokesmen and the reactions of the community generally to retardation. The parents' coping reaction is thus used as a paradigm to shed some light on what we are coming to view as the parallel, though not fully analogous, reactions of the community and the patterns of stress and trauma that run through the fabric of social and cultural attitudes toward retardation. We view this as an interactive phenomenon in which we ourselves are intimately involved. We then turn to further problems we have encountered in the development of services for the retarded as part of a comprehensive community mental health program.

A lack of coordinated effort had long been recognized as a major obstacle to orderly development of services for the retarded in San Mateo County. Formation of an ad hoc committee on retardation, composed largely of professionals who sought to combine and coordinate their efforts, was a response to this need for coordination. Planning could not be done without the direct involvement, active support, and leadership of the county government. Eventually the ad hoc committee produced a new avatar: the coordinating committee on mental retardation, which included relevant segments of the community, both professionals and lay citizens, interested in retardation; representatives of the county government; and representation from the county medical society, public schools, and county mental health services. This organization formed itself into subcommittees to attack the various segments of the retardation problem. There is a workshop committee, rehabilitation and residential committee, recreational committee, and a committee to make recommendations concerning the "mildly retarded."

In order to develop a plan for effective services, the committee had to have some data. A good deal of data available in a previous survey of a two-county area (San Mateo and Santa Clara counties) provided a starting point. In addition, it was decided that a developmental evaluation unit was necessary. This was to be a diagnostic unit linking in a close relationship a pediatrician and a child psychiatrist, both dynamically oriented. When I was placed in charge of this unit, a collection of statistics was requested, to aid in exposing gaps in services. These were supplemented by a review of individual cases to assure adequate information on which planners would base their decisions. The data collection later indicated a need for more respite and residential services, as well as a need for a day care school facility for the emotionally disturbed retardates of the county.

As a result of the foregoing study, counseling services to parents, long-term follow-up services for the parents of retarded children, placement assistance for state hospitalization of the severely retarded, and community organization and planning, as well as diagnostic evaluation, were incorporated into the service pattern of the clinic. In the process of forming this unit, the Director of Public Health and Welfare had to face directly a thorny question which had been debated in a California governor's Study Commission on Mental Retardation (of which the director had been a member): should a psychiatrist or pediatrician head such a retardation unit? In this county, the eventual decision was that a psychiatrist should head the program. San Mateo's decision was influenced primarily by the fact that such a service, under psychiatric administration, was eligible to receive state Short-Doyle reimbursement.

Whatever the decision concerning administrative direction, a closely coordinated effort between the pediatrician and the child psychiatrist is essential. Joint administration is usually not a workable arrangement, but cooperation is possible and crucial. The unit evolved through a series of meetings with the neurologist, the pediatrician, speech pathologist, and child psychiatrist. The first task was to decide under whose auspices this truly interdisciplinary team would function.

If the truth be known, no one wanted the task of administering such a multidisciplinary group. In the first place, it was to be a federation rather than a single unit under one administrative authority (the head of the unit does not have administrative control over the pediatrician, neurologist, or speech pathologist, all of whom are located in the appropriate departments of the county general hospital) and this, everyone correctly predicted, would cause administrative complications. Further, the stimulus produced by President Kennedy's interest augured considerable growth for mental retardation services in the coming years, and none of the professionals in our department was prepared to assume the additional administrative headaches of such a prospect. Least consciously admitted, but also operating in this equation, was the fact that mental retardation was still not a subject matter favored by most professionals.

The multidisiciplinary team which evolved included a pediatrician, a neurologist, a speech pathologist, a psychiatrist, a psychologist, social workers, and a public health nurse. The effectiveness of the clinic depends upon procedures to focus the input of diverse disciplines and several administratively distinct units of the multiphasic department. One such procedure, worth a special recommendation to the reader, is that the written reports of each observer are read *prior* to the staff conference at which a case is discussed by each team member. Therefore, meetings can be devoted to a brief review of these findings; this leads to a more thorough discussion of any differences of opinion about a particular child or facet of family problem and, finally, to the discussion of recommendations and their implementation.

Should one or more members of the team be absent due to unavoidable schedule conflicts, prolonged illness, termination of employment, or other unforeseen circumstances, the adverse effect is felt by every member of the team, and in time, by the community as a whole. This, of course, is an unavoidable price that must always be assessed against any multidisciplinary enterprise.

The initial multidisciplinary team met to discuss which population groups would be admitted for evaluation and diagnostic services. Because the unit was set up to serve the retarded, the AAMD classification of retardation became the intake cut-off point. It was realized, however, that some people evaluated by the unit would later turn out not to be retarded, and some would be borderline cases in which one could not make a reasonable decision without seeing the child and family.

Prior to establishment of the unit, the child guidance clinic had coordinated multiphasic diagnostic services. It had routinely supplied psychotherapeutic services to retardates with emotional problems. The new unit had to be very careful not to take over the responsibility of the child guidance clinic for children who had psychiatric difficulties. This would have diminished child guidance clinic staff involvement in mental retardation, thus occasioning a relative loss of effort by the community (substituting developmental evaluation unit effort for the child guidance effort which had been deployed historically to this activity would equal no real increase in mental retardation work). Moreover, the child guidance diagnostics of nonretarded (that is, the autistic children) realistically could not be assumed by a staff as small as was planned for the developmental evaluation unit. Even if these two reasons were insufficient, it was recognized that taking over a major segment of work being done by an active organization without excellent reason is always to be avoided, since it tends to be seen as a threat by the older organization and sets up a rivalry which leads to noncooperative efforts on the part of both units. Thus, through an early agreement, autistic children were made specifically the province of the child guidance clinic. When a known autistic child was referred for an evaluation, the family would be directed to the guidance clinic. Similarly, it was clearly understood that the developmental evaluation unit was not a treatment service and, therefore, was not offering psychotherapy; this function still resided within the child guidance clinic. Should there be a need, and we all felt that there was, for expansion of psychotherapeutic services to children, that expansion should be under the direction of and housed within the child guidance clinic rather than within separate therapy facilities set up exclusively for the retarded. This tended to keep the retarded within the mainstream of services whenever possible. At the same time, consultation around issues of retardation and to the general community were considered a responsibility to be shared with the consultation service.

### Family Coping Pattern

Having a retarded child presents to parents the problem of coping with a situation that is neither entirely known nor completely outside of their total range of experience (Group for Advancement of Psychiatry, 1963). They bring to this situation their own personality traits, their background and experiences, their current supports both emotional and material, as well as their expectations and desires. All of these things have an effect on the coping process, which, in general, follows a pattern. This same pattern, in an altered form, seems to underlie the community-wide responses to mental retardation, including the issues that impinge upon development of adequate local resources. To suggest what may be involved in the community coping pattern, it is first necessary to understand something about the general configuration of family responses.

Mrs. Jones, the hypothetical parent whose fateful encounter with the pediatrician was sketched in our first paragraph, first experienced a state of shock, a numbness, a lack of comprehension. After Mrs. Jones was once again able to think about the problem, her reaction was one of "denial." She said to herself and to others, "It isn't so."

That initial shock phase may have lasted for Mrs. Jones only a few hours, at which point the denial set in. By contrast, for another parent, the reaction of shock lasted perhaps nine months. The denial is usually almost complete at first, and parents are likely to say, "It is not so—the doctors don't know what they are talking about." In time this attitude softens, perhaps even reaching the point where the parents may use the word "retardation" or compromise by saying "slowness," "handicapped," or some similar euphemism. If the child has a known medical entity, the parents may learn to accept the name of that entity (phenylketonuria, microcephaly, Down's syndrome, or cerebral palsy) more quickly. Nevertheless, the denial persists, reaching more subtle forms of expression. "We have a retarded child, and she's quite slow to walk. As yet, she does not speak, but we are looking forward to the day when she grows up and graduates from high school." As the denial softens, feelings of guilt and thoughts of having been punished (by being "given" a retarded child) creep secretly into the minds of parents.

The guilt phase usually is rather hidden. Viewed from the exterior by the untrained observer, it might not seem to exist at all. The secret reasons for punishment, the fancied transgressions, the half-truthful remembrances are all kept secret from other family members and friends. The anger at the loss is thus turned inward as with other grief reactions. When allowed to come to the surface and gain verbal expression, as in a minister's office, it may be seen to turn suddenly to hostility. In one instance the mother accuses herself because she flew as a stewardess while carrying the retarded child or because she took drugs during the pregnancy. In another case the father might accuse himself for arguments with the mother or for premarital sexual relations with his wife. These are fantasies which the parents hold as a thought but without strong convictions. They have the quality of: "I'm guilty, and God is punishing me." Often they include a hidden death wish: "If I had not conceived this child, my life would be different; but I can't admit to that wish, so I must accuse myself of something which I can't really reasonably believe while concealing the real guilt (of wishing death)."

This hostility stage, which begins as a direct outgrowth of the guilt, signals that energies are more available than before. During the shock phase, parent energies were not available even for passive endeavors such as listening, remembering, and understanding. During the denial period, they were available only in a very defensive fashion to keep knowledge from the parent and to try to provide a way to disprove that which had been stated before. Their energies were used in an effort to destroy reality rather than to deal with it. The endless quest for better diagnosis, for a miraculous cure, is part of the denial phase. During the period of guilt there begins the overprotectiveness and oversolicitousness which will persist over a long period of time. The attempts to atone are fruitless, thereby contributing to the hostility which arises next. The anger may be expressed toward family members, spouse, siblings, or other children, but more often and eventually toward those external to the immediate situation: doctors, schools, and the community as a whole.

In the early stages of this phase, the aggressive energies cannot be made to "do work." However, the harnessing often comes next. The parents become interested in joining other parents in groups. They begin to organize to correct the lack of facilities in a community, mass their energies to build edifices and to staff programs on a voluntary basis. They may form groups which can exercise pressures on legislatures. Some turn their energies in an intellectualizing fashion toward educating themselves about specific or particular entities within the broad scope of mental retardation or toward becoming experts in different areas related to retardation. These energies, though sometimes irritating, can be highly useful to the community in contributing to the development of new facilities. If unharnessed, unchanneled, or unguided by less involved experts, they may go astray. The price of this sort of activity to the individual parent and perhaps to the family is high. The situation now is that energies are available which were once tied up in an intrapsychic process leading sometimes to apathy, as in the early denial stages, or to more frantic endeavors, auguring little, during the guilt phase. Nonetheless, these energies are specifically bound to the entire problem of retardation and are not generally available for solving other problems or meeting other personal or family needs, including especially the needs of other children in the family. This phase of involvement ideally melts into a stage called resolution.

Resolution probably never comes to completion. Some parents approach it when they can once again make use of their energies to deal appropriately with reality problems. That is, they neither have to overinvest nor underinvest their energy in any problem connected with the retarded child. They can allocate appropriately, then, their total resources to meet present and future needs. The acute grief process described by Lindemann (1944) and others probably takes place over less than a year's span; the acute reaction experienced by parents of a leukemic child (prior to the advent of newer treatment methods that prolong life) ran most of its course in six months' time (Chodoff, Friedman, and Hamburg, 1964); by comparison, the reaction in the unaided parents of the mentally retarded as described above, requires more than a decade. The chronicity of the retardation problem itself and the fact that the love object is not entirely lost (even when placed in an institution) probably contributes to the longevity of this reaction.

The coping reaction may be summarized (see diagram) as shock, the stage at which the parents first become aware of difficulties and react in a manner similar to an incident causing actual physiological shock. This leads initially to denial, which we will call *Type I* and which tends to be total ("It really isn't so!"). Next comes a softening of denial, which we will call *Type II*, in which the parents say something like, "I know my child is retarded, but we are looking forward to the time when he is able to go to college." This denial, Type II, may give way to guilt with all sorts of obsessive thinking and fantasies about having caused the retardation. The period of hostility represents that period in which the anger previously turned inward or repressed during the guilt phase, is now directed outwardly. In some cases this phase is modified by the following stage of intellectualization wherein the individual attempts to learn all he can about mental retardation.

The stage of involvement in which he puts his energy into some cooperative venture with the purpose of aiding the retarded usually comes next, and the stage of resolution is an idealized completion of the schema. The parents' reaction may slip back from one stage into another, and some of the most common reversals in the major trends are noted by the reverse arrows. The coping reaction may be schematized thus:

Shock → Denial I → Denial II → Guilt → Hostility → Intellectuali-

zation → Involvement → Resolution

### Community Reactions

In evolving a plan for meeting the manifold needs of retardates and their families in San Mateo County, this family coping reaction has been extended to propose a roughly analogous community coping pattern—that the community, too, passes through similar stages from shock through resolution. Like the family coping reaction which it parallels, this is, above all, tentative and subject to much more empirical study. It is probably seen most vividly in the behavior of groups of retarded children's parents' groups and their spokesmen, but is by no means limited to them, and, indeed, it explicitly includes all of us.

The difficult community organization task of working toward development of more nearly optimum services can be implemented most efficiently only if all concerned share some tentative vision of the mechanisms that influence community support and acceptance of, as well as resistance to, retardation services. This is no different from the importance—for the professional working individually with the family —of *understanding* the dynamics of the family's reactions rather than taking them personally (or stereotyping them) and reacting in kind. The coping pattern represents our tentative attempt to express in theoretical terms what lies behind the often curious and endlessly frustrating community responses and adaptation to these troubling disabilities.

First, the possibility that "strange" community behaviors actually correspond to familiar coping responses which are observed elsewhere (for example, grief studies) helps professional staff persevere in efforts to reach long-term goals.

Second, the possible existence of a logical community coping pattern removes much of the sting from what may otherwise seem to be unnecessary delays and useless conflict. The community, as a whole, can be helped to see that temporary stumbling blocks may represent essential stages of working through painful "hangups." Consequently, all concerned can be much more hopeful about future progress. This morale issue is most important primarily because we are trying to deal with disabilities which are, after all, incurable, and about which one can easily become profoundly depressed.

Third, individual services and agencies can perform in such a way as to feed into the process by which the community, over time, works through its denial and resistance phases and approaches the idealized phase of resolution. In other words, a theory about how the community adapts helps one to formulate long-range community organization goals and to design clinic and agency operations to enhance pursuit of such goals.

Fourth, having been armed with at least tentative understanding of such coping mechanisms, personnel can make some sense of phenomena that appear to defy logic or intelligent modes of behavior. For instance, the odd and rather dismaying choice of space for our new clinic (cramped quarters located across the hall from the county coroner's office) can be perceived as having a certain perverse but perhaps highly eloquent significance. It is a constant reminder of the community's wish to deny the extent of the problem and of ambivalent attitudes which hamper the community when it is finally moved to take action. Similarly, such a theory helps one to hazard an informed conclusion about the prevalence in communities of highly vocal, hostile individuals as chairmen and directors of retardation committees, services, and agencies, since it appears such individuals may carry the displaced or reflected affect of the community's own internalized response to retardation. In effect, these spokesmen symbolize a necessary and potentially productive phase of the community's coping pattern and, in working with such individuals, one can perceive, for example, that merely changing them (either by helping them to modify their styles of behavior or by contriving to have them removed) might actually impede rather than accelerate progress toward sound goals. The theory suggests that one must focus not upon these vocal and divisive figures but upon the climate and tenor of support and interest from which these spokesmen derive their sanctions and prohibitions. This can often be done through such organizations as our community's coordinating committee on mental retardation.

Finally, such a theory reminds one that he, too, is an active player in the drama. Objective as he may hope to be, professional as he is, he, too, is caught up in the community coping pattern. This knowledge does not prevent mistakes on his part, but it does arm him with a dimension of self-understanding that can help him perform more effectively.

In the discussion to follow, the reader is invited to keep this tentative coping scheme in mind. Clearly, if the theory is sound, it will require much more refinement. Nevertheless, one must emphasize that some attempt to make sense of community behavior patterns is an indispensable first step for any of us who hopes to engage in the kind and quality of community partnerships essential to produce improved local responses to the harsh and depressing problem of mental retardation.

With the above format in mind, let us now see what some of the community problems are, and how they have been or might be dealt with.

If someone asked, "What would a manual on developing services for the retarded contain in order to be most helpful?" the answer would be relatively simple. In the light of what has been said above perhaps the first thing would be some theoretical guidelines, like the community coping pattern, that one could employ as a tool in setting priorities and deciding upon alternative courses.

A list of the ideal services to the retarded necessary to the optimal function needed in this county should then follow. That description should be complete in detail to enable someone to develop those services, when possible. In addition, a list of already existing services should be juxtaposed to those which were ideal in such a way that one could see at a glance how existing services might be turned into ideal services. Next, the manual would contain data on quantities of need so that one might construct an ideal priority list.

This done, the manual would identify undeveloped resources. This list would include not only money but people, both professional and volunteer, who could support the effort, and both new and existing services. A specific list of names would be extremely useful, something about these people including their strengths, weaknesses, prejudices, and the points upon which they could be approached most easily. Next, the manual should respond to the question: what blocks the orderly development of these ideal services? This list would begin with the generalities often heard, for example, community apathy, revulsion, rejection, and denial of retardation; specifically, the wish of the community that there be no real problem of the retarded going unserved in the community, and that, if there is a problem, it not be considered their fault but someone else's. These generalities need to be understood in depth. In other words, the manual would analyze the ingredients that go to make up the shock, denial, guilt, and resistance phases of the community coping pattern.

For instance, it needs to be understood that rarely does the shock reaction phase of the coping pattern lead directly to effective action. People often have a shock-like reaction on their first exposure to the enormity of the problems of retardation. It may result from initial awareness of disgraceful conditions in state hospitals for the retarded or some other glaring local neglect. For many in the community, the reaction of shock stems in part from the sight of the retarded themselves. No doubt conditions for the retarded often are appalling. The disgrace is often attested to by those directly involved in the program, as well as by those external to the program itself. It is too easy for the community to make some token acknowledgment of the disgraceful conditions and thereupon recoil from the situation into a general denial, at which point the whole matter is forgotten and effective action is impossible.

For action to be effective, it must be sustained. That is not possible as an outgrowth of a shock reaction. Not that exposing these conditions is not useful. It is useful because with the progress of time the denial softens and the community as a whole will be able to look at the difficulties in programs for the retarded. However, community anger may be aroused in such a way as to come down most heavily on those who have administered the programs. This is true whether the deficiencies are directly due to the administrative ability of those involved or not. In this mood, the public sometimes throw out several good administrators as they attempt to revamp programs. Only later can cooperative efforts be more effective. That is when the community has passed this hostile stage and is involved in a cooperative effort similar to the stage of "involvement" that the parent passes through. Therefore, to understand the blocks to orderly development of services in a community, one needs, in this kind of process, an indication of where this particular community stands or, better yet, where various segments of the community might be along the spectrum "shock to resolution." We are pointing out that the community reaction follows a similar although not identical schema to the parents' coping process. The fact that the word *shock* is used in the first stage of the parents' reaction and in this illustration is not meant to imply that the reactions are the *same*. In extrapolation from the individual to the community level, these mechanisms are subtly modified, so that these words carry a modified connotation. The community is not an individual human being. Nevertheless, note the parallels in the processes.

Another kind of block paralleling the parent coping reaction is the tendency of local community leaders of parents' groups and retardation facilities to be aggressive, highly vocal, and prone to dissipate much energy in pointless feuding. For instance, one director in another county is described as "so hard to get along with that we have to put him on every committee just to keep him quiet." Or, this comment from an agency executive: "We are the only service providing care to the retarded in this community. We are the only ones who care about you as parents. We hope that you will continue to support us in our fight to obtain better services." This statement by a particularly assertive director of a mental retardation facility was meant to raise funds. This director was overtly reflecting the parents' hostile stage. Is it a coincidence that such individuals hold such positions? Is it not possible that groups of parents and the community as a whole preselect and use these directors in order to express their hostility toward those who they feel are not helping enough? Such incidents have important consequences later: cooperative efforts from those criticized and offended are needed at a later stage. These old wounds then have to be dealt with and resolved, sometimes months and years later. In this county the coordinating committee on mental retardation and the professional advisory committee to that organization provides a setting for doing just this; old arguments can be taken up in a semi-secluded atmosphere during which old feelings may be expressed and worked through. This may lead to some resolution, so joint action toward common goals may be undertaken. Without such a setting and without the unwritten agreement that such a setting can be used in that fashion, these hostilities are continued and allowed to be openly and destructively expressed in the community at large. In the community-wide sphere, they are misunderstood and, at best, "bought off" by token contributions to those who are most hostile. At worst, the entire field winds up by losing investment and interest which they have solicited from the population at large.

Pressure groups associated with retardation, both parents and professionals, act with such vigor at times that their hostility is thinly veiled. The community responds to that hostility negatively rather than reacting objectively to the specific propositions which it is requested to support. Essential to this schema is the concept that the community at large is not a passive or purely "reactive" element. It is *interacting* with these retardation groups. In the equation, then, one assumes the community is mutually responsible in determining the behavior of retardation-minded parents and their various representatives. This concept is fundamentally congruent with that of child psychiatry generally and, in particular, with the schema proposed in situational crisis intervention (Klein and Lindemann, 1961).

It is helpful, at this point, to identify what is facilitating or blocking the development of services. When the anger is sublimated in such a way that it no longer drives away uninvolved people but enables those involved in the work of mental retardation to join together in some stage of group involvements, the whole effort becomes tremendously more effective. It is then possible to go to local governing bodies, county health personnel, business organizations, and private agencies in a coordinated fashion. Only after these efforts are somewhat successful and a later stage has been reached is it possible for these groups to enlarge their scope (focused solely, in the past, upon the retarded) to encompass other handicapped and disadvantaged children.

### Financing and Related Topics

Financing decisions reveal significant clues concerning the nature of the interaction between the community and the problem-bearing groups. Enormous pressures to conform to or exceed the standards of service in surrounding counties are felt. The demonstration of an effective technique dealing with some facet of retardation in one county becomes quickly known to those in other counties. Whether the same means are developed to deal with the problem is somewhat dependent on the resources and imagination of those within the observing county. Similarly, if no such examples exist within a community or surrounding communities, their lack may be a block to developing services. Therefore, the development of the first such service is extremely important. For this purpose there have always been "seed monies" or grant funds available for "demonstration purposes." The problem is that these funds are time-limited; upon termination of funding a facility is often left in an untenable financial situation, unable to solicit resources from its own community in order to continue services. Examples of this kind of situation are legion; yet they have not led to realistic programming of demonstrations—which continue to fail to include adequate resources and methods to assure perpetuation of the demonstration on a new fiscal base in the community.

"Separate but equal" is an unwritten and almost unspoken doctrine to which pressure groups interested in mental retardation and pressure groups interested in mental illness subscribe according to the vagaries of the moment. It can be a major problem. Some say psychotics are too sick to be treated together with the retarded, that psychotic children and retarded children, as well as the funds and personnel deployed to serve them, should be separate. Is this a realistic decision? Or does it actually constitute a projection of underlying attitudes (for example, the community patterns of denial that have tended to deemphasize retardates and overemphasize psychotic children)? A local retardation agency cannot fund the placement of a child at a certain facility because the facility "accepts" autistic children and does not offer treatment for "mental retardation"—this despite the fact that the child herself is multiply handicapped (reduced visual acuity almost to the point of blindness) and has a very pronounced emotional disturbance, as well as being retarded. On the other hand, one hears from people in child guidance clinics: "We have enough of your retarded already." On investigation, it appears these are children whose IQ scores are in the range between 70 and 90. The tendency to exclude children with less than average intelligence can be pronounced. It should, however, be viewed as another clue to the community coping stage, rather than as a capricious (illogical or irrational) response.

In reviewing the statistics of this developmental evaluation unit, we see a high proportion of the moderately and severely retarded (Menolascino, 1968). About 50 per cent of our cases have an IQ of 50 or below. In the general population the ratio of mildly retarded (50 to 70 IQ) to moderately and severely and profoundly retarded (50 IQ and below) is more than four to one. Thus, we may expect to see probably four mildly retarded individuals in a school setting for every moderately, severely, or profoundly retarded individual we know to exist in this same age range (Group for Advancement of Psychiatry, 1967). Therefore, even in our unit, which is highly aware of the decreased attention to the mildly retarded, this population receives less attention than their sheer numbers would imply is needed. Of course, there are often factors in determining services such as the referring source, the need to evaluate the more severely retarded as they appear earlier in life, the relative effectiveness of the school psychologist in dealing with many of the mildly retarded, among others. Nevertheless, it is probably true that the mildly retarded have less of the retardation dollar than the moderately and profoundly retarded, and almost certainly less than their "share" on a purely statistical basis. The one-man-one-vote rule certainly does not apply at the present time in mental retardation circles. Perhaps there is some justification for this; perhaps it will always be that the moderately and severely retarded will require more expenditure of funds than the mildly retarded. However, there are hidden factors beyond the simple reality of severity. Mental retardation pressure groups are often made up of parents of the moderately and severely retarded. Parents of the mildly retarded are overwhelmingly from the lower classes (Group for Advancement of Psychiatry, 1967) and are rarely organized; when they do organize, their efforts are comparatively weak. Further, parental acknowledgment of mild mental retardation prior to school years is almost nonexistent. Sometimes obscured by the vocal upper- and middle-class parents of moderately and severely retarded is the fact that mild retardation, too, cuts across economic boundaries and affects all categories of social class—the disadvantaged most heavily. This discussion also demonstrates some of the subtleties of the coping patterns involved. Both parents and communities are, for many reality reasons, able to "repress" or deny the needs of the mildly retarded more successfully than is the case with the more visible and distressing populations.

### Developing Services

The developmental evaluation unit emanated from the embryonic ideas already enunciated. The parents and professionals worked together to bring about its origin, illustrating the "involvement" stage. But many professionals in the mental health field seem to have a distaste for mental retardation work. In part this attitude may be attributed to the lack of understanding by the professionals of the coping processes (parental and community). The professional is often at a loss to deal with the parent in the midst of a denial process. If this phase is hard for the professional to deal with, the phase of hostility may be even harder. Not recognizing this as a transitory step, the professional may become involved in the hostility and reflect it. Once this is done, he feels badly at his own loss of control and sees himself as inadequate to deal with that particular aspect of mental retardation work. This may lead the professional to exclude himself from the field of mental retardation work.

The frustration of being unable to "cure" can be a terrible burden. Some professionals may think that no amount of skill can lead to the "real" solution of mental retardation problems; therefore, it is best to put one's efforts in another direction. This is particularly true if one looks only at the process of retardation within the child and not at the total complex or how the retardation affects the family. When professionals begin to grasp the idea of the coping process as a longitudinal sequence of events and to see that they may be able to help the various family members over the rough stepping stones toward the idealistic stage of "resolution," the entire order of work takes on a new look. The support of the theoretical framework given by the "coping mechanism hypothesis" gives the professional a structure within which he can work more effectively with less anxiety and to greater purpose.

Recruitment for vacant positions continues to be difficult. Obtaining added positions has been a long, slow, uphill climb; but from the original gerrymandered team of pediatrician, neurologist, speech pathologist, and child psychiatrist a much more cohesive unit evolved still using borrowed pediatric, neurologic, and speech pathology time but now containing full-time social work services, a full-time psychologist, and a full-time public health nurse.

Acceptance of the unit's recommendations and ultimately its

status in the community was initially dependent upon the good will of the various portions of the community. In order to insure this good will the unit made extensive use of the individual key members to approach their particular segment of the professional community. The pediatrician spent a good deal of time with the local pediatricians, discussing the unit's developing program. Initially, the pediatricians were disturbed by the fact that the unit was going to be headed by a child psychiatrist rather than a pediatrician. When it was clear that none of the local pediatricians wished really to assume that responsibility, the opposition grew less intense. Subsequently when child psychiatry leadership proved effective, opposition dropped to a low level. Similarly, the social workers in the community undoubtedly felt their prerogatives were being diminished by the medical administration of such a multidisciplinary team. Experience with the unit quelled their fears, and eventually they felt a good deal more comfortable with the unit.

The unit's child psychiatrist worked with psychiatrists in the mental health services and in private practice. Many psychiatrists were concerned about so much medical involvement. Some visiting psychiatrists seemed appalled at the way we used public health nurses to make home evaluations. These psychiatrists feared that their public health nurses, who had little or no psychiatric training, could not see clearly the family's complex interpersonal machinations, which lead to overprotection or conflicts between the parents about disciplinary approaches, particularly if these patterns were at all subtle. This has not proven to be the case in San Mateo, partly, of course, because heavy emphasis has been placed upon consultative and educative work with these nurses (see Chapter 7); the information returned by the public health nurse on home visits has been extremely useful to the team as a whole. For example, our public health nurse was able to see clearly, in the feeding behavior of one mother, how she frustrated the child's attempt at manual mastery of tableware. This interference with mastery showed up in other areas, as well—in play with toys which would lead to increased coordination. In another instance, the public health nurse described how a father's rejection of his wife left her unsupported, and therefore less able to care appropriately for their retarded child. In still another instance, she reported how a sibling at times served as a mother, enabling the mother to get away for a few hours each week. We were then able to investigate the effect on the sister in this case.

The psychologist's liaison with school psychologists was remarkably helpful in establishing contacts necessary to make the clinic a service to the community. In addition, the interpreting of the unit's work to the schools has gone much more smoothly than we had expected, largely because the unit made use of school psychologists and its own psychologist as the liaison people. Some school psychologists have begun to use the team consultatively. In some instances, without referring a child or family for total work-up, a school psychologist will bring many of the materials to be reviewed by several members of the team, so that a conference may be held to discuss plans for management.

The team approach to evaluating the problems of mental retardation lightens the very heavy burden the professional may feel in dealing with the frustration of working with the retarded and their parents. Recently a school psychologist brought his school principal and the parents of an emotionally disturbed retarded child to our offices for a conference. The child functioned in the range of the educable retarded. The school supplied psychological reports. The child had been seen by a child psychiatrist; a social worker had been involved with the family; and a public health nurse had been making almost routine visits to the family home. But the school was intimidated by the hostility of the parents and had been hesitant to put pressure on the parents to follow the recommendations that the child be excluded from school and placed in a residential treatment facility. Both mother and child were known to be disturbed; there was concern about the child remaining at home without any outside activities. The mother of the child, more than the father, used her denial of the child's problems in a very hysterical, theatrical manner. She expressed anger at many different members of the community, by telephone and in person; although on days when she was feeling differently, she would call the school personnel and express to them her sincere feelings of gratitude for their work in her behalf. The conference had the effect of spreading the expressed hostility on the part of the parents to other members of the community, thus lightening the stress on any one agency, in this case the school. Further, the support given by staff members of the developmental evaluation unit to previous recommendations made denial less possible for the father of the child. The effect of the conference was twofold: first, it enabled school personnel to move ahead in excluding the child from school with a view toward increasing the opportunity for placement of the child in a residential treatment facility. The other effect was more dramatic. It occurred several days after the conference. Police were called to the home of the parents, because the mother was threatening to kill the child and herself with a gun. Various members of the community were involved; the local physician, the public health nurse, the school, and our unit were included. The mother had lost her tenacious hold upon denial, and psychiatric hospitalization had become necessary. This may be seen as an untoward result; but in fact, was this necessarily a disadvantageous result? It permitted the father to make some increased efforts toward the placement of his son in a residential facility. The mother's recovery and subsequent release from the hospital were also forthcoming. Such dramatic events are rather rare, and one would prefer not to go through such disturbances in order to obtain services for the retarded. However, one does not have the luxury of selecting the personalities and psychological makeup of the families with whom one deals. Under the circumstances, the conference proved useful both to the school and to the child and, in the long run, to both parents. The use of team members as support from an "outside expert"—the developmental evaluation unit—enabled the school to proceed toward the necessary goal.

Why should we use the community organization approach instead of attempting directly to control all services to the retarded through county auspices? The answer to this question is both simple and complicated; central control of retardation services has often been talked about. Without a doubt the integration of such services into a coherent network is necessary and central control would probably be, as it is in most things, most efficient until the organization (the machinery for providing services to the retarded) becomes too large and bureaucracy becomes self-defeating. Nevertheless, there is a cogent argument against direct control in one central authority which must be considered. If there is merit in the thesis that the community services and personnel involved in them will reflect certain aspects of the parents' coping reaction, then one would expect these institutions and agents to display and to receive a good deal of hostility.

This assumption quickly sheds new light upon some familiar (and frustrating) phenomena. For instance, in a meeting of one of the local boards—this one composed of professionals—one person speaks up forcibly: "There are too many people from the same agency voting on this question!"

Chairman: "How do you mean—I don't understand! There are people from all sorts of agencies—social service, family service, developmental evaluation unit, schools, and county government!"

The reply: "But there are too many people employed by the county!"

The different roles and different points of view are obscured for this critical person by the fact that they all are employed, with some exceptions, by the county rather than being paid through private funds or Community Chest.

Are his attitudes purely divisive and disruptive? Or are they an overt expression of deeper themes, currents of affect running through the inner life of the community? If so, does this suggest to professionals that, instead of responding with anger and dismay, there may be certain useful, task-oriented goals to be pursued in achieving the effect desired from the community organization endeavor?

If this hostility can be directed to a diffused group of recipients, all of whom share responsibility for serving needs of the retarded, and if it can be recognized as a reflected mechanism, then the chances of raw hostility interfering with the effectiveness of the programs is reduced. To have one central focus of power in retardation leads eventually to an attack on that central source of power. The attack would have to be rebuffed or the central power would have to submit. If, let us say, the power is vested in one county agency and a power struggle ensues which the county wins, then the resulting bitterness and loss of the opportunity for a broad base of community support would ultimately destroy the organization's effectiveness. If the central focus of power submits, there is immediately a power vacuum, disorganization, and confusion. It would seem this is a strong argument against centralization of retardation facilities. This author does not believe, however, that this precludes an organization which, more like a federation, can serve as an integrating force. Indeed, this has led to the evolution of the coordinating committee for mental retardation, in which professional and lay members are striving to integrate planning functions to expand and improve services to the retarded within the community.

But even enlightened members of the community are caught up in these complex reactions to retardation. For instance, as this chapter was being written, the coordinating committee met. During two years of regular meetings but relative inaction, we had not submitted one recommendation to the local governing body. Suddenly there was unanimous agreement on the need for immediate action. In retrospect these two difficult years had been taken up by our passing through the phases of shock, denial, and hostility, and reaching, at least, a partial resolution. By the end of the meeting we had evolved and decided to submit a plan to rectify one of the major gaps in services to the retarded in our county.

Thus, when seemingly nothing is being accomplished or when trouble brews within our coordinating committee for mental retardation people can be encouraged to pursue productive paths—rather than to resign in anger—if they know that these phenomena are symptomatic of a more pervasive process which can eventually result in more productive uses of the community's energy.

## PART III

*The chapters in this section are devoted to various aspects of the indirect services. These community-oriented services are relatively new; their principles and practices are derived from the social sciences as well as medicine. The evolving nomenclature is not yet sufficiently set to be uniformly understood. In general, however, the vocabulary is not new. Familiar words and concepts have been extrapolated into new contexts and imbued with special meanings, just as* prevention, *in public health practice, has been modified and extended to encompass concepts of treatment and rehabilitation. Thus a functional jargon has developed. This brief section provides a preview of definitions and local usage.*

284

# THE INDIRECT
# SERVICES

### Introductory Narrative Glossary*

The Short-Doyle Act *for community mental health services is the California state legislation, enacted in 1957 and amended in 1963 and 1968, which enables local governmental bodies to obtain state subsidy to develop comprehensive community mental health services. The initial legislation was permissive and offered approved programs matching monies. The amendments in 1963 and 1968 increased the state's potential share of the cost from 50 per cent to 75 per cent to 90 per cent. The 1968 amendments also included major substantive changes. Among these were integration of state hospital and Short-*

---

* This "glossary" is provided by Clarice H. Haylett.

*Doyle community service budgets, establishment of fixed program priorities, and revision of the reimbursable basic services. The spectrum of direct patient treatment services was increased, research and evaluation were added, and the indirect services were consolidated. Nevertheless, the basic services as defined in the original act were operative in the decade covered by this narrative. Furthermore, although the 1968 legislation reflects a shift in program emphasis toward treatment of manifest illness and the care of gravely disabled persons, definitions of the approved indirect services were little changed.*

*In 1957, five basic services were specified, of which three were clinical activities directly serving patients and two were aimed at preserving and promoting the mental health of the community by methods which did not usually involve direct contact with identified patients. The* direct *patient treatment services were (1) outpatient, (2) inpatient for up to ninety days, and (3) rehabilitation. The* indirect *or public health services were (1) information and education to the general public and to those professions and agencies whose work supports mental health; and (2) mental health consultation for the staffs of schools, health agencies, probation departments, welfare organizations, and other community agencies to help them deal more effectively with the mental health aspects of their primary tasks.*

*In contrast to the direct treatment services, the indirect services are prevention oriented and comprise the activities of mental health professionals as they work with individuals or organizations to expand their potential for the prevention of mental illness or the promotion of mental health. The educational method emphasizes the transmission of knowledge, whereas the consultation method is more specifically focused on problem-solving in work situations. Problems may relate to the mental health aspects of clients' cases, professional roles, or agency functioning. Consultation may sometimes include observation or other informal evaluation of an agency's clients to assist the consultee in his work. However, California Short-Doyle standards for indirect services exclude formal psychiatric diagnosis as an aspect of mental health consultation.*

*Consultation can be differentiated from other methods employed by mental health personnel by assessing primary intent and defined responsibilities.* Psychotherapy *is primarily for the purpose of increasing the patient's effectiveness in coping with his personal prob-*

*lems. Any sector of the patient's past or present living might be the subject of joint scrutiny. Consultation, in contrast, focuses on work problems and deals only with immediately relevant issues.*

Administration *involves executive functions and decision-making. The consultant is properly only a facilitator.* Supervision *involves responsibility for the work of the supervisee. As has been pointed out (Gilbert, 1960), a consultant brings only the authority of ideas.* Collaboration *involves shared responsibility. This can be at the clinical level where case data are shared and future actions planned. Agencies can also collaborate at the administrative or program level. Similarly, when agency representatives and individual citizens meet to deal with community problems, there is shared concern.* Community organization *covers a wide range of activities in which there may be definition of a community problem, plans for its solution, and implementation of those plans.*

*We define our* community *as the human ecology within the geographic confines of San Mateo County. We think of our community as a dynamic system of social systems. We use the term* social system *loosely to mean a collection of individuals drawn together in one or more agencies or organizations to further a common social function. Lindemann (1966) suggests that each community, whether geographically or functionally defined, has social systems to deal with such common community functions as governmental administration, education, health care, control of deviants, care of dependents, and transmission of moral and cultural values. In a comprehensive community mental health program, these are the systems with which we aim to establish consultative relationships.*

*In mental health consultation, the* consultant *is a mental health specialist who consults with* consultees *who are generally professionals from other socially relevant fields. In consultation jargon,* clients *are the people served by the consultee in his professional role. They may be students if the consultee is a teacher, patients if the consultee is a nurse, and so on. Before consultation actually begins, there should be an understanding between the consultant and the consultee and the consultee's organization about what is intended to be done and other details. Whether verbal or written, such an understanding has come to be called the* consultation contract.

*The indirect services are often linked with the goal of* primary prevention—*the actual avoidance of illness. This goal can be accomplished by educative, consultative, or organizational activities that render the environment less hazardous and that facilitate healthy growth and the development of adequate coping mechanisms. The indirect services can also be related to* secondary prevention *when they lead to attenuation or amelioration of disease; perhaps through early identification and referral for effective treatment. Similarly, the indirect services may be vehicles for* tertiary prevention *when they contribute to successful rehabilitation and limitation of disability. If one can help educate the community to greater acceptance of former mental patients, or consult with a potential employer, or help organize a halfway house, one is working at the tertiary level. Thus indirect service methods can support prevention at every level.*

CHAPTER **12**

# Evolution of Indirect Services

*Clarice H. Haylett*

California's 1957 Short-Doyle
Act, like the 1963 federal community mental health center legislation,
gave significant impetus to the development of indirect (non-treat-
ment) services. In addition to various traditional and innovative approaches to patient care, mental health education and consultation
were recognized as basic services. Local mental health administrators
were enjoined to take leadership in planning and developing comprehensive community programs in which there would be a broad spectrum of services. Principles and methods from public health were to
be melded with the best of hospital and clinic practice to provide
many-faceted prevention-oriented programs.

289

The rationale for a broader approach to the control of mental illness was certainly idealistic, there being no proof that public health methods would be effective. Nevertheless, since World War II, there was increasing awareness of the limitations of the traditional treatment-oriented, one-to-one, doctor-patient model. Even extending patient treatment services by providing ancillary therapists from allied professions (and more recently by the use of indigenous nonprofessionals), and by augmenting individual therapy with family and group approaches, did not appear sufficient to significantly reduce the incidence or prevalence of mental illness. Socially concerned psychiatrists, such as those who banded together to form the Group for Advancement of Psychiatry, public health officers, and other governmental officials who were concerned about the cost of mental illness as well as the humanitarian aspects of the problem, increasingly turned their attention to the possibility of prevention-oriented methods.

In the forties and fifties, private foundations such as Milbank, Commonwealth, and Grant subsidized a number of projects whose goal was the prevention of mental illness and social disability. Social scientists joined clinicians in a quest for techniques which could be used to study the epidemiology of mental illness. Biological, psychological, and social factors contributory to mental health as well as mental disorders were systematically scrutinized. Particular interest focused on the determinants of healthy emotional development in early childhood. In a field pioneered by Anna Freud, others such as Erikson, Spitz, and Bowlby also studied children and derived additional principles of normal and deviant psychobiological growth. Furthermore, Anna Freud gave lectures to parents and teachers on child growth and development, in the hope that enlightenment would facilitate healthier child rearing (Freud, 1931).

While Erikson (1959) was elaborating and extending his schema of developmental stages and tasks, Lindemann (1944) was studying the mental health implications of "accidental" crises. Major situational stresses such as bereavement also challenged the usual coping mechanisms. Adaptations and the assumption of new roles were required, if a crisis was to be weathered and perhaps even growth-enhancing. Failure, as with critical stages of psychobiological development, could result in susceptibility to later disorders as well as immediately apparent disability. People were seen to be more vulnerable, more susceptible to outside influence at times of crisis. They could be conceptualized as "at risk" and in need of enlightened emotional support at such times. In a more recent and comprehensive conceptualization Caplan (1967) also includes in the "at risk" category those people who experience chronic as well as acute deprivation of physical, psychosocial, or sociocultural resources.

The studies of the Joint Commission on Mental Illness and Health documented that most situational crises were not perceived as psychiatric matters (Gurin, Veroff, and Feld, 1960). The majority of troubled people turned first to their clergyman or family doctor rather than to psychological counselors for help with their personal problems. Clergymen, physicians, nurses, social workers, policemen, judges, and probation officers, school personnel, and many other community service professionals were clearly more strategically situated for sensitive intervention at times of life crisis than mental health clinicians. Thus, prevention-oriented programs that aimed to apply what was being learned about crisis intervention, as well as other potentially relevant psychological insights, needed to become allied with other community service agents. This task might be approached by a variety of educative, collaborative, and consultative techniques, assuming that the other community agencies and professionals shared an interest in and concern for the mental health needs of their clients and a willingness to work with mental health consultants.

Finally, from many areas came a reaffirmation of the importance of the social milieu and its potential for support, or failure to support, individual growth and meaningful existence. Not only the nuclear family, but extended families, work groups, religious congregations, and a vast constellation of dynamic groupings form the social matrix for human life. Both at the small group and at the community level, deficiencies and distortions were recognized as having the potential to fault character development, precipitate overt psychopathology, and limit rehabilitation potential. Thus mental health workers were needed with skills in social group work, community organization, public education, and other methods that might favorably influence the social environment.

Actually, most of the preceding rationale was unknown to us in 1958, when the San Mateo mental health consultation, education, and information service was initiated. San Mateo County, it should be noted, was unusually well-endowed and progressive in provision of public and private psychiatric services, well before the Short-Doyle Act was passed. Already operative under county auspices were an open-door therapeutic community inpatient service, an adult outpatient clinic, and a child guidance clinic. The child guidance clinic, at various times in its history, had provided mental health consultation to several child-serving community agencies. There were also two private psychiatric hospitals, a substantial number of psychiatrists and a few psychologists and social workers in private practice. In addition, most of the schools had at least rudimentary school guidance programs, the larger districts employing one or more school psychologists and occasionally school social workers as well. The enlightened administrators of the public health and welfare and probation departments already had well-established professional recruitment and staff development practices, including psychiatric consultation. Additionally, there were two private casework agencies and a number of other voluntary health and welfare agencies that shared a concern for the community's emotional as well as social and physical health problems. The Mental Health Association, which had been instrumental in promoting and supporting the child guidance clinic, welcomed the new Short-Doyle program. Finally, there was an unusually active and effective Council of Social Agencies which, at the request of the county health officer, H. D. Chope, had been working for three years surveying the mental health resources and needs of the county. Thus, there was an involved and well-informed citizenry as well as a wealth of existing public and private services when the Short-Doyle Act was passed. The state community mental health legislation gave a financial as well as philosophical incentive to consolidate the existing public services and to expand them into a comprehensive community program.

In San Mateo County, the new indirect service unit was initiated as a subsection of the child guidance clinic. This seemed natural, since the child guidance clinic had always performed some consultative functions. In anticipation of implementation of the Short-Doyle Act, additional staff were recruited; they brought with them a variety of professional training and experience, which proved fortuitous. Originally there were two child psychiatrists, a clinical psychologist, and a social worker. In addition to the usual diagnostic and clinical skills, our experiential repertory included public health administration, post-residency psychiatric consultation, school psychology, mental health consultation to schools, social group work, and community organization.

By administrative fiat we were told we were "the consultation service" and to go forth and develop a county-wide program. At that time the relevant literature was minimal and widely scattered. Actually there had been several pioneering mental health consultation projects in the San Francisco Bay Area by Mary Sarvis, Beulah Parker, Irving Berlin (1962) and other child psychiatrists and psychoanalysts. We learned that relevant work had also been done in Massachusetts and New York State. However, the doers were often not writers, and we turned to the Short-Doyle Act itself for an initial orientation to our new professional responsibilities.

Portia Bell Hume, then the Deputy Director in charge of Community Services for the State Department of Mental Hygiene, had written guidelines for the implementation of the act (Hume, 1957). Mental health education and consultation were described as two kinds of services that would "promote mental health in the community." Information and education were to be supplied to the general public and to professions and agencies concerned with mental health. Mental health consultation was to be provided to the staffs of schools, public health departments, probation officers, welfare departments, and the like, to "help them deal more effectively with their children's or clients' mental health problems before they become severe enough to require psychiatric treatment." Although the act named some of the major caregiving, people-serving organizations that should be recipients of mental health consultation, the guidelines encouraged sufficient program flexibility that there might be wide local variations in programs, in order that each might fit special local conditions to the greatest possible extent. There was not the precise template of action which we would have appreciated at that time, but there were suggestions indicating the direction and general method of procedure for our assigned work.

As we set about deciding what we would do, life was both complicated and simplified by the fact that we had been clearly mandated by our administration to take all of our available professional time to develop a county-wide consultation service and ourselves as consultants. Actually, protected time is essential for the cultivation of interagency indirect service relationships, and we had much to learn. However, we often felt guilty, being aware of the clinic's "waiting-for-treatment" list. Furthermore, when our initial overtures to potential consultee agencies were rebuffed or only ceremonially acknowledged, we often wondered whether the indirect services were possible or economically justifiable. It was nearly a year before we decided in the affirmative.

Our development as consultants was stimulated by occasional institutes sponsored by the State Departments of Mental Hygiene and Public Health. Gerald Caplan regularly participated, and William Hollister exposed us to concepts of mental health education. We also had county-sponsored in-staff training and secured Caplan and Irving Berlin for a few sessions. However, as each visiting expert shared his views and experiences, we found they were either too general or too specifically related to another situation to be immediately applicable to ours. Actually, at that time there was also considerable difference of opinion among the experts on several questions basic to program development.

In the absence of any clear authoritative patterns of procedure, we were forced to develop our own styles, relying heavily on our clinical and administrative experiences in other settings. In retrospect, this situation was probably fortunate. We developed a group supervisory practice. As problems arose in planning and later in various types of negotiations and consultation ventures, they would be presented at the weekly staff meeting. These interdisciplinary problem-solving sessions have continued as an essential aspect of staff development.

Within a year of the inception of the service, there began to be invitations to share what we were learning with other professional groups, especially with newly developing Short-Doyle centers. Although scanning the literature, attending institutes, and participating in ongoing group supervision had all contributed to our professional growth as practicing consultants, communicating what was being practiced required a different level of abstraction. Accurate description necessitated definition of terms and sophisticated study of a process involving oneself and others. These transactions needed to be placed in a meaningful context. Thus, research and teaching required conceptualization and became important adjuncts to our continuing education.

It was fairly clear from the outset that optimally the mental health consultant should be (or become) expert in two general areas: the content area in mental health about which he would be consulting and the process or technical aspects of the method he would be using. For example, consultants asked to function as mental health educators would need to know something of educational techniques. If the situation required community organization he would need either skill in this area or the ability to recognize this gap in his own training and delegate it to someone better equipped to handle the situation.

For several years consultation, as a method, was our primary interest, perhaps because we were called consultants and it was a logical extension of child guidance practice. As clinicians working with children, we were familiar with the importance of the family and social milieu for the understanding and treatment of children's problems. It was customary, as an adjunct to the treatment of any child, to work with the parents. Often we talked to parents in terms of the child, but with the hypothesis that at some unconscious level they might share complementary psychopathology. It was hoped that the parental problem might be modified or resolved by working through relevant issues in terms of the child, and that the parent would then be free to deal effectively with his child. The similarity of this technique to consultee-centered consultation is obvious. Child therapists are also accustomed to the use of parables and metaphors. They are sensitive to the possible need to facilitate better communication between the child and those people importantly involved with him. As therapists, they may catalyze a group meeting of interested parties to clarify issues and facilitate collaboration. They are accustomed to adjusting their tempo of interventions to the therapeutic situation. For instance, they may be quite active when the child is withdrawn and silent. Such sensitivity and flexibility is equally desirable in consultation.

The expert in consultation process must have a working knowledge of intrapsychic as well as interpersonal phenomena. He needs the kind of sensitivity that allows him to be a multidimensional listener— one who perceives nonverbal as well as verbal cues, who can follow content and process simultaneously, and who is aware of transference and countertransference as they affect the transaction. Since much indirect service activity takes place in group settings, a knowledge of group dynamics is also desirable.

In retrospect, it seems that our most effective consultants have been those who were interested in applying their clinical skills in a different way. They have been able to shift their focus of primary interest and responsibility from the case or matter being discussed to the consultee's dilemma. They have also been concerned with their own development as consultants and with the consultation process. Finally, they have brought with them or developed sufficient personal and professional maturity to allow them to understand and empathize with supervisory and administrative personnel as well as with workers and clients. It is likely that, as Marmor postulates for effectiveness in psychotherapy, the personal qualities of the consultant and the length of his professional experience are of greater import than the particular conceptual model which he professes to follow (Marmor, 1962).

In our service, the largest amount of time has always been devoted to consultation rather than to public information, general professional education, or community organization. This situation may be because of the close ancestral ties between consultation and the clinical methods. Stated another way, it is probably a reflection of the interests and competencies of incumbent staff. Not until an expert in community organization joined our group did we realize the potential as well as the complexities of that method. Only when a mass media expert joined the services as a "demonstration officer" were public information services greatly improved and expanded. Likewise, the addition of a mental health nurse and marriage counselor, and the periodic availability of a health educator and a sociologist has served to deepen our understanding of the community and how we may more effectively relate to it.

Diversification of staff has increased the variety of consultee organizations with which we can effectively work. Expertise in various specialized content areas, in addition to competence in the consultative process, is desirable. As child guidance personnel, we were awkward consultants to nursing homes for the aged. This work was improved when we recruited a colleague from our inpatient service. Although the essence of the consultation process is to help the consultee use his own expert knowledge more effectively, the transaction is significantly enhanced when the consultant is also an expert in the mental health aspects of the kinds of clients that are likely to be discussed.

Learning how to be consultants, and somewhat later, educators and organizers, proceeded simultaneously with program development. Coming from clinical work, the pace of the new community work seemed impossibly slow; we were organizationally naive. Building a new program, like building a house, requires a systematic approach and tedious groundwork. Actually, our foundations were firm, both legally in terms of the program objectives and methods defined in the Short-Doyle Act, and administratively in the sense of strong general policy support from our mental health director, mental health advisory board, and program chief. Only we and our former clinic colleagues seemed uncertain about procedure and outcome.

We started by orienting ourselves. We became familiar with all of our own mental health services and then set about defining the broader community. Census data were studied for demographic characteristics. We enumerated social functions and listed the professional groups and agencies that appeared to have active service programs. The Council of Social Agencies had recently published a comprehensive handbook and the League of Women Voters had an excellent synopsis describing governmental structure and functions. The annual county budget was also available and full of program as well as fiscal data. The County Superintendent of Schools issued an annual school directory, and the voluntary agencies all had some sort of brochure describing services. For a population of less than half a million persons, there was an amazing variety of community services.

The Short-Doyle Act had enumerated several general categories of agencies that should be recipients of our services. Those that were clearly eligible seemed to have as common denominators either that they served people at times of crisis or had significant contacts with children. In order to reduce the eligible list to more manageable proportions, we added some further qualifications. If we were to provide mental health consultation, it should be to agencies having professional staff who were actually providing direct services to patients or clients. Public agencies would have a higher priority than private, and we would not provide services where there seemed a reasonable possibility of obtaining comparable services privately. We did not then appreciate the difference between an isolated psychiatric case or ad-

ministrative consultation and the public health potential resulting
from the establishment of a network of indirect service relationships
throughout the community. Actually, piecemeal private consultation,
no matter how skilled, cannot have the same interagency impact as
mental health consultation which is part of a coordinated community
program.

Since clergymen and physicians were widely scattered and
usually in individual or small group practice, we tried to reach them
through educational, rather than consultative, projects. We obtained
a small NIMH grant with which we recruited men from the private
sector of psychiatry to serve as faculty in a year-long seminar on "psychiatry in general practice." Some private consultative relationships
evolved from this. The following year, the postgraduate extension division of a nearby medical school collaborated to provide hospital-
based weekend workshops to physicians. University extension divisions now provide a variety of courses and workshops each year. The
adult education and extension divisions of local community colleges,
as well as state colleges and universities, are also a rich resource for
mental health education. They may collaborate or take full initiative
and responsibility for presenting mental health subjects in TV panels,
lectures, seminars, workshops, and courses for both the lay and professional public. For three years, we have collaborated with a private
college to provide a postgraduate course on mental health for classroom teachers.

Although educational institutions are increasingly active in
community education, the Mental Health Association has been our
traditional partner. Through the years, we have co-sponsored seminars
for policemen and volunteers who will be working in mental health
facilities, as well as for clergymen. Mental health education to clergy
increased markedly after a marriage counselor with ministerial training joined our staff. He developed a short sequence of seminars on
pastoral counseling. He also consults with other staff when they have
occasion to work with clergy. Likewise, the addition of a nurse mental
health consultant greatly expedited educational work with nurses. We
often think of mental health consultation as a potential bridge between
two professional subcultures, namely, the mental health services and a
consultee system. A mental-health-oriented member of the consultee's
professional subculture can be an important link in such a bridge.

In spite of the foregoing on the evolution of educational activities, the bulk of our energies went into trying to develop consultative relationships with all of our defined major caregiving social systems. Some of our potential consultees already had psychiatric consultants. We invited these individuals to collaborate, and some joined our staff on a professional service basis. Other potential consultee agencies were not initially interested in psychiatric or any other type of consultation. Those who saw little connection between their professional work and the fate of persons identified as mentally ill often had concluded that their work also had little relevance for the much broader field of mental health. To develop a relationship with these organizations required a variety of overtures. Over several years, however, this was usually possible, if we were sufficiently motivated to follow up on any pretext for initiating a dialogue.

The question who should consult with whom arose very early and initially was resolved by asking who among us could work in a particular setting. We tried to take into consideration any traditional professional role or status variables, as well as personal preferences and relevant prior experience. On this basis, the psychiatrists tended to start work with health and social service agencies, psychologists with correctional systems and schools, and social workers with a number of less well-defined organizations and professions. The social workers also gravitated to the community organization projects. Once the initial consultant was well established in a system, however, colleagues with other professional origins could be introduced with greater ease.

To describe the initiation of mental health consultation in any particular system meaningfully, the process should be recorded in considerable detail. For instance, in 1958 in San Mateo County, there were thirty-one administratively separate public school districts, not including private, parochial, or nursery schools. Only a few of the larger districts had their own special services and guidance personnel. Only one of these had a school guidance program that included social workers, as well as a psychologist and consultation from a child psychiatrist.

The bulk of psychological services were provided by staff from the office of the county superintendent of schools. The county's director of special services was unusually interested in child guidance and consultation, and encouraged us to meet with his staff and the county school psychologists as a group. It seemed of primary importance to start work with the school psychologists, since we needed to clarify both how we could be of help to them and how we could work with other school personnel without being competitive or creating additional role confusion. Consultation to teachers and principals is, in fact, an important aspect of their functioning, and in each system we needed to explore how we might both facilitate their work and perhaps also extend mental health consultation to others.

However, before establishing more than casual information-sharing contacts with the school psychologists, we needed administrative sanction to proceed. Thus, we addressed ourselves to the district superintendents, both as individuals and collectively through their county association. Somewhat later we also secured an invitation to speak at the annual meeting of the county school boards association, in order to explain our program to them and to invite their understanding and sanctions at that level. All this took time.

Our initial approach to the school superintendents was to send an introductory letter and follow up with a personal interview. The first year there were many failed appointments. It was difficult to get through to some of the superintendents who were, in fact, very busy men and probably also wondering what mental health clinic personnel wanted with them. Eventually, all were seen and permission was obtained to explore in detail how we might function in their particular system. Usually the chief psychologist or director of guidance was officially designated as the person with whom we were to continue administrative negotiations. In many of the smaller districts, however, the superintendent himself continued the dialogue.

Their first interest was usually whether we would make available direct diagnostic and treatment services to their already well-identified disturbed children. A few had feared that this was what we would propose to do in their schools, but most were disappointed that it was not. Some then questioned any other useful function except, possibly, serving as clinical consultants to the guidance staff. A few were interested in trying out the usefulness of consultation to themselves, and some proposed consultation for principals, guidance counselors, and teachers of special classes. Some proposed that we conduct group therapy with parents of handicapped children; others urged training for staff in group counseling techniques. (The current pressure is for sensitivity group training.) Some of the younger psychologists wanted technical assistance and supervision of their projective testing and ongoing counseling and psychotherapy.

Clearly, we needed to define for ourselves role limits that were consonant with our abilities, service responsibilities, and the school setting. Since other clinic and private patient services were potentially available, we unequivocally and consistently excluded any diagnosis or treatment. We might, occasionally, jointly observe a child, but there was no pretense that this constituted an adequate clinical examination. We also declined to provide in-service training on group methods or to advise on how to set up a model school guidance program. We did, however, consult about these proposals to the point where the administration had clarified what was wanted and where they might find more appropriate experts.

It became a general principle that we would do what we could to enhance the mental health effectiveness of incumbent professionals in the furthering of their assigned functions. Thus, we consulted about problems involving psychodiagnostic testing or counseling in the school setting, if this was part of the consultee's official duties. However, we declined to offer indoctrination in clinical methods, if they were not clearly appropriate to the consultee's work assignment or when it was clear that an occupational transition was desired and formal education in a training center would be more appropriate.

When an experienced social group worker joined our staff, we did offer to co-lead some parent groups. This was for the primary purpose of helping school staff devolop sufficient confidence and competence in themselves to continue such programs. There was no premise that we could provide this service wherever it might be desirable. Similarly, we have, at times, made an experienced school social worker available on a demonstration basis. However, even if philosophical and ethical issues were not sufficient to militate against the county mental health service actually contracting to deliver a comprehensive school guidance service program, the administrative impediments, in California at least, are almost insurmountable.

The roles of our mental health consultants in the various school settings were grossly defined by initial administrative negotiations. They were subsequently refined in discussions with intermediaries and, most importantly, with those professionals who chose or were assigned to work with us. (We soon learned to request participation on a voluntary basis.)

In the first few years, we tended to deny or feel guilty that we were not often in a position to provide consultee-centered case consultation directly to the classroom teachers, who were most immediately involved with disturbed children. As we became more experienced in school work in this particular area, we recognized that consultation with elementary school principals, secondary school deans and chief counselors, teachers of the handicapped, and central office specialists in guidance, curriculum, and nursing could easily absorb all available consultation time. Furthermore, we are now satisfied that in schools, as in other consultee systems, scarce consultation time may be most effectively deployed in collaborative relationships with middle management and any designated special services and training personnel. These echelons appear to be the professional culture carriers for their organizations. Elected or designated directors can declare policy, but how it is translated into action seems to be vested in the intermediate supervisory strata. Thus, if we hope to introduce or reinforce principles of mental health practice, we need the general sanction of top administration and hope for more than occasional consultative sessions with line workers. However, our highest service priority will be to be available for work with the training and intermediate supervisory echelons.

Actually, we became associated with different agencies and professional populations in different ways. What there was in common was a willingness on the part of the potential consultee agency to talk with us and see if there might be some way in which we could be of appropriate use. In some instances, this involved jointly collaborating on a research project, such as the pre-employment screening of deputy sheriffs (see Chapter 13). In other settings, consultative relationships evolved from an information or education project, such as a seminar series on the psychosocial development of children.

Where the supply of diagnostic and treatment services is limited in relation to demand (which seems to be universal), it is our experience here, as it was Eisenberg's in Baltimore, that social agency collaborators may increasingly use the scarce time for consultation instead of direct client services (Eisenberg, 1958). Thus, the child guidance clinic's service program to the juvenile hall, juvenile probation, and the juvenile court has moved from a primary mission of direct service to one of considerable consultation (see Chapter 10). Similarly, the adult courts and corrections unit soon redefined its optimal usage and transferred its administrative affiliation from the adult clinic to the consultation service. Direct clinical services to patients or clients will always be a natural base for the development of indirect consultative relationships. However, as will be discussed later in more detail, there are both advantages and disadvantages to the consultant's being available for both kinds of services.

The organizational and administrative negotiations which were necessary to prepare the way for consultation were tremendously time-consuming. Our psychiatrists and psychologists, more than our social work colleagues, were sometimes insufficiently prepared for the exquisite complexities of the task we had so cheerfully undertaken. As Howe (1964) has pointed out, if one is a layman in community organization and ill-informed about the facts of life in social systems, it is easy to invite system rejection by improper timing or procedure. Fortunately, potential consultees are usually charitable when the would-be consultant seems to have something to offer and is sincerely desirous of learning to be helpful in their settings.

Regardless of the niceties of preparation, actually beginning consultation with an individual or group is generally a stressful time for all concerned. The neophyte consultant may be fortified if he appreciates that he may have to deal with any of four levels of defense in regard to any particular issue. The consultee's work problem may be based in some personal or cultural "hangup" having to do with insufficient knowledge, skill, self-confidence, lack of sensitivity, or insufficient objectivity, to define and cope with the situation. Professional values and traditions may also interfere with his understanding and doing the human thing. Sometimes co-worker or supervisorial conflicts within the "work family" result in problems with clients, as well as in perplexities for the consultant. Finally, the institution or social system itself may have socially assigned functions as well as policies and regulations which are conflicting, dehumanizing, and otherwise dissonant with the mental health consultant's own values and operational practices.

The more the consultant is perceived as critical and alien, the more difficult will be his task of establishing a viable working relationship. He is bound to be tested in many ways. With each consultee, he will have to enact and so redefine their individual contract. His role limits and trustworthiness will surely be tested, and he must demonstrate that, as a consultant, he will not play psychotherapist or decision-maker. He must prove a trustworthy confidant and helpful associate. After the initiation rites have been weathered, a working relationship based on mutual respect and trust generally evolves. Such relationships are a potential vehicle for increasing interagency understanding and cooperation, as well as for dealing more effectively with the mental health aspects of a particular client or agency problem. The consultation service aims for the development and maintenance of such relationships with all major caregiving social systems.

CHAPTER **13**

# Issues of Indirect Services

*Clarice H. Haylett*

There are a number of possible patterns for developing and administering an indirect services program. From the outset our designated indirect service personnel were administratively separated from their patient treatment service colleagues. At the same time all identifiable indirect service functions were relegated to the new consultation unit. It was soon apparent there were both advantages and disadvantages to separation and specialization.

Of course, there is bound to be some overlapping with direct service functions. What is considered direct and indirect must in some instances be an arbitrary decision. This is exemplified by the academic niceties of separating screening and client evaluation activities, which are to aid a consultee in his work, from direct diagnostic services and case collaboration which may also aid a consultee in his work.

Furthermore, there are situations in which both direct and indirect services are most economically performed by the same personnel. This seems especially to be the case in institutional settings where the clients—whether patients, prisoners, or boarders—are controlled by the institution. Even diagnostic services require recognition of the dependent status of the client and some familiarity with the institutional subculture. Treatment, in such settings, necessitates the cooperation and preferably the active support of the establishment. Where a clinician has learned to collaborate effectively with institutional staff, he is likely to be far more acceptable to them for indirect service functions than an unknown and relatively unknowledgeable outsider. Thus, as earlier mentioned, an operation that begins as an extension of an outpatient service may, in time, change its primary focus and character of service (compare Chapter 14).

Finally, staff on all of the direct, as well as the indirect, services tend to accumulate special knowledge as they mature in their work. Thus direct service staff are often the most appropriate educators on many mental health subjects such as suicide prevention, drug abuse, and so on. Furthermore, as they become aware of community problems that have relevance for the care and rehabilitation of their patients, it is natural and logical that they collaborate with other agencies and individuals to ameliorate such problems. Thus, in an active, responsive community mental health program, a completely rigid separation of the direct and indirect services is probably neither possible nor desirable. Whoever is responsible for the overall administration of the indirect services should, however, know what his direct service colleagues are doing in the community services area and coordinate, but not necessarily control, major involvements with other community agencies.

A significant advantage in having an administratively separate service is that time is more easily protected. It takes time to develop as a consultant, educator, or community organizer. Mastering these methods is enhanced by being a member of a dedicated interdisciplinary staff that shares experiences and works together over time. It also takes time, and flexibly available time, to develop the kind of relationship with a consultee agency that permits fruitful collaboration and consultation. Months and even years may be required. Besides the formal overtures, the would-be consultant must be alert and available to pick up on any opportunity for a dialogue with the administrators of the potential consultee agency. With even the most guarded and aloof organizations, sooner or later there are opportunities for the would-be consultant to become known to his potential consultees in some nonthreatening capacity. If, however, he has no free time to make an occasional speech, attend an occasional community meeting, or visit his potential consultees at their offices and at their convenience, he probably does not have the kind of time necessary to develop a new service.

Even after a consultant has been accepted into a consultee system, it takes time for him to learn a particular agency's subculture, its primary functions, professional values, methods, and jargon. It takes time to understand typical work problems and the administrative structure that should facilitate the work of the agency. Only when the consultant has shown himself trustworthy and generally useful can he negotiate freely with a consultee system. Much is invested by both the mental health service and the consultee agency in the on-the-job education of such "system specialists."

We use these senior system experts as coordinators who keep track of all of the indirect services being desired, offered, and used by their consultee organizations. System coordinators are generally responsible for the administrative aspects of negotiating an annual contract for services, reviewing the services rendered annually, and other aspects of the interagency relationship. They are also centrally involved in recruiting, training, and generally supervising new consultants who are brought into the system. Optimally, a system coordinator should be a mature professional person who has consulted and negotiated with his system for some years. To have done so reflects a liking for and competence in both the indirect services and working with that particular system. An administratively separate consultation service seems more likely to attract and retain such staff, at least on a part-time basis, than a service in which staff have a variety of patient and agency responsibilities.

The third advantage of an administratively separate service is that the would-be consultant is more clearly presented as available only for indirect service functions. The consultee agency may then find it easier to accept the consultant's role limits when he declines to diagnose or treat clients in the agency setting or when he does not directly intervene to obtain preferential services for their clients. Actually, consultants do have many other professional roles. In the clinic and in private practice they may diagnose and treat agency clients and hold collaborative case conferences with agency personnel. They may also be educators, organizers, administrative negotiators, research associates, and so on. Where direct patient services are in exceedingly short supply or difficult to arrange, the consultant may provide brief client evaluation and screening service. If he is the only mental health professional in the area, obviously he will do whatever he can that is professionally appropriate.

However, if an agency begins to experience consultation as simply a means of obtaining clinical services for their clients, the spectrum of consultation issues will be narrowed to whatever the consultees consider their most "mentally ill" clients, and the increasingly ambivalent consultant may see little advantage to initiating an intake with agency staff in their establishment instead of with the clients themselves in his office. Where consultants are generalists who do both direct patient services and consultation, the use of consultation solely as a referral gambit has been minimized by establishing the policy that there will be no connection between presenting a case to the consultant and having it picked up or not through the clinic's usual intake procedures.

There are also disadvantages to an administratively separate indirect services unit. We look upon the indirect services as reciprocal processes: we share information, knowledge, and concerns with our consultees. As consultants, we become bridges to different community subcultures and periodically become privy to insights that have relevance for colleagues in other branches of our service. Administrative separation of the direct and indirect services reduces opportunities for a natural and informal flow of information. Separation promotes estrangement. Eventually, the full-time consultant may lose his clinical identity unless he has other direct service outlets such as a part-time private practice.

The question of promoting specialization in indirect services is also related to the availability of other mental health professional staff and the size of the population to be served. Where staff are few, generalization is the usual pattern. Where staff are more abundant (and this usually presumes a greater population to be served), some degree of specialization may be not only more feasible, but more efficient. In San Mateo County indirect services are presently provided by generalized staff in one regional office who do both direct and inrect services, by specialized staff from the central office, and by two central special units that provide both direct and indirect services to circumscribed populations in correctional settings.

As regionalization proceeds, our county plan calls for delegating many more indirect service functions to generalists in the regional offices. Where consultee agencies are wholly within regional geographic boundaries, for example, some school districts, police departments, recreational districts, and churches, these will be serviced definitively by regional office consultants. Consultation in regional offices will be coordinated by a full-time specialist on the regional office administrative staff. A cadre of central office consultation specialists will be maintained, however, to provide in-service training and ongoing support to generalist staff. They will also continue to be available for consultation to the administrative echelons of county-wide organizations and to coordinate the indirect services to major functional groupings.

Although initially our consultation staff were all full-time employees, we soon found that most able consultants wanted to maintain and improve their clinical skills. They also wanted to make more money. Thus, after a year or two, most of the psychiatrists and psychologists reduced their service time and expanded their private patient practices. Some experienced consultants have been hired on a half-time basis and some for as little as four hours per week. For overall service objectives, however, at least half-time initially is desirable, since it permits an adequate orientation, regular staff and supervisory meetings, and an opportunity for identification with the service as a whole. Our consultants often remain with the service for many years and thus contribute a sense of stability and continuity to the consultee systems they coordinate. Consultants who are hired for only a few hours per week generally work only as case consultants and tend to remain relatively isolated from the administrative mainstream.

### Training and Research

Another administrative issue of current concern is the optimal balance between research and training and community service obligations. In recent years, both training and research functions have burgeoned. In 1967 a twelve-month introductory course was offered on the principles and techniques of mental health education, consultation, and community organization. Biweekly lectures and supervised field experience were provided. Trainees included third- and fourth-year psychiatric residents and staff from all the clinical disciplines. This course is being repeated and will probably become a regular service commitment. The service also provides field placements for trainees from many centers. (See Chapter 16, on training, for more details about this course and other training activities.)

In addition to the considerable staff time now spent in training and supervision, the senior psychologists spend 40 per cent of their time in research. In the absence of additional staff, the net result has been a significant lessening of community service. Trainees under the supervision of experienced staff meet some of the service demands, but short-term trainees are not freely interchangeable with regular staff. Our experience suggests that the service gain is not really significant unless the trainee is sufficiently committed to involve himself half-time or more for at least one year and preferably two. Although field work in mental health education can usually be arranged on a piecemeal basis, the process of interagency consultation requires time for preparation and relationship building. Most of last year's trainees lamented that after six months they were just beginning to get a good sense of the process and to take satisfaction in their work when it was time to begin termination.

More important, from the perspective of a service agency, consultee systems frequently do not welcome annual replacement of consultants, regardless of trainee or staff status. They invest considerable time in the education of the consultant and do not like to lose him just as he becomes knowledgeable and effective in their setting.

There appears to be a natural evolution in the development of a consultant's usefulness to a particular system in a particular capacity. For a consultant new to such systems it may take a year or two to attain peak effectiveness. Then there is a plateau period followed by a lessening of the contribution that he can make to the same consultees. However, in most of the settings where we consult there is a growing edge with new programs, new positions, and new staff. Thus, a consultant experienced in a particular system usually moves where the need is greatest. Consultants always being in short supply, the possibility of stagnation, or of developing overly dependent relationships, is usually avoided.

Continuity over time is required for the natural evolution of consultation experience. Consultants in a system tend to move upward from lower staff echelons to higher supervisory and administrative strata. Given time and effective working together, consultants also tend to shift from mental health education and case-oriented consultation to consultee-centered consultation about administrative and program issues, as well as clients. This type of increasingly rich relationship between the consultant and a whole consultee system is predicated on the growth of mutual respect and trust.

In addition to the limited continuity of service that is inevitable with transient trainees, both training and research can threaten the foundations of trust which are basic to our community relationships. To build these ties there needs to be confidence that the consultant is unfailing in his discretion. Most professional matters discussed with consultees are understood to be privileged and, unless the consultee wishes it, not discussed with others within the consultee's organization, and rarely in any other setting. (Occasionally, very complicated issues are reviewed in consultation with a senior colleague in the consultation service. However, strict confidence is then maintained.) Unlike clinic patients, consultees often have many other personal and professional contacts with mental health personnel. Consultee agencies are difficult to disguise. The safest practice is to observe the prescription which concludes the Hippocratic oath: "Whatever things I see or hear concerning the life of men in the attendance on the sick or even apart therefrom, which ought not to be noised abroad, I will keep silence thereon, counting such things to be as sacred secrets."

Written, as well as verbal, communication should be considered and guarded. Individual consultants' records of ongoing service are a personal matter. A few make detailed records of their work in order to understand the process better. Others make none. At the service level, only minimal administrative data are required. There are agency folders with identifying data on a face sheet. There is an activity record which documents the fact of contact and the general nature of the service. Finally, a brief summary is required on initiation of service, annually, and at transfer or termination.

Trainees, obviously, must study process in detail, sharing their experiences with their supervisor and often with other trainees. They may wish to dictate voluminous accounts of the interaction and the hypotheses on which their interventions were based. Such dictation may go to a typing pool and pass through several nonprofessional intermediaries in the course of transport and transcription. Thus, the chances of violating confidentiality are greatly increased.

The preparation of papers, especially for publication, can pose additional problems. Consultation service staff are deeply aware of their responsibility not to let mischief or harm come to their consultees because of their association. Even in those extreme and unusual instances where the consultant has serious question about a consultee's values or practices, the consultation bond must be protected. Transient research or training personnel may not fully understand the fundamental importance of remaining discreet and trustworthy, even after they have left the scene, if the interagency relationship is to survive.

Furthermore, short-term participant-observers are likely to underestimate the complexities of what they see. In writing for publication they may easily not anticipate consultee sensitivities. Consultants with long experience in a consultee subculture are also quite capable of misunderstanding and misinterpreting, but the chances of being unintentionally offensive are probably less.

We have mentioned our concerns about the issues of quantity and quality of community services and in regard to confidentiality and basic interagency trust. On the other hand, there is need for orienting and training increasing numbers of clinical staff who will be extending their roles and functions as they move into the new regional mental health centers. Our administration has also been sensitive to our responsibility to share what we have learned with psychiatric residents and others who come from training institutions where there is little likelihood of comparable supervised field experience. Besides, we have a cadre of experienced consultants who find professional satisfaction in teaching and research. Furthermore, because of generally helpful service in the past, we still have cordial working relationships with many caregiving systems, which facilitates the rich variety of field placements. Thus, as long as there is a brisk demand for this type of training, it seems likely that we will continue to find time to provide it.

### Evaluation

Evaluation is another perplexing problem to the administrator of an indirect service program and to those who fund such programs. We have tried to document some rationale for these services, and we recognize there is still much to be learned. In the original guidelines for the implementation of the Short-Doyle Act, "action research" was encouraged. The problem of "scientific" evaluation, however, seems as complex and unmanageable as it did ten years ago. Subjective data from consultees and consultants are easy to collect, but their usefulness is limited. Statistical facts, which will define the frequency and duration of contacts with consultees as individuals and in groups, can be collected. One can even define the extent of potential consultee populations and the percentage of the defined population with whom one has had some type of codable indirect service contact in a given period of time. The difficulty, of course, is in assessing precisely what the service was, and what difference it made to the consultee, to his clients, and to the mental health of the community in general.

We are still without a commonly understood nomenclature or conceptual framework for the indirect services. Erickson discovered an appalling diversity of usage in 1961 (Erickson, 1966) and Parker, in 1967, still finds significant variations in theory and practice in California (Parker, 1969). Some consensus at the descriptive level must precede objective attempts to evaluate the impact of these services.

We may anticipate eventual descriptive agreement, but this essential preliminary step hardly guarantees that useful evaluative procedures will follow. Unfortunately, most indirect service activities occur in situations which are subject to multiple variables which may be unknown or uncontrollable for other reasons. Thus, it seems likely that attempts at cause-and-effect research in this field may be so oversimplified as to be meaningless or become so complex as to be unresearchable. Even meaningful or useful statistical procedures would, of course, be a welcome development.

### Ethical Considerations

Philosophical and ethical issues also arise in the course of service administration. Some are common to public professional practice;

for instance, the consultee who wishes therapy for himself, a relative, or friend. Others seem more unique and have to do with some basic consultation role ambiguities. Inasmuch as there are abundant public and private resources in San Mateo, those consultants who are in part-time private practice do not accept their own consultees or their close associates as patients. This prohibition exists primarily because of the inevitable change that would result in the consultation relationship. However, clients of consultees are sometimes accepted in private practice or by the consultant in his clinic work when referral is appropriate.

There are also occasional opportunities to consult privately on a fee-for-service basis. Here, the policy has been not to accept as private consultees those agencies who are clearly eligible and might reasonably expect to obtain the same type of service from us in our role as mental health consultants in the county Short-Doyle program. Where consultants are requested to give lectures or speeches and honoraria are involved, schedules are adjusted so this can be done on their own time. Whenever there is any question about proper professional stance, we generally review the issue at a consultation service staff meeting and arrive at some consensus about principles of practice.

Much more complicated are the issues unique to the practice of consultation in general and mental health consultation in particular. Can (or should) the consultant strive for a neutral, non-judgmental, teacher-helper, participant-observer stance, in contrast to public commitment and even overt activity as a social change agent? Few consultee systems would tolerate a foreign agent who could not empathize with their avowed goals and primary functions. Some difference of opinion is usually acceptable regarding the means by which their basic system objectives are accomplished. In well-disciplined community agencies consultants are generally welcomed if they offer the possibility of expediting the primary work of the agency by the essentially indirect consultation techniques we have described. However, as Lindemann (1968) has pointed out, the more diffuse social action groups now emerging in conjunction with interracial and poverty programs may demand that a consultant be identifiably one of them. Simple neutrality may not be enough to separate the consultant clearly from his origins in the allegedly hostile establishment. Deviations from the dialectic of the group would be further proof that the would-be consultant could not understand or be of use. Lindemann suggests that we use a chain of intervening agents, including indigenous subprofessionals, in order to establish a bridge of communication to such target populations.

Underlying the foregoing tactical problem of establishing entrée and developing a dialogue with a group that merely suspects our motives is the real dilemma when the consultant, in fact, has significant ideological differences. Can he, or should he, even try to consult with such a group? To resolve this question, the consultant must consider the context of his work and what would be implicit, as well as explicit, in any consultation contract. To begin with, the mental health consultant is not a management expert who is employed simply to further agency efficiency. The justification for his employment as a community mental health consultant is the premise that his professional work will somehow extend mental health principles and practices. This public health mission should not be a secret hidden agenda. The mental health consultant is not, in practice, a neutral scientific observer. However, his methods for influencing policy and procedure are through education and help with problem-solving. Thus, if his own biases are not so strong that they preclude any professional work together, and if the consultee system will allow him access, they may find some basis for collaboration and, perhaps ultimately, modification of those practices which the mental health consultant perceives as deleterious. If there is no possibility of working together in some context, then it is unlikely that the would-be consultant can have any impact on that system's programs and practices.

Another kind of philosophical and ethical concern lies in the potential role conflict that results from the fundamental ambiguity of the mental health consultant's allegiances. Is he, simply because he is a "professional" and a "consultant," exempt from the usual employee loyalties and responsibilities to the organization that pays his fee? Should he, or can he, be a completely free agent rather than a collaborator with the administration of the system that employs him or sanctions his presence in a consultee system? Obviously, he must define the limits within which he can function both ethically and effectively. Even when he learns something that might greatly expedite the work of his colleagues or the administration of his own or his consultee's agency, he must try to steer this intelligence, via his consultee, into appropriate channels.

Some consultants, especially those employed by industry as management consultants, are clearly identified and identifiable as agents of the establishment. In the mental health field, clinical personnel may be employed by the court to examine and make judgments about the mental status of prisoners. In other situations, as in the Peace Corps, clinicians may be hired to examine candidates and make prediction about future adjustment. However, whenever trained clinicians are hired to examine clients and use their particular knowledge and skills in other than clinical settings, there are latent ethical questions (Halleck and Miller, 1963). How can one neutralize the impact of status, transference, and the traditional role of the doctor-healer confidant whose primary responsibility is to help and protect his patient? Clinicians, of course, also have obligations to society which may require violation of patient confidence, as when restraint is necessary to prevent harm to the patient himself or to others. However, short of dire circumstances, the clinician does not initiate discussion of his patients' disclosures. Even where permission is given by the patient to share information with a social agency, the ethical clinician must be guided by what he perceives as the best interests of his patient.

In contrast, a consultant's primary responsibility is to his consultee. When a consultant is employed by a social agency such as the court, or even when a patient asks for an examination to fulfill employment requirements or to document eligibility for disability benefits, the consultant's responsibility must be at least as much to the agency as to the patient.

Yet, as Halleck cautions, there can be disquieting ethical ambiguities when the consultant uses his clinical skills for purposes other than healing. For instance, in interviewing a prisoner for the court, verbally cautioning against self-incrimination and even urging that the prisoner not say anything that he would not want the judge to hear, does not necessarily stem a flow of damaging data. A sympathetic and skilled interviewer may draw disclosures which would not have occurred with ordinary interrogation techniques.

At the same time, being a clinician does not wholly exempt one from social responsibilities. Especially in these unsettled times, it would seem quixotic not to contribute what one can from the clinical spectrum of the behavioral sciences, to those who seek to provide community services more humanely and effectively. Thus, in theory and in practice we make well-intentioned compromises while seeking greater understanding and wisdom.

## The Future

Finally, there is the question of the future of the indirect services in the California state-local community programs. Prior to the Short-Doyle Act, state hospitals had some community contacts via the Bureau of Social Work which provided aftercare services to "parolees." County hospitals generally had at least emergency and detention services for psychotics until they could be moved to private or state mental hospitals. Outpatient psychiatric services for indigents were generally minimal except for scattered child guidance services. Mental health education and consultation were only sketchily available, often as pilot ventures which were funded either by private foundations or with federal "seed money" channeled through the State Mental Health Authority. Prior to the Short-Doyle Act, the State Department of Public Health, not the State Department of Mental Hygiene, was that authority. Child guidance and consultation projects were generally seen as prevention-oriented public health services.

Since the passage of the original Short-Doyle Act of 1957, there have been subsequent revisions and amendments which increase the state's financial participation but which also shift the program emphasis in the direction of local assessment, treatment, control, and rehabilitation of chronically as well as acutely mentally ill persons, especially of persons sufficiently disabled to require hospitalization. At the same time, the economics of medical care have been rapidly shifting to third-party payment for medical services, including psychiatric services. Health insurance, Medicare and Medi-Cal increasingly cover outpatient and inpatient diagnostic and treatment services. In San Mateo County, the county manager has proposed closing the county hospital in order to "get the county out of the medical care business."

One has the feeling that we may be rapidly approaching roughly the same deployment of services and personnel as existed before the Short-Doyle Act was passed over a decade ago. Although the 1963 federal mental health center construction and staffing grant legislation followed Short-Doyle precedent in defining mental health education and consultation as basic services, the 1968 California amendments to the Short-Doyle Act clearly place highest priority on work with persons who are already seriously ill. Regardless of what other services are offered, there must be elaborate provisions for the screening, care, and conservatorship of persons who are gravely disabled by their mental illness. Other outpatient and indirect service programs may be maintained at present activity levels, but any expansion has low priority.

Increasingly, it appears that brief, crisis-oriented treatment services in quasi-public regional centers and private offices will provide the bulk of adult outpatient psychiatric services. Preventively-oriented services such as child guidance and consultation are not likely to be self-supporting if they concentrate on trying to provide services where most needed, instead of to those individuals or agencies who are willing and able to pay the actual cost of service. If present trends continue, it might be logically consistent to move both the child guidance and the bulk of the consultation service back into the public health sector.

Actually, mental health education, consultation, and community organization can be used to further preventive goals at all levels. Depending on the character of the work of the consultee agency, and the case or matter brought for discussion, consultation often supports maintenance of chronically ill adults in the community. Consultation with public health nurses, nursing home operators, social agency workers, vocational counselors, and many others, may help to minimize environmental stresses for known disabled clients. Furthermore, educational and organizational campaigns can be undertaken to increase community tolerance for former mental patients. With or without screening evaluations, consultation to police and other agency personnel may help to determine which clients should be referred to treatment facilities and which would probably not benefit from a clinical course. Thus, the indirect services will continue to support Short-Doyle objectives, even though the state's program emphasis has shifted in the direction of community care for severely disabled persons.

However, if in the future the financing of the direct services shifts to a private model, the indirect services might properly be moved back to public health auspices. They are clearly public health oriented in terms of goals, aims, and methods. Theoretically more possible of attainment than in the adult clinical services is their goal of primary prevention by facilitating the development and conservation of mental health. Shared with the clinical services are goals of prevention at the secondary and tertiary levels. Their methods all involve educative and collaborative approaches to the general public and to essentially healthy colleagues in community caregiving agencies. The dissemination of information and community organization activities are pursued in a manner completely analogous to public health education in other subject areas. Epidemiological surveillance, casefinding, and screening projects for early identification of pathology are well-established public health practices.

If mental health consultation and education were solely for the benefit of a particular consultee or his organization, it would then seem logical to charge a fee sufficient to cover the cost of services rendered to those requesting them. However, we see the potential impact of the indirect services in a broader context which has implications for their placement in a public agency and support by public funds.

The indirect services seem to have the potential for furthering public mental health goals in many ways. By sensitizing our community colleagues to the mental health aspects of their work and by increasing their knowledge of mental health principles, we aim to make them collaborators in the health education of their clients. As in maternal and child health programs, for instance, our consultees may be in a position to offer anticipatory guidance. Enlightened consultees may also be better able to help themselves and to help others to be supportive to their clients at times of life crises. Hopefully, their assessment of the mental health needs of their clients will become increasingly sophisticated, and they will then be better able to judge who might benefit from referral to specialized mental health resources and who might profit from other approaches, such as remediation of educational, general health, or social deficits. It is recognized that referral to a mental health treatment service may not be the most desirable course of action, even for a clearly mentally ill client, if there are more urgent issues involving other aspects of his life. Ideally, referrals should be made because there is a knowledgeable assessment of the total situation and it has been concluded that such referral is timely and will result in services which cannot be provided equally well in some other setting. Mental health consultation aims to help increase a consultee's diagnostic acuity and to improve his counseling skills. Thus, after consultation services, he may come to feel more confident and competent in his work with those disturbed and disturbing clients for whom he is in the best position to provide ongoing counseling services.

Mental health consultation also provides an opportunity for the consultant to pursue informal epidemiologic studies. He can observe the mental health predicaments which face the clients of his consultees and perhaps secure community collaboration in minimizing environmental stresses. Thus, mental health consultation is a vehicle through which the consultant can keep contact with a significant segment of the population. Optionally, this contact should be spread through all the major caregiving systems and professions in the community. Where his observational network is widespread, he may gain valuable insights for program planning.

If mental health consultation and education were available only on a fee-for-service basis, it is unlikely that all major caregiving systems would pay to participate in what they might see as primarily the work of the mental health services. Especially during the period of administrative negotiations, it seems unrealistic to expect a fee for service even though considerable professional time may be involved. Furthermore, a public health oriented service can deploy scarce consultant time where it seems most needed and most productive in terms of mental health objectives.

Agencies willing to purchase their own consultation and education services may not be those who should have the highest priority, as viewed from a public health perspective. Furthermore, they might logically expect to control that time, so that the consultant would be the agent of their administration in respect to whom he sees and how he functions. This is not to say that agencies should not employ case consultants or experts in other content areas for the purposes of staff development, in-service training, and other special services. However, privately employed professionals, whether in the role of consultant, educator, or clinician, then become agents of the organization rather than representatives of the community. Furthermore, independently contracting consultants rarely are able to function in a community-wide context. For these reasons we believe the indirect services are important public health services. Whether they are administered from mental health or public health auspices is not crucial. We believe, however, that they can only fulfill their potential if they are part of a coordinated, community-wide, public mental health program.

# CHAPTER 14

# Consultation to Courts and Corrections

*Leah B. McDonough, Theodore I. Anderson*

𝄢𝄢𝄢𝄢𝄢𝄢𝄢𝄢𝄢𝄢𝄢𝄢𝄢𝄢𝄢𝄢𝄢

The adult offender, a foreign body in the flesh of the community, has rallied around him a social inflammatory reaction consisting of a magnificent array of social organizations. These organizations vary widely from community to community; for purposes of this discussion they primarily include the various city police departments, the county sheriff's department, the adult division of the probation department, the district attorney's office, the municipal and superior courts, private attorneys, the Legal Aid Society, various voluntary organizations (Northern California Service League, Friends Outside, halfway houses, and so on), the state correctional facilities, Atascadero State Hospital (for therapeutic detention of sex offenders and "criminally insane"), and the California Rehabilitation Center (for civil therapeutic commitments in lieu of criminal sentencing for convicted narcotic addicts). These organizations themselves constitute a "community" defined by their relevance to the offender's behavior. It is the offender within this relevant community, along with the community of these organizations within the broader social context, that is the focus of attention for the courts and corrections unit of the mental health consultation service.

Mental health professionals working with social-offender-oriented systems encounter many situations requiring creative and often unconventional responses. Participating in these ways raises questions of professional appropriateness and ethics and often creates new dilemmas for participants from both mental health and correctional systems. Nevertheless, correctional agencies, faced with increasing numbers of problem citizens and spiraling costs, are turning to mental health specialists for help in devising methods of increasing effectiveness and decreasing costs.

Could a convicted felon safely and effectively be granted probation, sparing the state the costs of incarceration and sparing the felon unnecessarily demoralizing estrangement from his community? Can probation officers and deputy sheriffs learn group counseling techniques? What new probation techniques and supportive community programs can be invented to increase the probationer's chances of successful correction? Cannot mental health professionals, skilled in recent years in techniques of group therapy, therapeutic community perspectives, and community organization, add something to these correctional agencies' efforts?

As mental health agencies grapple with these questions still more peripheral problems are brought up. The district attorney's office wonders if any evidence is available to support their contention that pornographic literature, sold by a local bookstore, is actually damaging the community. This question, posed to the mental health unit and rife with implications for the development of future interagency relationships, is described in detail in the following paragraphs. Should a psychotherapist reveal to his patient information from the probation office that the patient is being shadowed by a plainclothes deputy sheriff? How could this situation be used to strengthen trusting and collaborative relationships between the mental health system, the sheriff's department, and the probation office? What are the relative responsibilities of the therapist to his patient's quest for health, the therapist's own mental health system, the quest for effectiveness, the requirements of interagency collaboration, and the considerations involved in long-range program development goals?

Expensive and elaborate maximum security jails are used to house large numbers of alcoholics and other misdemeanants. The sally-port and the bullet-proof glass in the visitor's room cleave the prisoner from the community. Can the sheriff's department utilize honor camps, work-furlough programs, and counseling programs run by deputies to reduce the cost and to minimize the stress of estrangement to these clients? Can their programs augment the mental health of significant groups, lessening their potential for incapacitating reactions? The evolution of these programs and the additional questions they generate will be discussed.

Racial and civil rights issues impinge daily upon law enforcement personnel. Can a mental health worker help ease unnecessary tensions in these encounters? The 1964 Republican National Convention in San Mateo County presented the sheriff's department with special problems related to these issues and presented an opportunity for the mental health consultant to work intimately with them. This activity, with its implications for future interagency relationships, is also discussed below.

Needs perceived by the correctional systems themselves were the initial factors leading to the creation of the courts and corrections unit. Adult probation had for many years been aware of the emotional disturbances in many of their clients. Some of these clients needed treatment. In addition, problems of increasing crime and recidivism rates demanded of all correctional systems new points of view leading to new solutions. Should all criminals be considered mentally disturbed? Could "treatment" by "experts" accomplish what probation surveillance had not? In keeping with the Zeitgeist, the probation office expected that mental health professionals had techniques which would reduce these stresses if only they could be made available. They attempted to obtain these mental health services for their clients. Frequently they requested pre-sentence mental health evaluations and post-sentencing psychotherapy as a condition of probation. For some time these requests had been routinely referred to privately practicing psychologists and psychiatrists and to the tax-supported adult clinic. Occasional difficulties arose due to the frequent inability of the mental health staff to perform evaluations as promptly as required by the legal notions of due process. In addition, the unfamiliarity of most mental health professionals with the unique social and legal forces impinging on the offender prevented optimal intervention or consideration of the alternatives available.

Furthermore, the evaluation and treatment services of the adult clinic at that time were designed for clients who met the traditional criteria of internal motivation and "psychological mindedness." These offenders, on the other hand, were often "ordered" to seek and maintain psychiatric treatment by the courts and the Probation Department. They were clearly patients not by choice or because of any self-acknowledged need; consequently, these offenders were often passed over, because coercion was frequently needed to ensure their presence at therapy appointments. The clinic staff selected first from their waiting list those who expressed strong motivation to use the services and who presumably had a better prognosis. The sophistication and willingness to coordinate the psychotherapeutic and legal coercive forces were at that time rare. Certainly, in many cases exemplary mental health evaluations and treatment were provided. However, the director of the adult probation office became increasingly convinced that improved services to his clients could be provided by a mental health team devoting their entire energies to his clients.

While the director of the adult probation office was requesting more available and prompt mental health services for his probationers, the sheriff's department was also working in directions which involved mental health concepts. Increased awareness of a need for more selective screening of personnel had evolved during informal collaborative work on law enforcement problems between a county psychologist and the sheriff's department. This interest in psychological screening became critical after an incident in which a deputy sheriff misused a weapon in a public situation. A program of psychological testing and psychiatric interviews for all applicants in the sheriff's department was therefore initiated, with the understanding that subsequent evaluation of the effectiveness of the screening would permit refinements and improvements in the procedures.

In addition to being interested in staff improvement, the sheriff's department was also concerned about the rehabilitation of its incarcerated prisoners. Could the work farm for jail trustees be transformed into a rehabilitative honor camp based on therapeutic community principles? Could these ideas relevant to mental health be transposed to a correctional setting? How could the sheriff's staff be provided the training, support, and supervision required by such a transition? Only with the assurance of continual collaboration with the Mental Health Services Division was the sheriff prepared to attempt these innovations.

These requests were of such priority to the county that the Board of Supervisors approved the establishment of a special mental health unit. The courts and corrections unit was established in 1961 as a special section of the adult clinic. The unit was provided office space in the adult probation facility in Redwood City (the seat of county government), in close proximity to the other major legal departments, the courts, the district attorney, the sheriff's department, and the jail.

All the other county mental health services were located in San Mateo, a city seven miles to the north. Being housed within adult probation facilities has had advantages and disadvantages. It is important, even vital, for this kind of unit to be close at hand to the legal centers with easy access and the kind of informal familiarity this breeds. Being housed within one of the recipient departments has confused certain issues. Questions of autonomy, resentment of time spent elsewhere in other facilities, feelings of proprietary interest are among the negative features. The positive features are apparent in the uniquely free and spontanous relationship between the probation staff and the staff of this unit. The ease with which they can drop in, the frequent informal types of consultation possible, the development of a level of consultative relationship not easily achieved are among the benefits of the physical arrangement. With the intensification of the relationship to both the sheriff's department and the probation department, however, some difficulties arose.

The probation office and the sheriff's department were both eager to put these newly available mental health "experts" to work and were especially aware of the relative allocation of time to their departments. Minor interdepartmental rivalries between the sheriff's department and the probation office had antedated the arrival of the mental health unit. These rivalries became focused on the mental health staff and considerable sensitivity was required to assure each department that its needs would be attended to. Moreover, the proximity of the mental health staff to the adult probation office lent identity diffusion problems to the mental health professionals and the unit staff felt isolated from their mental health colleagues. The courts and corrections unit staff, facing unique flexibility requirements, irregularly attended the adult clinic's staff meetings, which were devoted to maintaining a more traditional outpatient identity. What kinds of additional probation office and sheriff's department tasks could the mental health staff participate in, and with what priority? In what ways and for what purposes were the mental health staff "better trained," "more expert" than the probation officers and the deputies, and in what ways were they less well trained and less expert? How were the inevitable excessive expectations and consequent disappointments of the probation officers and deputies to be managed?

From the outset, attempts were made to adhere to the original agreement to provide direct service to clients. As this work began, however, previously unrecognized problems became apparent. With some clients, the probation officer would shift the burden of his responsibility to the therapist, since the therapist was "more expert" in human behavior problems. In self-defense, the therapist would declare difficult probationers "unmotivated for treatment," shifting the burden back again. The relevant discussions between probation officers and therapists emerged as imperative in order that collaboration could continue. These discussions were reflected in administrative meetings, as well as in meetings among line staff.

Other questions arose. What confidential information could the therapist discuss with the probation officer? What were the effects on the patient-probationer of such sharing, and what were the effects on the interstaff relationships? Could the probation officer, therapist, and client all profit from a relationship in which no secrets were sanctioned? Could the judge, on the advice of the probation officer, "order" the therapist to treat the probationer as a condition of probation? If the therapist refused, what problems would emerge in his developing relationships with the probation officer and the judges? Again, discussions among staff members began to take precedence over the prompt provision of direct service.

In time, probationers needing treatment which was independent of their need for correction were encouraged to apply for treatment through customary channels (privately or through the adult clinic). Limited time was set aside for treatment of probationers whose illness and criminality seemed to be related and in whom successful treatment could be expected to augment successful probation supervision.

Even by the time the unit had actually begun operations, the philosophy of the mental health program had shifted sufficiently to cause a subtle, though unacknowledged, change in the focus of the unit; thus the staff, from the outset, intended to provide mental health education and consultation to the probation office staff, as well as direct treatment service to their clients. Indirect services had become recognized as a desirable method of intervention, and the focus of energy was therefore reduced on direct service to the offender. Instead of the offender as the sole focus of interaction, the people having legal responsibility for him were now also considered the clients of the unit. The multitude of problems, as well as the undeniable benefits resulting from this different approach, were not wholly predicted.

The staff was concerned not only about the identifiable mentally ill population of offenders but also about the entire offender population. This group, operating marginally and at great community cost, was considered to be a population in high risk of developing emotional problems. Successful preventive programs required that the unit staff work with the probation officers on issues relating to management of probationers *before* they needed referral. The unit staff, then, encouraged discussions about any probationer and gave special priority to those discussions in which ultimate referral to mental health services was not the issue. At times, these concerns of the unit staff ran counter to the concerns of the probation office, which was looking for more direct assistance. Furthermore, case discussions which did not result in referral of the probationer to mental health evaluation services led the probation officers to feel that they, themselves, were the target of the mental health experts. This was a service which they had specifically not requested. The director of the adult probation office, concerned lest the identified problem for which he had originally requested assistance be ignored, maintained a steady request for less involvement with his probation officers and more involvement directly with their clients. The supervising probation officers wondered if these mental health "experts" were to be better teachers and supervisors than they, and the probation officers themselves often voiced complaints about being "psyched out."

Consistent with the general direction emphasizing preventive services through mental health education and consultation, the administrative relationships of the courts and corrections unit shifted. In 1963, with a change in leadership of the unit, the administrative connections of the courts and corrections unit were shifted from the adult clinic to consultation, education, and information service. This shift acknowledged the changed mission as seen by the unit staff, but was accomplished without the participation of the correctional agencies involved. Role definition was unresolved at that time and continues to be an interprofessional issue, as does the disparity between the mutual expectations of the mental health and the correctional staffs.

As these developments were unfolding with the probation office, the relationship with the sheriff's department was also leading in unforeseen directions. The sheriff's department initially requested assistance with the transformation of the work farm into an honor camp with a therapeutic community milieu. Fulfilling this request for program consultation and collaboration was a major responsibility of the courts and corrections unit from its inception. In this activity, as well, a number of questions arose. How could a deputy, trained in his primary role in the jail as a custodian, shift from that responsibility at the honor camp and adopt a "counselor" role? What principles derived from mental hospital therapeutic community experience could be translated into a correctional setting? How could the deputies be trained as counselors and supported in their emerging identity?

Before the opening of the honor camp, the consultant arranged for the deputies to spend some time on the county psychiatric inpatient ward and to visit other therapeutic community programs. This brief orientation to mental hospital therapeutic community work provided a basic model for the honor camp staff. The deputies and their supervisors were engaged in many staff discussions in attempting to increase their tolerance for greater expressions from the inmates of their dependency, hostility, and affection. When the camp opened, the psychiatrist led the therapeutic community camp meetings and held seminars for the deputies on group process and counseling.

As the relatively diffuse community meeting became more comfortable for the inmates and deputies, small counseling groups were started. The seventy-two inmates were divided into six groups of twelve, each with a deputy assigned as its leader. Again, the psychiatrist participated in this, initially as a co-counselor and later withdrawing to a consulting role. More seminars were provided to discuss small group and individual counseling.

This withdrawal from active participation precipitated other questions. Was the mental health unit relinquishing its responsibility for the honor camp milieu? Could the sheriff's department really take the responsibility for the conduct of the meetings and the camp atmosphere? Crises arose. Would the psychiatrist be available to treat the inmates if they became mentally disturbed? Should the sheriff's department have started this kind of honor camp in the first place? The ensuing staff discussions often reflected the problems the deputies were having with the inmates. Many inmates who were used to just "doing time" wondered if they really wanted to be counseled. Others, unused to a sense of self-determination in a correctional setting, sought to have limits imposed. As the deputies struggled with these problems, they reflected their distress to the psychiatrist in consultation sessions.

The developing educative and consultative role of the psychiatrist coincided with the previously mentioned administrative shift. What had begun as an extension of the adult clinic was shifted to the consultation service. The unit staff identified itself now as primarily consultative with prevention its primary concern.

As with the honor camp, the jail also experienced some difficulty with the shift from direct service to consultation. The jail staff wondered if the unit could assist them with their disturbed inmates. Previously, they had relied upon the visiting jail physician and the county hospital emergency room for assistance. In responding to this request, the unit staff attempted initially to act in accord with their identity as treating professionals. Crisis treatment was offered. Brief psychotherapeutic intervention was tried and medication was dispensed. As these attempts were made, the mental health staff discovered the crucial elements of the jail milieu, which augmented or diminished their objectives. The jail staff, originally requesting treatment services for the inmates, learned that an important part of the treatment involved their own behavior. A "problem" inmate might not continue to be a problem if the staff could understand him differently and modify their management of him. The unit staff soon learned that a jail is not a mental hospital. Any modifications of milieu and management leading to minimizing the disturbance of inmates had to take place in a busy jail where the primary business was not the mental health of the inmates. The jail was discovered to be a busy community in which the secure custody of the inmates was paramount. The jail staff was concerned with booking new arrivals; transportation of inmates to and from courtrooms; supervising visits of attorneys, friends, and others; and performing many other tasks in extremely crowded quarters. The jail staff was obligated to ignore management suggestions from well-meaning mental health professionals, who sometimes underestimated the urgency of these primary penal needs. As the contact between the unit and jail staffs continued, however, increased understanding of these difficulties became possible.

The jail commander felt that the women's jail, a small, isolated twelve-bed unit at the main jail, was affected by intrastaff problems. If these could be minimized, it was hoped that the women's jail might provide a more constructive experience for the inmates. The unit psychologist agreed to initiate group therapy within the women's jail and to meet with the staff to facilitate coordination of their inmate-focused activities. Initially, adherence to the clinical model of psychotherapy led to the exclusion of the matrons from the inmates' meetings, and the intercommunication "bugging" device was turned off during meetings to insure privacy and facilitate freedom to talk. It soon became apparent that many potential advantages were being sacrificed for this attempt at privacy which could never be fully guaranteed anyway; there was no way of knowing that the intercom key would not be accidentally left on during any particular meeting. The inmates were often able to continue projecting blame on the staff, a problem-avoidance exercise which did not really serve a useful function; they needed to learn to cope with these problems more effectively; without practice in dealing with them directly, they were deprived of the maximum benefit. Also, the matrons were being denied the opportunity to sit in a relatively objective setting and listen to the inmates in a way not often possible. The matrons were left with a feeling of secrets having been discussed and, even more important, with the feeling of having to deal with heightened tension and anxiety as a result of the meetings. Clearly, the psychologist entered, stirred things up, then left, and the staff understandably experienced this as adding to their problems.

These factors led to a changed structure for the women's jail meetings. All matrons on duty were invited and expected to attend the meetings. The advantages for both the inmates and the staff became clear. A major goal of the meetings was to enhance the sense of self-direction and autonomy of the inmates, to help them learn to think of themselves as active participants in the events of their lives rather than as simply passive recipients of whatever society chose to do to them. The sense of control and responsibility fostered by this development was considered more important than any typical intrapsychic approach to understanding; they needed, first of all, to see themselves as having some say in their destiny. These inmates were generally not the type of clients seen in a clinic asking for help in changing themselves; they saw the cause of their problems as lying in society and its abuse of them. These goals for inmates were explicitly explained to the matrons, because it was essential for them to understand their role in the interaction with the inmates. The matrons' emotional responses to inmates, both positive and negative, their acceptance or denial of responsibility for certain aspects of their role were necessary components of the process. The importance of staff involvement in this shifting perspective was highlighted in one occurrence early in the meetings.

One day the jail matron decided to impose certain punitive restrictions on the inmates because of some infractions of jail rules. In order to allow the "community" meeting to proceed smoothly without disruption, she decided to announce these restrictions immediately after the meeting. The meeting proceeded as usual with the inmates giving voice to some frustrations and complaints. At the end of the meeting, the announcement of the restrictions convinced the inmates that they had been tricked into talking about themselves and then were being punished for it. This experience had a sequel four years later when it was recalled by an inmate who returned to jail charged with another offense. She felt obligated, then, to warn her cellmates bitterly of the trickery involved.

Separate weekly meetings between the psychologist and the matrons were initially focused on the group meeting and the individual inmates. As the relationship matured, the discussions shifted to more general work problems within the women's jail. The matrons wanted to discuss ways to implement new programs, ways to improve relationships with the deputies in the main jail, and with the sheriff's department administration. The fact that the consultant was close at hand, spent at least two hours a week in the women's jail, and was readily available for consultation about any problem inmate, certainly facilitated the rapid development of a useful relationship here.

Innovations in the unit's therapeutic interventions progressed. Occasional probationers were taken into long-term treatment as a condition of probation, and attendance was enforced by close collaboration of therapist, probation officer, and the patient-probationer. In one case the therapist agreed with the probation officer and his client that he would assist the probation officer with the task of correctively applying coercion and force on his client and that he would then attempt to treat the coerced patient. In order to do this, the therapist excused himself at the outset from any privileged communication. Both probation officer and the patient knew that the therapist would be talking with the other. All three participants met together at the initial meeting, periodically at crucial stress points, and at the termination of treatment eighteen months later. This contract posed several problems. For example, the sheriff's department, on the basis of other data, became suspicious of the probationer and assigned a plainclothes officer to shadow him. Unaware that the suspect was involved in the above therapeutic contract, the deputy sheriff routinely advised the probation officer that his client was being shadowed. The probation officer told the therapist but objected to the therapist telling the patient on the grounds that this would destroy the relationship between the sheriff's department and the probation office. The therapist, respecting this relationship, requested the probation officer to ask permission of the deputy in order to tell his patient that he was being followed. To the probation officer's surprise, permission was granted, and the therapist was then able to share this information with his patient.

In collaboration with probation officers interested in group counseling, the unit staff started a number of probationer groups. These groups were explicitly not mental health projects and the clients were not patients. The unit staff were participant-consultants, enabling the probation officer to learn new group skills and attempt group counseling as a part of his role. The sanction of the probation office administration was required for every phase of these developments. A group of probation officers was involved in the design of the first groups, and later in observation of the group through one-way mirrors. Subsequently, several probation officers started groups with varying degrees of support from the unit staff.

Although the initial expectation had been that the unit staff would assume responsibility for these groups, the probation officers' growing awareness of their own capabilities and the satisfaction of achieving an independent professional role reduced the necessity of direct intervention by the unit.

The unit staff became increasingly enthusiastic about preventive indirect services—case, administrative, and program consultation. Having joined the consultation service, the unit was further encouraged in these directions. Perhaps more importantly, however, the approach and emphasis on indirect services have often reflected the professional attitudes and personal inclinations of the succession of administrators of the courts and corrections unit. The variety and changes in these approaches have resulted in interesting and predictable reactions both from the probation department and the sheriff's department.

Whereas the acceptance of the direct service function had earlier led to willingness to treat jail inmates even to the point of establishing jail rounds and the provision of direct service to honor camp inmates, a more puristic concept of indirect services evolved under a new unit chief. Jail staff were encouraged to take disturbed inmates to the county hospital emergency room rather than to ask for even preliminary consultation with the unit. Inmates at both the honor camp and the newly established work-furlough facility were similarly sent to the emergency room, because the unit viewed its role as almost exclusively indirect. The emergency room staff and the jail staff expressed dissatisfaction with the cessation of direct services.

In the probation department there was an increased focus on indirect service with the resultant dissatisfaction on the part of the director and some of his staff who felt that they were again in the position of being unable to obtain evaluations of their clients or adequate services for them.

The frequency and fervor of these complaints about this shift in focus eventually resulted in a softening of the line, a reversion to contacts with clients as a legitimate aspect of the courts and corrections role. It seems apparent that in this particular unit a puristic concept of indirect services is inappropriate and often not helpful and results in serious breakdown of constructive communication.

While these relationships with the probation department and the sheriff's department were developing over the years, other activities with the district attorney's office and the courts had been taking place. Some of the municipal court judges have asked the unit to be involved in a variety of ways, from assessing an inmate's suicide potential if he were released on bail, to determining need for hospitalization and suggesting community resources for problem cases.

Assignment of the criminal court docket is rotated among the twelve superior court judges every twelve months. Each judge has required a uniquely different relationship with the unit staff. One judge found mental health professionals not at all useful. Another judge requested the mental health staff to provide psychotherapy to the probationers on his order, as a condition of probation. Another judge wished the probation officers to gain "expert" (mental health) opinions on the advisability of granting probation to offenders. Still another judge found it useful for the unit to preview defendants to evaluate the appropriateness of seeking formal psychiatric evaluation of their suitability for trial, for referral as a "mentally disordered sex offender," or for referral to the California Rehabilitation Center for narcotics addicts.

If convicted of a sexual offense, a defendant may be examined by two court-appointed psychiatrists who assess his suitability for a civil commitment to Atascadero State Hospital, where he will be treated as a "mentally disordered sex offender." One judge wished the unit to examine such defendants to help decide which ones would warrant investigation as described above. In other cases, defendants convicted of any crime who are current or potential narcotics addicts may be certified on civil commitment to the California Rehabilitation Center for treatment in lieu of penal incarceration. Again, several judges requested the mental health staff to help in evaluating which defendants would probably satisfy the eligibility and suitability requirements of such commitment and would thus warrant formal determination.

In these cases, the unit psychologist or psychiatrist has frequently been called upon to testify in court as a friend of the court. In this role, he has been requested to add his opinion to those of the formally appointed medical examiners. In evaluating the appropriateness of a referral to the California Rehabilitation Center, the mental health staff has been able to provide special knowledge unavailable to the usual medical examiner. The unit staff members all have made personal visits to the institution (located four hundred miles away), resulting in an informed acquaintance with the institution and its program. Data from examination of the defendant, and from examination of the files of the district attorney and the probation office, are available to all examiners. This body of knowledge and experience enables the consultant not only to evaluate the overt question of suitability for such commitment but to function as an educational bridge between the California Rehabilitation Center and the local courts, district attorney's office, and probation office.

When issues have arisen regarding competency to stand trial and responsibility for the offense, the unit staff members have often been asked to contribute their understanding of the offender, although formal court testimony has been solicited from private psychiatrists. In establishing this policy, the judge advised the courts and corrections unit that their prior relationship with the judge as a friend of the court and the prior relationship as a consultant to the district attorney and probation office might raise the question of mistrial due to the court having appointed a psychiatrist who might be biased. Thus, in order to respond adequately to some needs of the correctional system, the unit has excluded itself from other roles.

These functions are adapted to the requirements of the judges, and they demand great flexibility on the part of the staff and judicial system. The relationship with each judge must be established as he arrives on the criminal bench and must be maintained with him during his tenure. Naturally, an attempt is made to carry over to incoming judges programs which have worked out well with outgoing ones. For example, several judges assigned in rotation to the domestic relations docket have similarly utilized the unit staff as consultants.

As mentioned above, requests for screening evaluation and consultation about the advisability of proceeding with commitment hearings involves the criminal and civil court, the probation department, and the district attorney. The district attorney has at other times requested information about more general community issues. In 1966, several citizens were bringing pressure upon the district attorney's office to prosecute a "pornographic" bookstore owner. This bookseller had been acquitted of similar charges two years previously. In deciding how to enforce the laws, the deputy district attorney raised several questions for the psychiatrist. What is pornographic, lewd, or lascivious literature? Is the material intended to be so, or is it incidental to the author's purpose? Is there a danger to the community from such material? Would the mental health professional testify in support of or against such a bookstore owner? If the prosecution were to be unsuccessful, could the bookstore owner be dissuaded or controlled in ways other than by a formal legal proceeding? Could the complaining citizens be dealt with in other ways?

The psychiatrist was pleased to become involved with the district attorney's office and was willing to help with their problem. As he listened more closely to the request, however, it became clear that the district attorney wanted his expert testimony to be the key evidence in the potential prosecution. In the view of the deputy district attorney, if the psychiatrist failed to testify in cooperation with the prosecution, the store owner probably could not be convicted, and the community would continue to suffer the consequences of having pornographic literature sold on the street corner.

Again, many questions were raised for the psychiatrist. Was it appropriate for him to testify at all, thus setting a precedent that the courts and corrections unit would take an adversary position on legal issues involving establishing and controlling morals? What would be more appropriate—to assist the district attorney, court, and jury in reaching their own decision, or to try to persuade them, as requested by the district attorney's office? The district attorney's office wanted to provide the court with persuasive testimony. If testimony were agreed to, what was known to the psychiatrist to be fact about the effects of pornographic literature, and what was held as his personal conviction? What expert knowledge did he really have? How could the psychiatrist best acknowledge his inability to satisfy the district attorney's request directly? How could the psychiatrist best continue the interagency dialogue? If he himself could not offer persuasive expert testimony based on facts, should he offer the district attorney something else which was needed but unasked for, for example, suggesting a local psychologist, expert in the field of learning and attitude development and patterning of behavior, who could offer empirical and experimental evidence on such topics? In the end, the psychiatrist confined his role to consultation to the deputy district attorney.

Some other examples of the unit's participation with correctional agencies are worthy of mention. In the probation department, a special unit was recently established to provide intensive services for offenders who would ordinarily be sentenced to a state correctional institution. The state's interest in maintaining these serious offenders in the community, through intensive probation supervision, was in response to disappointment in the effectiveness of the prisons and the exorbitant cost of building more prisons and maintaining inmates in them. With smaller caseloads, special funds for training, and encouragement to seek and devise newer and creative uses of probation, the special unit, partially financed by the state, has worked closely with the courts and corrections unit. Providing consultation on new programs, such as family therapy, staffing of problem probationers, and collaborative treatment services between courts and corrections unit and the probation officers have been included.

A learning theory approach has been implemented with some of these clients, working with certain probation officers, as well as jail staff, if the offender was serving time in the county jail as a condition of probation. The importance of the client understanding the contingencies, of his awareness of the specific behavior which leads to specific results is explained. Too often the offender has only a vague idea of the reason for his punishment. It has been pointed out to the responsible person (jail staff, judge, probation officer) that in order to have the punishment effective it must at least be associated with the offense in the eyes of the offender. Random negative reinforcement or punishment which is viewed as resulting from some entirely different behavior than that actually causing it is worse than useless, since it impedes the learning of the desired behavior. Similarly, the clear evidence that positive reinforcement is more effective than negative reinforcement in learning (with any population, but especially with offenders) is one part of the scientific body of data which can be usefully employed in the correctional process. Toward this goal, some consultations have focused specifically on seeking adequate rewards for certain clients and determining the contingencies for them. Obviously with a late adolescent boy, the type of reward used as a motivation will be different from what may be appropriate in motivating a middle-aged housewife. The engagement of the jail staff, the probation officer, and, less frequently, the judges, in the pursuit of implementation of scientific theory has been rewarding. It is an area which deserves considerably more attention.

Another aspect of this approach has been used in attempting to heighten the awareness of the staffs in their dealings with citizens. For example, the sheriff's department has had particular problems with some minority groups of the county and vice versa. Hostility, suspicion, and distrust are prevalent on both sides, and each unfortunate incident increases the intensity of these emotions. Attempts to help the law enforcement officers become more professional in their role have focused their increased awareness on the effect they have on the community. Carrying out one's duties with deliberation, pursuing goals rather than being distracted by minor harassment, being aware of the responses elicited on the part of the community—all are stressed as necessary components of a professional self-concept and role. The maturity to ignore less important features of a problem (for example, name calling) and to focus on what is identified as the main problem is stressed as a positive trait rather than as a sign of weakness. The extremely difficult and defensive position the law enforcement officer is often forced into can easily lead to a reflexive type of response to assert one's authority. If the assertion of this authority diminishes the opportunity to settle the problem, clearly it was an unprofessional action. The sense of dignity and self-assurance required to withstand harassment without responding blindly and impulsively is not easily acquired, but to maintain it as a desirable goal is important.

Community organization has been a primary channel for facilitating changes in hiring standards and procedures in the sheriff's department. The sheriff was enabled to specify more clearly the real requisites of the job and eliminate requirements and procedures which interfered with his obtaining the best candidates; the county civil service people were eager to participate in these changes once the rationale for them became clear.

As a final example of the work of the courts and corrections unit, one consultation with the sheriff's department will be discussed in greater detail. The sheriff's department had been concerned about social and minority problems for several years and had, of course, pro-

fessional training in maintaining order in large crowds. It was prepared, therefore, for the situation presented by the Republican National Convention, held in the Cow Palace in San Mateo County in
1964. This convention was expected to bring together the forces supporting Senator Goldwater and the forces supporting the increasingly
vigorous civil rights proponents.

In preparing for this confrontation, the sheriff's department
was planning to minimize open conflict and disorder. While mindful
of the necessity of supporting the orderly convention process, the sheriff's department hoped that civilly disobedient demonstrators could be
controlled by means other than mass arrests leading to overloading of
the judicial and correctional facilities. The undersheriff began early to
work with the Republican Party representatives and the multitude of
civil rights organizations. He shared his law enforcement plans with
them and asked them about their plans. He helped the many civil action groups organize themselves. He hoped thereby to reduce the
number of civil action leaders with whom he would negotiate. He attempted to find areas of agreement among themselves and his department. He attempted to establish with their leaders trusted lines of communication which could be maintained during the convention. And he
attempted to communicate to his deputies and to other local law enforcement personnel his idea of a way of maintaining peace during
the convention. He was hoping that his line staff could withstand the
provocative situations they were sure to encounter and that they could
negotiate administratively with the demonstrators. This goal was an
unusual one for his staff, who were trained to see negotiating with
provocative civilly disobedient citizens as a sign of weakness.

The psychiatrist, participating as a consultant to the sheriff's
department, was initially seen as an "expert on crowd control." It was
also expected that he might provide on-site emergency brief treatment
for anyone experiencing acute emotional stress reactions during the
convention. These initial expectations were unrealistic, but the request
led to discussions which revealed possibilities of participating in still
other roles. The consultant observed a series of planning meetings between the sheriff's department and civil rights groups. He agreed to
address a large orientation meeting in which all the deputies and other
law enforcement personnel were brought together a few days prior to
the convention.

Participating in these early activities raised many questions. Could the psychiatrist assist the undersheriff in his task of planning the convention at all? Did he have any expertise on "crowd control"? What facilities, if any, should be planned for psychiatric emergencies at the convention site? Could he anticipate the stresses to be encountered by these deputies as they attempted to behave in an unfamiliar role in a highly emotionally charged setting? If so, how could he help prepare them for these stresses? Could he help the administration in maintaining communication with and support of the deputies? Would it be worth the consultant's time to attend the convention itself? If so, what would he do?

It was decided that the consultant would attend the convention and would seek out areas in which he might find an appropriate function. As the convention began, the consultant discovered many deputies posted around the convention hall in isolation from each other. He began to function as a traveling information center, answering questions about the nature of activities elsewhere inside the hall and outside in the demonstrators' line. He inquired about the deputies' perceptions of their tasks, seeking to identify strengths and convictions, as well as faulty perceptions, conflicts, and distress.

During one contact, he encountered an immaculately uniformed deputy standing at his isolated post high in the bleachers of the Cow Palace. This deputy related his fatigue, boredom, and an envious suspicion that his relieving deputy was "goofing off over a cup of coffee somewhere." Inquiry revealed that this isolated deputy had worked eight hours prior to this voluntary, extra ten-hour shift, that he had not spoken to any person for at least an hour, that he had been standing uncomfortably trying to maintain the appearance of an alert, friendly officer. Prepared for the excitement of conflict, he assumed the "action" was taking place without him somewhere else. The consultant responded by acknowledging the difficulty anyone would have in carrying out this assignment. Having talked with a number of other deputies, the consultant assured this one that his feelings were not only genuine but shared by most of his colleagues. The consultant added that the demonstrations of the civil rights groups outside the convention hall were going very slowly and there was not only "no action," but that a cold wind and light fog outside the building made the deputies' tasks out there difficult, too. Upon leaving, the consultant mentioned that he would be back again in a while and would continue the conversation, if the deputy's relief had not come by then.

Outside the convention hall, the problems were different. Deputies were standing in the fog, protecting a roped-off area in front of the main entrance. This area contained the demonstrating civil rights activists, as they marched in a circle. As their numbers grew and as they began to feel hemmed in and restless, the sheriff's captain worked out plans with their leaders to lead them out of their roped-in area, to march throughout the parking lot, and then to return. Time and again, throughout the four days, the captain walked at the head of the line, clearing a way through the busy parking lot traffic for the demonstrators' marching column. Although this sheriff's department support of the demonstrators led to a continuation of the open communication and trusting relationship between the civil rights leaders and the sheriff's department administration, many deputies were disturbed to observe their captain actively collaborating with "the enemy." Many of the consultant's contacts with the deputies revealed their discomfort, their questions, and their reluctance to accept the new goals of their own leaders. The consultant repeatedly attempted to work with both the administration and deputies to bridge this gap. The consultant sought ways to help the deputies discover elements of strength, assertiveness, control, and self-esteem in their leader's new efforts. The deputies, often caught up in the intense emotions involved, responded with personal vigor to the provocations offered them. The consultant sought ways to reinforce their professional armor and to assist them in delaying expression of their personal frustrations until a less sensitive setting was available.

Confronted with a large crowd chanting "lily white cops," one deputy in line muttered in four letter words of desperation what he would like to do to those "beatnik bastards," if one would only give him a chance. The consultant, free to move around among the demonstrators and deputies alike, stopped to talk with this deputy in an attempt to help him verbalize his impulses and discharge the burdensome affects.

As the consultant learned of the relevant factors confronting the peace officers, other questions were presented to him. Immediately after the nomination of Senator Goldwater, the demonstrators became increasingly agitated, defiant, and obstructive. The undersheriff wondered if the demonstrators were going to demand that a few arrests be made to call attention to their distress. Furthermore, he knew that these openly defiant and provocative people were being tolerated with increasing difficulty and tension by his deputies. Would a few arrests satisfy the demonstrators and mollify his deputies as well? If so, the undersheriff was prepared to make the arrests. The undersheriff used the consultant at this time to review objectively the issues relevant to this decision. As it transpired, no arrests were ever made.

On other occasions, direct suggestions were offered by the consultant. Late one evening, as the civil rights leaders were bringing the demonstrators together to close their activities for the day, the last group of public buses was preparing to leave for nearby San Francisco. The consultant, aware of the tasks facing the civil rights leaders in controlling the mood of the demonstrating crowd, predicted that the buses would leave before the demonstrators were ready to go home. He advised the undersheriff of this prediction. The undersheriff was then able to delay the departure time of the buses a few minutes until the demonstrators were ready to board the buses unhurriedly.

These few examples are intended to illustrate a variety of problems confronting the consultant and his responses to them. Opinion was not uniform that the consultation was worthwhile. Some consultees questioned whether the consultant had canceled his appointments with them and their clients during the convention activities in order to "goof off." The consultant himself had questions about his activities. Would the sheriff's department have done as good a job without his intervention? Could he have consulted effectively with the sheriff's department if it had adopted a more militant, rigid stand regarding the enforcement of the laws? Was the sheriff's department able, as a result of negotiating the convention crisis successfully, to use this new identity as a growth experience? Did the deputies really accept the principles they had practiced at the convention, and could these principles be implemented in other settings? Answers to these and to other questions are still forthcoming as more educative, consultative, and collaborative activities follow each other.

As in so many mental health endeavors, program evaluation is a major challenge for the courts and corrections unit. The problem of asking questions which can be meaningfully answered, of establishing valid criteria, of objectifying subjective impressions, all are at least as problematical in this setting as in any other.

One effort in this direction took the form of a survey of all actual and potential consultees of the courts and corrections unit: superior and municipal court judges, adult division of the probation department, district attorney's office, and the sheriff's department. An attempt was made to learn what they felt was available to them, what they availed themselves of, and what they would like to have available from the unit. For a twelve-week period surrounding this survey, the unit recorded all of its activities, and the content of each contact, and then compared their account of its activities with those of the consultees.

The discrepancies between the consultees' and the consultants' perceptions of activities were of major interest, and the areas of misunderstanding, of expecting services never intended by the unit, as well as the revelation of unmet needs, proved extremely useful. One of the main values of the survey, not fully anticipated, was the expression of dissatisfactions and expectations and the ensuing improvement in some areas of service. The discontinuity in direction of the unit, due to frequent changes in leadership and the necessity of renegotiating a contract with each new administrative head with his unique philosophy and approach were considered major impediments to maximum utilization of the unit.

Appointment of the clinical psychologist to administer the unit —a departure from the prior custom of psychiatric administration— was based upon a variety of factors, each with some relevance to this discussion. Most important perhaps were the practical considerations of experience and administrative continuity. The psychologist had been with the unit from its inception; her sensitive knowledge of this highly specialized sphere of community mental health work was augmented by the longitudinal experience of knowing the consultee agencies and their relationship with the mental health program during the important formative period. Moreover, as this discussion reveals, the unit has increasingly engaged in the application of behavioral science theoretical formulations and techniques in delivering both direct and indirect services. This infusion of new skills is potentially shared by all mental health disciplines and has significantly enriched community mental health practice at many levels.

Another result of the survey concerned the sheriff's specific request for training for his department. Mutual efforts to define the needs ensued, and this has become a major focus between the two departments.

An overlapping concern with this latter one involved the evaluation of the program of screening of deputy sheriff applicants. The search for what is considered desirable by that department in their deputies has been mutually pursued. The appraisal of each of the deputies hired, based upon three different sets of administrative criteria that have been made available to us by the sheriff's department, is being compared with the psychological and psychiatric data which were collected on each applicant. The comments, predictions, and descriptions of traits whose relevance for law enforcement was unknown at the time of screening are now being compared to the progress the man made within the department. The data thus far suggest some specific areas of validity and will be reported elsewhere. The overall results will permit modification and refinement of the screening procedures. Only if these extensive and expensive screening procedures prove valid should they be continued. Too often a program is perpetuated without ever being justified. However, one argument for continuing this screening, even before the positive results were known, was the fact that the initial encounter with mental health personnel by every man entering the department facilitated further positive transactions between them. Certainly, the fact that the applicant considers himself to have been favorably rated by the mental health staff enhances future communications between the two departments. This initial encounter also gives the new man the message that mental health concepts and contributions are valued by his own department and are, therefore, all right to pursue, contrary to the more defensive stance of some other police jurisdictions.

The unit has participated in training psychology trainees and psychiatric residents who come to San Mateo to obtain training and experience in mental health consultation, education, and community organization. The unique experiences available in the unit have been actively sought by trainees who, under supervision, provide a specific service to a correctional agency.

Most assuredly the courts and corrections unit has eschewed the role of the mental health expert treating psychopathology expressed as law violations. The consultees are sophisticated enough themselves to recognize that this simplistic approach is neither valid nor useful. The offenses which lead to arrest may in fact be due to some pathology in the offender, but it is frequently an interaction of social forces, involving the expectations of the individual, the neighborhood, the legal system, the mores—all leading to the particular result in any one case. For example, the fact that youths from middle-class neighborhoods are allowed to avoid entering the legal system, without the stigma of a record, whereas in the lower-class community the luxury of such parental help is often unavailable is an aspect of the system which must be understood and acknowledged if meaningful consultation is to occur. The courts, the law enforcement agencies, the probation agencies, and the legal resources may be enabled to work toward some more equitable and economic (in both financial and human terms) manner of extending this concept of family support and informal handling of problems. Similarly, if the expectations of the community lead citizens to avoid calling the police for help, if police are seen only as the enemy or cause of trouble then these citizens are not only deprived of the same level of protection that others enjoy but are almost guaranteed to end up in legal difficulties. The potential benefits of a program to counteract these expectations, of associating the police with something positive in the experience of the community, aiding in the development of such a program, are aspects of consultation which clearly see beyond the "psychopathology" concept.

In summary, the overall task of the unit has been to establish functional relationships with each of the organizations rallying in response to the adult offender and to assist these organizations in coordinating their energies. Community organization in the establishment of future programs focused on these social issues is one aspect of the current program which is being emphasized. Implementation of the body of knowledge in social issues and psychological theories of human behavior is timely.

## PART IV

*I*nnovation is a cardinal characteristic of community mental health. Because it asks conventionally trained workers to consider new methods of service delivery and new roles, there is an urgent, often understressed need for solid evaluation and new training formats. Because today's programs do represent departures from many of the models and assumptions that have been complacently accepted for a generation or more, both program evaluation and training are on the leading edge of the community mental health transformation. New values require the kind of operational testing that can occasion what can only be termed anguish among professionals who sincerely and, it must be conceded, reasonably question the desirability of certain changes. This is vividly portrayed in Chapter 15.

348

# PROGRAM EVALUATION
# AND TRAINING

ᔑᔑᔑᔑᔑᔑᔑᔑᔑᔑᔑᔑᔑᔑᔑᔑᔑᔑᔑᔑᔑᔑᔑᔑ

*Developing a program to meet community mental health needs is a complex and often extremely difficult process, as other chapters in this book have amply demonstrated. With all the pressures that accompany such a process, and without clear and widely accepted evaluative techniques, it is frequently too easy to neglect the objective evaluation of the effectiveness of mental health programs. Indeed, program evaluation and research are not a luxury, but rather a crucial aspect of program development, as we also learn in Chapter 15.*

*Training, offered in new patterns reflecting the emerging value system of community mental health, is of vital importance for the community programs now springing up. Chapter 16 shows how, in the course of developing our training program, we have found that training becomes an integral part of each service in which it is offered. Further, a reciprocal relationship exists between the training function*

*and the service function, as both functions mutually influence one an-*
*other. Recognizing these factors, we feel that training requires special*
*attention and personnel specifically assigned to it. As described in*
*Chapter 16, we have come to see training not simply as a way in which*
*mental health personnel can be better prepared to do their work within*
*their own centers, but as a function which serves the mental health*
*field in general and the community at large.*

CHAPTER **15**

# Program Evaluation and Research

*Gary M. Heymann*

$\int$•$\int$•$\int$•$\int$•$\int$•$\int$•$\int$•$\int$•$\int$•$\int$•$\int$•$\int$•$\int$•$\int$•$\int$•$\int$•$\int$•$\int$•$\int$

$P$rogram evaluation and research in the San Mateo County mental health program have taken place in the context of the changing times of our society in general, and of the mental health field in particular; simultaneously, they have contributed to these varied changes. This work is inseparably part and parcel of the development of the psychology service, which itself participated in the evolutionary process our program has undergone over the past ten years. The psychology service and the clinical psychologists comprising it have changed, both in number and in function. A staff that was once one full-time and two part-time psychologists, working in two separate clinics, is now an independent service staff of eleven full-time and two part-time members plus a full-time service chief. Another full-time and five part-time psychologists are adjunctively working in our program through research grant and various contractual arrangements. The function of this staff is no longer to be merely a handmaiden to clinic cases, but to evaluate the program itself at various levels of operation, to introduce new treatment methods into the system and, hopefully, to be a general catalyst for change. The division has been transformed from a loose confederation of traditional psychiatric services, focused on the psychopathology of certain identified patients, to a comprehensive community mental health center, committed to meeting the mental health needs of its half-million county residents.

When it was organized in 1958, the Mental Health Services Division was set up with program evaluation and research built in as part of the total operation (see Chapter 1). Two decisions were made at the outset: (1) to find out how scarce professional time was being used on behalf of patients in the two outpatient clinics, and (2) to make already easily available operational statistics useful at the local level. Nobody really knew how professional clinic time was invested, so a two-week time study was designed to focus on three major categories of activity: (1) time spent with patients, (2) time spent in activity directly related to patient contact (case collaboration and conferences, progress notes, and so on), and (3) activity indirectly related to patient contact (clinic staffing of cases, for example).

All other aspects of this study were overshadowed by the sobering finding that for every hour spent with patients or collaterals, two hours of staff time were spent talking or writing about this contact. Probably most other outpatient psychiatric clinics around the country had similar time investment patterns, since the San Mateo clinics followed the standard operational procedures of the mid-fifties. Nevertheless, this investment was regarded as unsatisfactory for a clinic with virtually no other assignment than patient evaluation and treatment. A goal of 60 percent of staff time at work to be invested in patient or collateral contacts was set by the program chief. Data relevant to this issue were included in the monthly service reports. Later, charts showing percent of time spent with patients and collaterals were prominently displayed on the wall in the program chief's office. The two outpatient clinic chiefs chose to keep their respective charts out of view, which proved to be an early clue of the extent to which they and the program chief failed to share a common view of program goals.

The percent-of-time-spent-with-patients issue has never been satisfactorily resolved in the outpatient services. Genuine concern about possible reduction in quality of service became confused with maintenance of ritualistic behavior, so change was not experienced as freedom from meaningless activity. For many reasons a positive atmosphere in which to assess the percent of time spent with patients did not develop. Many unfortunate attitudes, some of which have been reinforced many times and persist to this day, were set in motion by this study and the handling of its findings. They were not confined to the administrative protagonists but brushed off on program evaluation and research as a realm of activity and concern.

A further finding that considerable time was invested in elaborate progress notes and other paper work eventually led to a revision of the record-keeping procedure for the entire division. Also, our considerable time investment in case staffing procedure pointed to the need for a closer look at that activity, which eventually led to a reorganization of internal clinic structure.

The California Mental Health Act (Short-Doyle), which authorizes state reimbursement for a part of the cost of local services, requires that we provide the state with certain basic information regarding patient characteristics, patient activity, and patient movement. Feedback of these data was often sporadic; moreover, the data were organized to meet state-level needs rather than the needs of local jurisdictions. It was decided to add a few locally meaningful items and use the about-to-be-revised data gathering system to yield monthly and annual reports that would describe this program independently of the use to which the state put this information. Further, we began to request specific data tabulations from the Bureau of Biostatistics, State Department of Mental Hygiene. This combination of data was our first gross approach to continuous program evaluation (Heymann and Downing, 1961). Two distinct informational systems gradually developed out of this approach, the operational charts and the fiscal year data analysis reports.

The time study findings had already raised many questions about our mode of operation. A further assessment of things showed that the application-intake-admission procedure in the adult clinic usually took six or seven weeks. Things were little different in the child guidance clinic. All this stimulated our attempts to find a staffing device which would utilize staff time more effectively and simultaneously provide better service to the people who sought our help. A three-member team was put into operation on a demonstration basis to function on a processing-within-twenty-four-hours-of-application procedure while the rest of the clinic continued to carry on as usual. This approach seemed so satisfactory to those involved that it was adopted in modified form by the entire adult clinic even before the data being gathered for comparison with the standard procedure could be analyzed. (They never were.) Eventually the child guidance clinic also adopted the team approach.

Significantly, the combined use of study data, clinic personnel in a demonstration project, and active support by the service chief concerned had made real change possible. A traditional procedure, no longer effective in terms of changed conditions confronting the clinics, had been shed. Nevertheless, only the structural aspects of the clinics had been changed. Still cherished was our staff's general treatment philosophy orientation—that the clinic was there for people with long-standing, internalized neurotic problems which require strong motivation and a willingness to participate in a long-term therapy process.

A uniform division-wide record system was obviously needed if we were to achieve smooth functioning in keeping clinical records required for patient care, in data collection for program evaluation and research purposes, and in financial management of budget requirements and patient billing for services rendered. To shape such a system, an independent research psychologist and a small staff were brought in to carry out a records review study. This group did a thorough job of looking into everything in our recently formed division. They compiled a "Manual of Forms and Definitions" which has served us well with little major revision to the present time. Subsequently they wrote a book about the whole experience (Blum and Ezekiel, 1962).

Perhaps the greatest impediment to this study was intrinsic to the arrangement itself—the fact that the study staff were "outsiders." This maximized the opportunity for a renewed era of "we–they" feelings. The program office and research were once again paired as the bad guys. A general feeling of resentment toward the record-keeping system prevails in only slightly muted form to this day. Records are still seen as something imposed from above and serve as a convenient vehicle for the displacement of all sorts of unproductive feelings. It is interesting to note that new professional personnel learn these negative attitudes very effectively, despite the fact that the major function of these records is to provide useful clinical information for staff about their patients. Nevertheless, a later time study (1965) showed that a reduction of staff time spent in record keeping had, in fact, been accomplished.

One of the consequences of division organization was the establishment of a uniform fee system. Thereafter outpatient services staff were regularly confronted with the need to refer financially ineligible applicants to private practitioners. This generated staff concern about the fate of these people—did they go through with the referrals or were we unwittingly creating a pool of untreated people in the community? A follow-up study was quickly designed, the social workers in both clinics participated willingly in making out a standard telephone interview schedule, and for several months the outpatient services were a program evaluator's delight. When the data were in, we knew that two out of three cases had followed through with our referrals, a ratio considered satisfactory by local standards. The important thing we learned here is that a staff-generated study has a good chance for survival and its findings a fair chance for acceptance.

In 1960, program evaluation and research were considered to be of such importance that funding was approved and the organizational structure was amended to create an independent psychology service. Allan Goldfarb, a highly competent psychologist with an additional doctorate in public health, came in as our service chief and began the long and difficult task of developing this service into a new entity. He began by extending the continuous evaluation idea through the medium of wall charts to be provided and maintained for the program chief and each service chief on a monthly basis by the psychology service. The purpose of these charts is to keep the decision-making people up to date on what is happening in their respective services. They display such operational information as number of applications; admissions and discharges; number of cases on the waiting list; backlog on intake process; size of active and inactive case loads; number of individual and group treatment interviews; day center attendance and inpatient bed occupancy rate; percent of treatment work invested in individual and group therapy; and so forth.

Of course, our ability to deliver this information reliably and validly is completely dependent upon a well-administered and effectively monitored record system. This is accomplished almost entirely at the clerical level under the direction of the administrative coordinator who reports directly to the program chief. Coordination of such a manual data-gathering effort is no easy task and requires clear and open communication between a considerable number of people in different locations throughout the county. From time to time this requirement has provided spectacular interpersonal fireworks between almost all of us. Beware, particularly, when a clerk and a professional decide to act out their temporary animosities through the medium of the record system. Whether electronic processing of these kinds of data will reduce the human interaction risk factor appreciably is by no means certain, but one can look forward to this next step in the interest of quality control.

The wall charts can and do call attention to what is happening in a persistent sort of way that takes obvious effort to ignore. Equally important are some things the charts cannot do. They usually cannot indicate why something is happening, unless it is obviously a seasonal phenomenon. They also cannot insure receptivity in the beholder, or suggest solutions, or insure implementation of proposed solutions. They are a tool; their use, non-use, or misuse is a function of the people in the system. Major problems have become apparent over the years. The psychologists assigned to the various clinical facilities were to have functioned as representatives of the psychology service in interpreting the charts to their respective clinic service chiefs and educating the clinic staffs to their usefulness in guiding clinical operations. Some of the psychologists themselves turned out to be ambivalent about this task, but perhaps the most important interfering factor was the fact that this would have alienated each psychologist from his clinical colleagues. The opportunity to make program evaluation data useful is seriously hampered in the inhospitable atmosphere which results when a service chief fails to act in concert with the division goals of the program office. It was difficult to be enthusiastic about the function of providing information which not only made you unpopular, but which did not include much real prospect of implementation.

By this time the psychology service staff had increased considerably in number. We had established the idea that psychologists could legitimately invest 10 per cent of their time in research work, and several program evaluation studies were launched under various auspices.

The program administrator posed the question, "What percent of the patients being admitted to our inpatient service (twenty-four-hour bed-occupying care) could instead receive adequate care in our now well-established day center (seven-hour non-bed-occupying care)?" The ensuing study showed that an appreciable percent of the hospitalized patients could indeed be treated successfully in the day center. This finding had a variety of consequences, both short- and long-term. Patient care was changed to allow for presumably more appropriate treatment at the point of entry into the mental health program. Staff attitudes were changed on both the inpatient and day hospital services, we assume for the better. In planning the next major change for the division's operation, administration felt sufficiently encouraged by these study findings to authorize establishment of our first regionalized mental health center (north county) without its own adjacent inpatient ward. Finally, when San Mateo submitted its projected long-term needs to the State Department of Mental Hygiene, the estimate of future psychiatric bed requirements was significantly reduced from earlier estimates. The study was later published (McDonough and Downing, 1965) and is further discussed in Chapter 5.

This study clearly made important contributions toward shaping division programs and planning; however, certain non-occurrences should be noted. A proposed cohort study to allow "outcome" comparison between the patients treated in the day center and those treated on the ward never got off the ground. Consequently, we do not know how much patient and staff time was invested in the recovery effort, or how effective these two treatment approaches were in terms of postdischarge adjustment in the community—return to job, need for additional mental health care, rehospitalization, and so forth. While the staffs immediately involved in the study, as well as their colleagues on their respective services, had acquired different attitudes and behavior regarding dispositional alternatives for the seriously disturbed who came to the emergency room for help, no training procedures were instituted to maintain these changes over time, particularly for the new psychiatric residents who enter our staff system several times a year. Also, nothing further was done to clarify and refine the criteria which separate the successful participants in the day center treatment program from the unsuccessful.

Once the division-wide operational statistics reports and charts were set up, it was possible to give closer attention to the annual state statistics. With the help of the biostatistics bureau in Sacramento, we cut our teeth on the 1959–60 data, from which we learned some interesting things about ourselves. On the basis of that experience, a revised format was designed to give us a better look at the ways age, sex, diagnosis, length of stay, and condition on discharge were interrelated on the various services. Aiming for routine fiscal year reports from the state, we expected to use the findings as self-corrective information for the division, as well as clues for further investigation. However, for a variety of reasons beyond the control of the state biostatistics staff, they were unable to provide this service at that time and could not predict when in the future we could reasonably expect them to do so. Our solution was to request a duplicate deck of their IBM cards, which we continue to receive regularly. After much trial and error, we managed to work out a program for the desired data analysis at our county electronic data processing unit.

This analysis of the annual statistics has found many piecemeal uses over the years. On the inpatient service, for instance, the data told an identical story four years in a row. Alcoholics made up one-third of all admissions; their average length of stay was two to three days; needless to say, their condition at discharge was not much improved. In a sense, this was no great news. The ward staff knew they had no real treatment program for alcoholics, and the rest of the country had no better story to tell. The repeated exposure to these unhappy facts made it more difficult to keep the problem hidden from ourselves at the decision-making level and introduced a measure of dissonance in those administrators who were in any serious way committed to the notion of a community mental health approach. It was not enough to trigger a dramatic change, but it had alerted the system to some extent.

The outpatient services data also told a self-repeating story.

A majority of the admissions to the adult clinic, for example, terminated their contacts with five interviews or less, and a majority of these were considered unimproved at termination by their therapists. The general orientation of that staff was the psychiatric-psychoanalytic model, so there was little surprise in the fact that the "motivated" minority of admissions were being seen for a year or more. Most clinics throughout the country showed similar statistics. But the question arises whether this orientation is a useful one within the context of a program aimed at broader community mental health needs. These data helped to remind the decision-makers once again of the real discrepancy between the orientation of the program office and some of the service chiefs. Around this time a new psychologist was assigned to the adult clinic. She was a highly competent person, experienced in crisis intervention methods, and readily saw their applicability to the problems brought to this clinic by the public. She was unsuccessful in affecting clinic policy at that time and soon took her leave.

We are all in the midst of change and these were our growing pains. It is not equally easy for all mental health professionals to make the difficult transition to a community mental health orientation. It is not easy for them to experience program evaluation data as useful cues for improvement instead of criticism of themselves for what they have inherited from their predecessors. Moreover, the making of program policy is a complex, multi-determined process. No matter how persistently research identifies problems, other considerations may prove more persuasive. The follow-up studies which could throw further light on what happens to the people who have had our best are yet to be done. Nonetheless, we had made a start.

The operational statistics charts had been showing a gradual, continuous increase in the readmission rate on our inpatient service. When this reached a plateau at around 35 per cent, a staff psychologist was assigned to evaluate this phenomenon. A restrospective statistical study was designed to determine how certain patient characteristics of the readmission population differed from those of the nonreadmission ward population (Chin, 1965). The variables studied were age, sex, city of residence, diagnosis, length of stay, and condition on termination, all of which could be retrieved from data already gathered in previous years and quietly reposing on the duplicate decks of IBM cards we were now receiving from the state. This study showed quite clearly that it was the alcoholics who were the major component of the ward's readmission rate, particularly in the multiple readmission group. With this study, we had taken another modest step toward identification of a special high risk group which could then be studied further to the point where appropriate treatment programs could be developed for specific subgroups of patients going through our division program. From this standpoint the study was a success, but implementation fell into a long coma.

Meanwhile, Goldfarb addressed himself to the division's objective of dealing with the community at large and began work on a casefinding instrument which could become the vehicle for a genuine public health approach to community mental health care. If successful, we would have an objective basis for determining incidence and prevalence in the community, to identify high and low risk areas in the county, study these to learn what makes them so, and eventually apply appropriate remedial and preventive programs to entire geographic areas. We were heading in the direction where the census tract, or something like it, would be the "patient." The Leighton casefinding procedure was finally selected and with NIMH support the Cornell-San Mateo project was on its way. Reliability and teachability studies of the Leighton scale were completed (Goldfarb, Moses, and Downing, 1967a,b). A grant renewal had been submitted for the next step, a validity study, when Goldfarb died suddenly in the prime of life. Various loose ends were sadly gathered together, and the project closed down six months later.

The concepts involved in this project were at the forefront of our field and had excited the imagination and participation of some of the best qualified researchers in the country. Except for the program chief and our departmental director, there was little understanding or enthusiasm for this project within our division. There was still a wide gap between those who conceptualized the role of the services and those who envisioned the direction of the division.

In the child guidance clinic a series of statistical program planning and evaluation studies were being carried out (Mlodnosky, 1964). Various demographic characteristics of the families applying to the clinic for help were examined as a first step toward identifying special high risk groups in the community. These studies also focused on the effectiveness of some of the clinic's operating procedures, such as the relationship of waiting period to dropout rate, length of diagnostic evaluation, and outcome of diagnostic evaluation.

One study had shown that the majority of applicants to this clinic had to wait from three weeks to two months between the family's initial call and their first clinic appointment (Mlodnosky, 1964). It also showed that there was a 40 per cent dropout rate for this group of families, while only 15 per cent dropped out when the wait was less than two weeks. Clinic administration decided to introduce a group parent orientation meeting as the first clinic contact experience, this to occur no more than two weeks after the initial call (see Chapter 10). This procedure did succeed in cutting down the initial waiting period to less than two weeks (the median duration turned out to be five days) and achieved the predicted 15 per cent dropout rate. However, the parent orientation meeting procedure itself generated a high dropout rate; people did not go on to the individual appointment which would have initiated the diagnostic evaluation which the family sought and which the decision-makers of the clinic considered their major definitive service. Consequently, the dropout rate between initial call and start of diagnostic evaluation after introduction of the parent orientation meeting, which was the very means chosen to reduce dropout, increased to 62 per cent of the original applicants.

From the standpoint of program evaluation we had done a good job. A deteriorating situation in the child guidance clinic had been clearly and continuously reflected by the operational statistics charts and the studies had identified some of the problem areas and even indicated the consequences of the clinic's first attempt to correct the intake and evaluation situation. Unfortunately these program evaluation findings were not utilized by clinic administration to solve the problems confronting the clinic. They may, however, have helped to bring about the change in clinic leadership which subsequently took place. These same intake process problems were tackled with imaginative innovation by the new administration.

Continuing discussion of time-use problems led to the 1965 time study. This began with a small data gathering effort needed to meet some new state requirements. When this was brought up at the weekly administrative meeting, there developed a sudden and pervasive interest in expanding this task into a full-fledged division-wide time study. Each service chief wanted to know something special about his service; all chiefs wanted to have certain information in common. They wanted to know time spent with clientele, time on the phone, time in travel, time in various categories of staff meetings, time invested in various types of clinical activities, in supervision, and in training. There seemed to be an active interest in the study on the part of the chiefs, and in the course of several meetings with them a uniform coding system was developed and a remarkably smooth operational procedure worked out. Even the clerical staff, who monitored the paper work, were relatively enthusiastic about their involvement. For the five weeks of the study, staff morale was remarkably high and good-natured study-hostility jokes crackled in the California spring air. All the study forms were completed on schedule each week. The reliability of the data was 95 per cent, certainly a sound basis for confidence in the findings. Each service chief received the findings for his service in a packet containing a study summary plus a summary sheet for each staff member, showing his or her contribution to the work of the service. The program administrator received similar summaries yielding a division-level overview. Everyone was now in a position to know exactly how the division's time was being invested.

The operation was a big success, but the patient was dead as a doornail. In the three years that have elapsed since, there has not been a word of feedback from any service chief. The silence which has prevailed regarding the study has been as remarkable as the apparent initial enthusiasm. Whatever the many-leveled reasons behind these remarkable phenomena, it seems evident that the decision-making group was not yet ready to deal with certain aspects of the division's work from a strictly task-oriented, problem-solving point of view.

With the passage of another year the general framework within which the division's program evaluation and research was being carried out had become clarified. Studies could be classified according to the focus of their activity: intraservice, interservice, division-wide, and community. The situation then prevailing was described by Goldfarb (1967) in a paper written shortly before his death. Responsibility for initiating appropriate studies still rested with each service chief at that time. Some chiefs implemented this responsibility; others did not. One conflict of interest inherent in this arrangement was between giving direct service to patients or consultees and investing precious staff time in evaluative research about which there was still considerable ambivalence.

The chief of the rehabilitation service wanted to explore the possibilities of developing appropriate services for maintaining chronic psychiatric patients in the community rather than perpetuating their chronicity in state hospitals. In reviewing one year's admissions to our day center, he found that almost the same per cent of chronic and non-chronic patients successfully completed the center's treatment program, although it took the chronic patients roughly twice as long (Lamb, 1967). The next step was to determine the characteristics of all our chronic patients still in the state hospital. This second study focused on all the chronic patients in our county state hospital wards over an eighteen-month period (Lamb, 1968). It indicated that the percentage of patients characterized by long-term hospitalization and organicity was systematically building up in the hospital, even though the total number of these hard-core patients was decreasing. Follow-up of those chronic patients discharged into the community showed a heavy reliance upon sheltered work and living situations. A third study, funded by a Department of Health, Education, and Welfare grant, is now under way, evaluating the extent to which our comprehensive community mental health rehabilitation program can shift the treatment and maintenance of this hard-core group of patients from the state hospital to the community.

After the North County Mental Health Center had operated for about two years as our first regionalized area, some measure of the effectiveness of this new service delivery pattern was wanted by administration. One of north county's mandates was to implement the continuity-of-care concept, particularly as this applies to county residents returning to the community from the state hospital (Agnews). North county's way of doing this was to send a staff member to Agnews to contact all north county patients in the San Mateo wards, participate in their discharge planning, and take responsibility for the returnee's contact with the appropriate staff people back at the north county center (see Chapter 17). The nonregionalized remaining three-quarters of the Mental Health Services Division had not been able to work out comparable arrangements, so the burden of contacting anyone for aftercare service remained largely with the releasees, who are generally believed to be poor bets for making or maintaining such contacts.

This development seemed to present a natural laboratory situation. A psychologist was hired half-time and the aftercare study was on its way. The attempt to harness patient-related data from such disparate record systems as the state hospital, the state bureau of biostatistics, the state bureau of social work (a state-operated aftercare service), the county public health nursing service, and our own Mental Health Services Division turned out to be quite a soul-shaking undertaking. We hope to determine whether there is a significant difference between north county and central county aftercare service delivery as regards coverage (whether contacts were made and what kind) and effectiveness (rehospitalization rate). This information should be helpful in guiding the future operations of the north county mental health center, as well as in planning the imminent regionalization of the remaining division services (see Chapter 19).

Another study nearing completion attempts to evaluate the mental health screening procedure employed in the hiring of deputy sheriffs. These peace officers are in contact with an appreciable segment of the citizenry under a variety of stressful circumstances, an example of which would be the task of bringing someone into the emergency room on a seventy-two-hour hold for psychiatric evaluation. The sheriff's department wanted its applicants screened to select personnel whose own emotional problems would be unlikely to interfere in the performance of their duties. A discussion of this screening procedure and the evaluation of it is found in an earlier chapter (see Chapter 14). It is worth noting explicitly that this study represents an important step in the division—the fact that a service unit planned for evaluation from the beginning of this screening activity, and what is more, that this plan has been implemented.

In the adult outpatient clinic a study now nearing completion represents the collaborative efforts by the psychologist and the service chief on that unit. This study focuses on the expectations of applicants regarding treatment and therapists. Over the past two years all applicants (with few exceptions) to the clinic have taken the project test battery (some standard tests such as the MMPI and some specially designed questionnaires) before admission to the intake appointment. Each admission is then followed through his clinic career and at time of discharge classified as an "early terminator" or a "remainer." At the conclusion of the study, the investigators hope to have useful predictors for early termination from the individual and group psychotherapy treatment programs available at that clinic. They would then be in a better position to introduce timely modifications of the treatment programs for the persons so identified.

Our developmental evaluation unit has the task of early identification, evaluation, and referral of people with deficits in intellectual functioning (see Chapter 11). From the very beginning there has been a close collaboration between the psychologist and the other staff members regarding systematic evaluation of the unit's operating procedures. The unit psychologist provides built-in feedback information pinpointing the factors which interfere with the unit's ability to render maximally effective service to its clientele and relevant agencies in the community. For example, when certain school referrals were spotted as dropping out of the unit's evaluation procedure, staff began to make consultation visits to the schools and to participate in the schools' referral process. Consequently, the incidence of incomplete evaluations was reduced. It is a genuine pleasure to see applied research efforts utilized so constructively.

There are times when a public program, such as ours, has sudden and often instant need for data to meet urgent administrative issues. This sort of "evaluation" is quite different from systematically designed studies to answer specific questions. For example, a political situation arose suddenly a couple of years ago, requiring that our departmental director have available local cost-of-treatment figures for display at a public meeting. Our program was suddenly, publicly and politically being "evaluated" for cost effectiveness vis-à-vis other local programs and state programs. We patched together what figures we could lay our hands on that were in any way relevant to the issue. What data we were able to extract from our reporting systems and previous studies were more a matter of chance and remembering who had seen what in which report, than a matter of foresightful planning. Of course, our "foresight" improved somewhat with each of these kinds of crash efforts, but a certain amount of the unanticipated can never be prepared for. A more recent instance was triggered off by sudden events in our state legislature, which provides the major funds for our division's operation. We were confronted with the need to demonstrate the extent to which we provide local services to those county residents who, but for our program, either would have gone to a state hospital or could not have been discharged back to the community. Fortunately our data bank is now sufficiently versatile to allow us to provide some data reflecting our contacts with these patients. The legislature may reasonably conclude that we have, indeed, provided services to these patients. Whether they might otherwise have become and remained residents in state institutions remains a matter of speculation rather than a demonstrated fact. Nevertheless, our ability to provide data of this kind can have real survival value for the mental health program.

About two years ago the psychology service agreed to accept division-wide responsibility for program evaluation, research, and innovation encouragement. As a starter, all psychologists were to invest 40 per cent of their time at work in applied research and, whenever possible, to combine this with "new" treatment methods thought to be appropriate to the problems brought by the public to the mental health units where they worked. Some psychologists have used this opportunity to acquire or enhance new skills by participating in training workshops in family therapy, behavior therapy, encounter groups, and the like. When the chance to use these procedures arises, we can evaluate their effectiveness.

Some psychologists pursued their respective research interests and produced a number of pilot studies. These covered such divergent areas as (1) analysis of operational procedures on two north county city teams, (2) alternative statistical reporting of staff activities (consultation service), (3) estimating the magnitude of certain problems in our adolescent populations (self-destructive behavior, illegitimate pregnancy, drug abuse), (4) preventive mental health action (for example, anticipatory guidance) at time of entry into kindergarten, and (5) relationship between the staff goals, consultee expectations, and actual use made of certain consultation services (adult courts and corrections unit). In many respects this seems a lively and encouraging beginning, though coordination is still to be imposed, whereupon the inherent conflict between the need to establish priorities and the need to nourish freshness and unfettered inventiveness will be upon us.

Another important corner was turned something over a year ago when we added to our staff the skills of an experienced full-time research psychologist. His first assignment was to review the program evaluation and research needs of the division and to make his recommendations regarding them. He met with each service chief and other relevant personnel; his resulting report was reviewed with the program chief, and priorities were assigned to the proposed studies in line with division objectives during the coming fiscal year. These were tasks for which we could feel a genuine sense of responsibility, accountability, and commitment, which made the going noticeably easier. For example, a descriptive study of admissions to the emergency room was done effectively, in close working cooperation with the inpatient service chief. This study is now being prepared for publication. The next high priority study will be our first real attempt to evaluate the effectiveness of a program vis-à-vis its clearly stated goal. In collaboration with the vocational rehabilitation unit, the research psychologist is now planning a study to measure changes in employment status of those psychiatric patients who have gone through their vocational rehabilitation program. This priority procedure may well set the tone for future research work in the division.

### Decade in Retrospect

Program evaluation began to evolve in an era of relatively rapid change throughout the entire mental health field. The major shifts were from evaluation focused on an individual patient's progress during psychotherapy to evaluation of the treatment methods themselves, for short- and long-term effectiveness. Later the focus shifted to include unmet needs in the patients coming to clinics; it then widened to include unmet needs in the community. Finally it broadened still further to encompass evaluation directed to preventive measures applied to the entire community.

Early program evaluation efforts were carried out primarily by our clinical psychologists, who had only their academic training as behavioral scientists to guide them. These psychologists were able to adapt fairly readily to the public health–community mental health frame of reference of this new era. Their vested interest in the psychiatric-psychotherapy model was less than that of their psychiatrist and psychiatric social work colleagues, and their training as behavioral scientists gave them a frame of reference in which evaluation and change are natural parts of their professional discipline.

The program description level of program evaluation was our major initial approach. It proved useful and was sometimes able to lead to change. Evaluation of pilot or demonstration procedures was also carried out and also led to change. From the prior sections of this chapter, the reader may have observed certain turning points in the development of the San Mateo program to which specific program evaluation projects made major contributions. The organizational structure of the outpatient services made for unwieldy and inefficient service delivery. Our original study of how time was invested, the studies showing an excessive time lag between application and admission, and the record-keeping studies all led to a reorganization of the clinics into team patterns. These studies also helped to focus on the necessity of rendering more effective service as a part of the ongoing concerns of the clinics and the division.

The day center study produced another key turning point. It broadened the use of our daytime facility to treat acutely disturbed patients and, consequently, accelerated plans for regionalization. This led to the establishment of our first regional mental health center without the immediate availability of twenty-four-hour bed facilities. The corner we turned was that of accepting the relative independence of regional center programming from hospital bed requirements.

The operational statistics reporting system and the annual data reports focused the division's attention on unmet needs of a significant proportion of those seeking help from us. This applied particularly to alcoholics and people in need of crisis intervention type of care. This type of program evaluation work served to alert our system and the persistent nature of data presentation initiated some steps toward change.

We have tried to take note of conditions under which program evaluation findings were accepted or rejected by division personnel. Research findings were generally accepted when the study was staff generated, when a service chief was personally interested, or when the program chief insisted on implementation. Results were usually rejected when findings reflected negatively on existing staff practices and treatment philosophy, when findings threatened the existing power structure, or when change was desired by the program chief but opposed by a service chief, whatever the underlying reasons.

In one of his last papers, the late Allan Goldfarb (1965) drew upon his San Mateo experiences to comment on the problems of implementing research findings in our service-oriented setting. He concluded that the program director's response to research findings is crucial to implementation. Appropriate implementation of findings by the director can make or break the usefulness of study findings and the attitudes of staff toward the value and priority of doing research. Finally, Goldfarb pointed out that prior agreement regarding implementation can avoid mutual frustration and should be arrived at whenever possible.

One of the major problems confronting the division over these years has been what to do about the amply documented fact that new and different services and treatment methods were required to meet the real needs of the community. Our experience in the outpatient services is a good demonstration of the conflict, rather than the problem-solving, that developed around this issue. The program chief wanted the various clinical services to change in the direction of meeting more of the community's needs. The outpatient service chiefs, on the other hand, wanted to maintain the integrity of their traditional psychiatric clinics. The operational essence of this position was that the clinics would, in effect, be helpful only to those clients who could fit the psychiatrically preconceived concepts of psychiatric illness. Program evaluation efforts, alone, were not effective in bringing about enough of the required changes. In the final analysis, it was easier to create new services with new staffs than to persuade existing professionals to change their orientation and treatment skills.

We have seen that the vicissitudes of program evaluation and research work are to a considerable extent a function of powerful factors beyond the realistic control of the evaluator. The final determination of policy is the responsibility of administrators. Lest one forget, they do not function in a vacuum and they are people, too. Yet program evaluation and research can and do help to shape policy, sometimes quickly, sometimes very slowly. As a person, a psychologist, and an administrator of program evaluation work, I now have definite convictions, shaped by the experiences described throughout this book. Clearly they are shared by some, but hardly by all, mental health professionals.

As regards treatment programs, I think the job that needs to be done and the conditions necessary to do it have been clarified in the course of our San Mateo experience. We need to combine evaluative research and innovation in the service of the public health policy of providing appropriate mental health care for the entire community, not just those "motivated" for our traditional methods. We must systematically develop and refine usable criteria for an appropriately broad range of mental health treatment methods, then evaluate the effectiveness of these criteria and methods. We must identify those subpopulations in the community with special needs for which our available treatment methods are not really helpful, then innovate new methods and evaluate these. This is an immensely tall order, but it must be achieved if our communities are to make any meaningful headway in the mental health field. If these are truly to be our program's guiding policies, then the role of program evaluation is clear enough. It is equally clear that the ground rules for such an operation must be those of the behavioral scientist.

As for preventive programs, we have hardly scratched the surface. The development and introduction of preventive mental health procedures into the operation of other agencies, public and private, such as schools, industry, various governmental agencies dealing with the public (police, poverty programs, and many others), all these are still at the frontier. Those who carry out the pioneer work should do so with evaluation built in step by step from the start, both for the methods of introduction and the results, in terms of measurable aspects of the community's mental health.

If we really want all these things to come about, I believe they can be ours for the doing during the coming decade. The San Mateo experience, to which the work described in this chapter has contributed, plus the tide of the times, have prepared the way.

CHAPTER **16**

# Evolution of a
# Training Milieu

*Paul I. Wachter*

$ſⱷſⱷſⱷſⱷſⱷſⱷſⱷſⱷſⱷſⱷſⱷſⱷſⱷ$

From the very inception of this community mental health program, there has been a pervasive interest in the function of training. This has been manifest in many ways. As our various service programs have evolved, they have each served as full- and part-time field placements for trainees at various levels in almost all of the mental health professions. Within the entire program, there has been extensive involvement in inservice training activities of all kinds. Many of our professional staff, aside from teaching within our own services, serve as clinical faculty and engage in teaching functions within the various training centers in this area.

With this degree of involvement and commitment to training,

we might well have assumed that it would be a relatively easy step for us to assume more responsibility for basic training programs for the various mental health professions. However, as we embarked upon the development of our own three-year psychiatric residency training program,* we discovered that providing an excellent clinical field experience for trainees whose formal didactic program is provided elsewhere is quite different from assuming the full burden of academic responsibility for the development of a trainee's professional identity. In this chapter, we will review the process by which our program has begun to assume this responsibility, its difficulties, and its rewards in this particular setting. We will also discuss the implications of our experience for this and other community mental health programs for the training of not only psychiatrists but other mental health professionals and subprofessionals.

At the outset, we should review the factors that led us to a deeper involvement in training. It is not surprising that a taxpayer-supported, service-oriented community agency should find itself reluctant to embark on an expensive formal training program. Nevertheless, as our service program developed and matured, a number of critical issues forced us to move toward developing training for mental health professionals: (1) We found increasingly that the traditional training programs in the mental health disciplines did not sufficiently prepare our staff for the kinds of functions that we were asking them to perform. (2) Furthermore, we began to feel more and more the pressure of increasing demand and competition for trained mental health professionals nationally. (3) With the diversification of our services and our venturing into new areas (for example, consultation, education, work with disadvantaged populations) we felt the need for new kinds of skills. (4) With the increasing demand for services, we felt the need and opportunity to fashion new and different programs and patterns of service (for example, regionalization). (5) With all these changes, we have felt a concern about the place of the role and skills of the clinician in this new orientation. (6) With increasing use of nonprofessionals, and our nontraditional use of the various professionals, we have raised questions about what skills and what training backgrounds are needed for which tasks, and who can best offer them.

* The work described in this chapter was supported in part by NIMH Training Grant #T01 MH-10533.

It is interesting that these are the same needs and concerns raised in virtually every conference devoted to the developing field of community mental health (Goldston, 1965; Hammersley, 1964; Group for the Advancement of Psychiatry, 1967). Most of these issues boil down to a single basic question: what are the skills that will be required of the professionals working in the developing comprehensive community mental health programs, and how and in what settings can these skills best be learned? It was to this question that we addressed ourselves when, in 1965, a separate training service, with a full-time chief of professional education, was established.

Initially, the main focus of this service's activity was on planning and implementing a basic three-year psychiatric residency curriculum, taking the fullest advantage of the special qualities of our community mental health program. To our knowledge, this was the first instance of such a community, public-health-oriented mental health system attempting to establish a basic residency program. During the previous years, our program had become intimately involved, through extensive exchange of faculty and trainees, with Stanford University Medical School and the Berkeley Center for Training in Community Psychiatry. C. M. Bryant, our first training director, worked to extend and deepen this involvement with these centers and also with Mount Zion Hospital's department of psychiatry. These reciprocal relationships were extremely valuable in fostering the development of our own residency training program. In 1965, we received approval by the AMA Council on Medical Education for a three-year residency training program and were awarded a seven-year NIMH training grant to support this program (Bryant, 1967).

During the course of our becoming involved in the process of implementing the residency program, we have found our horizons expanding from a narrower preoccupation with residency training to include a much broader involvement with all areas of training in community mental health. Hence, this review is divided into two separate parts: the development of residency training within our program; and the overall development and integration of our many training activities as we evolve toward what we call a system of continuing education in community mental health.

To list the advantages of exposing the resident to community psychiatric practice during his basic clinical training would seem to imply that we have a choice in this matter. This is not the case. In recent years, considerable concern has been voiced by psychiatric educators about the challenge of unmet needs and growing manpower problems in the field of community psychiatry (Caplan, 1964; Bernard, 1964; Hume, 1964). There seems to be a consensus that exposing trainees to this area of skill and experience is an urgent responsibility of all training programs. This theme was predominant in the 1963 Conference on Graduate Psychiatric Education (Hammersley, 1964). The Group for Advancement of Psychiatry (1967) states: "The resident needs opportunities to identify himself with a faculty which is actively engaged in the practical application of community psychiatry concepts to patient care in the ordinary clinical settings in which the resident customarily works. The objective is to bring about more 'community psychiatry mindedness.' " Indeed, this is the greatest single advantage and most eloquent rationale for structuring residency training within a sophisticated, operational community mental health setting.

Since 1959, San Mateo's inpatient, adult, and child outpatient services, and later the North County Mental Health Center have each served at various times as clinical field placements for psychiatric residents from Stanford Medical School and other institutions. In the course of our experience with these residents, we have discovered several additional advantages to training within the community setting.

Even during his work with inpatients, the resident is forced to pay more attention to the social matrix of the patient's family and the community. This more intimate acquaintance with the painful psychosocial realities of the patient's life serves to broaden and deepen the resident's clinical understanding. With our total responsibility for our geographic catchment area, the resident has an opportunity to become more acquainted with the longitudinal course of his patients, as there are no other public treatment resources for them to go to. Even if they enter the state hospital, their presence is usually known to the local program since they are admitted to the regional unit. Thus, the resident gets a more realistic picture of the whole course of the patient's illness rather than a time-limited segment of it.

In his work with agencies in the community, the resident gets a more intimate acquaintance with the various community resources and with all facets of the care of his patients. This gives him a much more balanced perspective about possible alternatives and adjuncts to patient care. He learns that individual and group psychotherapy and full or partial psychiatric hospitalization are only part of a vast complex of resources that contribute to the emotional well-being of the community.

One cannot overemphasize the value of the trainee acquiring, early in his experience, a firm grasp of the public health principles involved in community mental health practice (Bernard, 1964; Hume, 1964; Caplan, 1964). We have seen our own residents develop an intuitive awareness of the social context, an appreciation for the basic concepts of primary, secondary, and tertiary prevention, a readiness to grasp such concepts as "populations at risk," and so on. They seem to take for granted that there are many resources within the community which can be used and strengthened.

Despite these advantages, a number of issues are often raised with regard to a community mental health program undertaking a primary responsibility for the basic training of psychiatric residents (Kubie, 1968). One category of problems usually raised is related to the fact that a community program is of necessity service-oriented and that the pressure of service demands presents the danger of the needs of training being overlooked. When the primary responsibility of a system is to provide service, the values and priorities differ from those in a training institution. For instance, in our program, although each individual staff member has a strong interest in and commitment to teaching, he finds that this is not always in accord with the overall priorities of the service system in which he works. The demands of time and energy for teaching purposes often conflict with service-related responsibilities.

From the trainee's point of view, in those parts of the system where there is a necessarily rapid turnover of patients (that is, in acute services), there is less opportunity for him to get to know his patients in depth. Also, it is no doubt strikingly apparent from the content of this book that our community system is necessarily a very fluid one, with changes in program in response to the changing realities of the community (service needs, legislation, budget changes, and so on). These changes can be expected to cause some disruption in the stability of the trainee's experience. Furthermore, in a setting where the roles of staff members are often blurred, diffused, and even changing, we can expect some difficulty in the trainee's development of a solid role identity for himself.

It is important to note that, while each of these problem areas may pose an obstacle to a training program within a service setting, they can at the same time present distinct advantages. Within such a community setting, the trainees are indeed exposed to *all* the realities of the community and the many possible ways of dealing with them. Along with the conflicts posed by the service responsibilities of our staff, is the advantage to the trainee of having functional role models committed to providing the best quality of service for him to identify with. Along with the danger of overlooking the needs of trainees, there is a special need and opportunity within this setting to listen to the trainees and to encourage their participation in planning and evaluating the program offered them. Along with the less extensive genetic understanding of patients in the more acute phases of our services, comes a broader sample of experience and confrontation with a wide gamut of psychiatric disorder, leading to a heightened degree of comfort and competence in dealing with the many difficult problems presented by patients. Along with the dangers of lack of stability in the program and changing role models, there is the advantage of the trainee acquiring a certain degree of flexibility early in the formation of his own identity.

In anticipation of the problem areas outlined above, our services sought to deal with them in a number of ways. A curriculum committee of senior psychiatrists was organized to plan and review the curriculum of residency training and the optimal placement of residents within our services. We sought to involve as many of our staff as possible in the training program itself, in order to incorporate more explicitly into our system the values and priorities of training. Administratively, we sought to shelter the residents from excessive service demands insofar as possible. We sought to place residents in the most stable and established parts of our program, particularly during their early training. In addition, we worked to develop further our reciprocal ties with other academic institutions in order to strengthen our formal teaching program.

Another legitimate area of concern expressed by many psychiatric educators is that the public-health-oriented philosophy of the community mental health program differs considerably from the philosophy and goals of the individual-psychotherapy-oriented clinician. This might interfere with the learning of the basic skills of intensive diagnostic understanding of the individual and a capacity to understand and deal with the vicissitudes of long-term individual relationships. In this setting, the focus is on communities and populations rather than exclusively on the disordered individual. There is an emphasis on prevention, rehabilitation, and environmental manipulation as well as on an in-depth understanding of the individual patient and his illness. To the extent that there is a focus on social adaptive processes rather than on an intensive study of the individual, there is considerable opportunity for a defensive avoidance by the trainee of an intimate encounter with the patient's inner pain. This is particularly true early in the resident's training, when his anxiety is the greatest. Hence, special efforts are necessary, if there is to be adequate development of basic psychotherapeutic skills within a strongly public-health-oriented program.

In our own setting, we sought to provide (through supervisors, seminars, teaching conferences, consultants, and the training staff itself) competent and experienced clinicians and psychotherapists to serve as useful role models for identification. We have also encouraged, exhorted, and demanded that the resident seek for himself a small number of patients whom he might follow under supervision over a prolonged period and with whose inner experience he might become more intimately acquainted.

Hence, our program sees its training task as twofold: to provide adequate opportunity for the acquisition by the trainee of basic clinical and psychotherapeutic skills, while at the same time exposing him to the realities and helping him learn some means of coping with them so that when he enters the real world of private or community practice, he will not feel overwhelmed and helpless.

It has been gratifying to note that, perhaps in some measure because of these efforts, our residents do acquire an identity as psychotherapists as well as a competence in the other areas of community psychiatry. They have shown a high degree of interest in working intensively with individual patients and groups of patients during their second year, and we have found them to be unusually comfortable (a comfort they seem to take for granted) with the most seriously disturbed patients, even on an outpatient (or emergency room) basis. Perhaps more important, however, are their recognition and acceptance of the realities of mental illness—the chronicity, lack of "cures," and the need for multifaceted approaches to many of their patients.

So much for the problems we anticipated and the efforts we expended to resolve them. During the course of these efforts, however, we encountered yet a third category of problems which, in our naiveté, we had not at all anticipated, but which we feel should be shared with those who may be planning to embark on a similar venture.

Shortly after our own residents began their first year, the honeymoon was over. Relations between training and the clinical services became more and more strained. The director of training was chagrined to find not only an absence of the priority commitment to the goals of training which he had naively taken for granted, but even a distinct resistance to the burdens and restrictions that he found himself imposing upon the already overworked services. The spectre of training versus service was heatedly raised and haggled over, and sentiments to the effect of "Who the hell needed a training program anyway?" were more than once expressed.

We have since come to understand, in retrospect, that during this period we were engaged in the painful process of working through a major change within the mental health services, namely the integration of a new component—training—into our social system. Indeed, it can be anticipated that the process of establishing a training program within any system where there had been none before will inevitably be fraught with considerable turmoil until the whole system establishes a new equilibrium.

Throughout this process, it was very important that a firm administrative decision to develop a training program had been made and received firm and consistent support. However, the fact that training was not given any direct administrative power over the clinical services meant that achievement of training goals had to be through negotiation and compromise, rather than by administrative edict. In retrospect, though at times burdensome, this helped make it a process of mutual interaction and two-way adaptation and was therefore very useful.

The residents, too, felt the strain of this process. At times they felt like outsiders—not respected and not listened to—and responded with their own degree of hostility and passive-aggressiveness. The process of working through these changes took almost the entire first year of our residency program. There was a gradual accommodation on both sides and training progressively became more of a shared responsibility. Feelings among staff around the issues of training became more positive and the residents were able to identify with the system and feel a part of it. They became more aware of and interested in larger issues within the entire program, besides those involving training. By the end of this first year, a resident representative became a regular member of the curriculum committee and other ways of involving the residents in on-going program planning and review were being considered.

During this period, the training service itself underwent considerable change. Whereas it had previously seen itself as an initiator and developer of the residency training program and had been involved in the various demands and confrontations necessitated by that responsibility, the training service now began to work more closely with several of the clinical services and saw itself as a facilitator of the development of other training functions within these services. Its task became more to facilitate the exchange of ideas and discussion of training issues, to develop committee efforts with regard to training functions and to advise the services about matters of training. Thus, we have seen a process of mutual interaction, accommodation, and transformation by which training as a function has been incorporated to become an integral part of the overall system. This process has been a dynamic and at times painful one, but in the final analysis quite gratifying.

While discussing this process of change within our system, it is worth noting its particular relevance to our field. Community mental health is often seen as working toward major changes within the social and institutional systems comprising the community. To have taken part in such a process of change within our own mental health system and to experience personally the vicissitudes of this process has in itself been a learning experience for the training staff, as well as for the residents.

As is probably apparent from the rest of this book, there is a basic conviction in our mental health program that a sound foundation in basic psychodiagnostic and psychotherapeutic skills is essential for effective community psychiatry practice. It was for this reason that the program chief explicitly sought people who were committed to psychotherapy to plan and administer the training program. Thus, the residency program has a strong orientation toward learning the basic skills of psychodynamic diagnosis and treatment during the core curriculum of the first two years. The emphasis is on an empathic involvement with our patients, leading to a dynamic understanding of intrapsychic, interpersonal, and sociocultural processes.

During his first year, the resident is assigned to the inpatient service and the day hospital. The formal teaching curriculum focuses on interviewing skills and a dynamic understanding of personality development and psychopathological entities. It also focuses on other treatment approaches, such as somatic therapies and milieu therapy and on the role of the psychiatrist in relation to other mental health professionals that comprise the treatment team. During the second year, the resident works primarily with outpatients. The formal teaching emphasis is on long-term individual and group psychotherapy, psychoanalytic theory, and diagnosis and treatment of children. There is also exposure to such fields as neurology, mental retardation, and public health. We anticipate that with the consolidation of the regional centers, the resident will find increasing opportunity to relate his psychotherapeutic work with outpatients to other kinds of community intervention and a more intimate acquaintance with the sociocultural context of the community.

It is our hope that this two-year core curriculum of clinical work and didactic instruction will prepare a resident to carry forth his skills and interests into a largely elective third year. Work required in the third year consists of continued long-term psychotherapy with selected patients, some clinical and preventive work in the community setting, and advanced seminars. There is considerable exposure to child psychiatry during the second and third years. During the second year, the resident spends six to eight hours a week in seminars, diagnostic and therapeutic work with children, and supervision. During the third year, it is expected that some of the resident's work in the community will be directly related to child-oriented systems such as schools and juvenile probation, either around case collaboration or in consultation to these systems.

There are some broader implications for residency training in general that may be derived from our experience. In discussions regarding psychiatric education in recent years, there has been an increasing preoccupation with the question of how to make room, in an already overcrowded curriculum, for the explosive increase in new subject matter and skills which have to be learned. There is considerable uncertainty as to how, when, and to what degree in his training the resident should be exposed to the concepts of community mental health (Caplan, 1964; Hume, 1964; Gaskill, 1968). With regard to these issues, it has been our experience that in a community mental health setting such as ours these concepts permeate the program and become an integral part of the resident's professional identity. Thus, we have come to feel that as psychiatric educators we should look not only to the *curriculum* which we offer our residents, but also to the *models* with which they are confronted, to the philosophical attitudes of the program in which they grow, and to the style of the program which nurtures them. These are what stimulate the trainee's interest, openness, initiative, and readiness to apply his clinical skills to a constantly changing model of practice. Indeed, this very flexibility, adaptability, and readiness to apply skills to new and different situations and circumstances is the very essence of a style that is most important in working in community mental health.

### Continuing Education

During the academic year 1967–68, the mental health services served as a significant field placement or a full-time training site for over one hundred professionals. This included first-, second-, and third-year psychiatric residents; advanced residents and some staff members studying community psychiatry; medical interns; undergraduate and postgraduate social work, psychology, and nursing students; and trainees in mental health education, vocational rehabilitation, and public health. Various training experiences have been developed for volunteers, college students, and medical-student clerks who spend time in our program. In addition, our NIMH-sponsored demonstration office has become deeply involved in developing films as instructional aids and curricula for use in short-term educational experiences for the many professionals who come to visit our services from other programs throughout the world.

In an effort to pull together this complex network of training activities, an interdisciplinary committee for training was formed consisting of representatives of psychiatry, psychology, nursing, social work, and our demonstration officer. The purposes of this committee were: to encourage interaction between the various disciplines at the training level and to acquaint them with the training backgrounds of the various subspecialties within each discipline; to become informed about all the levels of training experiences being conducted within each discipline throughout the services; to evaluate the different kinds of experiences offered in the various settings and to encourage thinking and discussion among the staff about possible additional learning experiences for trainees; and to foster as much interaction of the trainees of different disciplines with each other as possible. It might also become a forum to discuss academic standards of our various training programs and to advise the training service and program administration in this area.

It is our hope that by establishing such a committee, we will avoid the usual widening gulf between the disciplines, as each goes its own way with proliferating education programs. We hope this will foster cross-fertilization of ideas among the faculty, as well as among our present and future trainees within the various disciplines.

Along with the proliferation of training activities described above, there has been an increasing involvement of all staff in such activities as teaching, supervision, and coordination of the work of trainees. For example, in our North County Mental Health Center, it became necessary to form a training committee to take responsibility for planning and coordinating the experience of the many trainees placed there. A staff member was given the responsibility, on a part-time basis, for administrative coordination of training within the regional center and to relate to the central training office. With the development of the three other regions within our mental health program, a similar pattern of local coordination of training will eventually be established.

A striking example of the extent of staff involvement in training activities is the development, by the staff of our consultation service, of a course, "Introduction to Indirect Service Aspects of Community Mental Health." This course is a natural outgrowth of attempts by our staff to conceptualize their experiences and to share them. Its antecedents can be traced back directly to our staff members' participation as lecturers in neighboring training institutions, and to their production of an early monograph on mental health consultation (Kazanjian, Stein, and Weinberg, 1962). In 1966, a formalized course offering an introduction to community psychiatry was developed by our staff in conjunction with the Stanford University department of psychiatry. It was subsequently expanded and since 1967 has been located within our consultation service at San Mateo. It now consists of three basic components: didactic lectures and seminars, coordinated field work, and supervision of the field work experience. It runs from July to June of each year, and requires a commitment of six hours per week of the trainee's time. It begins with a didactic sequence on the various approaches to understanding human social systems, along with a one-month field experience, in which each trainee visits and studies an agency within the community. By September, each trainee is assigned to an agency or system within the county and his work is coordinated by a consultation service staff member, who has an established relationship with that system. The trainee's task is to develop a consultation relationship (or fit into an already developed one) with a significant person or group within the system. He receives biweekly supervision, generally in small groups of three trainees. On the alternate weeks, there is a series of lectures about principles of mental health consultation, mental health education, and community organization. There is considerable exposure to experienced professionals from within and without our mental health services, who share their experiences in their various roles.

Besides coordination of field experiences and supervision of the work of trainees, those staff members who function as faculty for this course meet weekly for one hour throughout the year. During this meeting, administrative problems are dealt with but, more important, it is a forum for development of the identity and skills of our staff as teachers and supervisors. This reflects an important assumption: namely, that pedagogic skills are not necessarily acquired in the course of extensive experience and skill in the field itself. We see this systematic attention to the development of necessary teaching skills within our staff, as well as careful preparation and coordination of course material, as a prototype for the development of systematically programmed learning experiences of various kinds and at various levels within the entire mental health services.

While it is still too early for a systematic follow-up of the effects of this training experience upon the trainees, our impression is that it has had considerable impact upon them. A number of residents have sought further supervised experience in consultation and at least one has gone on to a full-time fellowship in community mental health at the fourth-year level. Those staff members who took the course have shown much more comfort and readiness to involve themselves in working in indirect services. When the course was offered again the next year, it was oversubscribed and enrollment had to be limited to nineteen trainees. It is noteworthy that among the current trainees in this course are many experienced staff members from other services, some at an administrative level. The chiefs of various services have requested slots for many of their new staff members—in some cases even before the staff had arrived.

Based on the sucess of this program, we are currently planning the development of similar programmed curricula in other specialized areas, either in which our staff has become proficient enough to teach or for which there is a need felt by the developing services. Currently, a sequence focusing on community organization, similar to the one described for mental health consultation, is being developed. Our child guidance clinic is developing a "training track," as an introduction to work with children, to consist of didactic seminars and supervised clinical diagnostic and therapeutic experience with children. Initially, this will be for the training of second-year residents in the child psychiatry field, but the expectation is that this course, perhaps with some modifications, will be very useful to staff members who will be working directly or indirectly in children's services within the regions. Tentative proposals are being entertained for sequences in special therapeutic techniques (behavior therapy, family therapy, and the like) as needs arise, as well as for sequences in research, program evaluation, psychotherapies, and rehabilitation techniques.

The extent of time required for teaching and coordinating these courses, as well as the skills in certain areas, will certainly require the hiring of outside faculty. However, an extremely important step in the development of this program has been the administrative sanction and support for this extensive involvement of our staff in training activities. Indeed, it becomes apparent that, as this process develops, almost all of the professional staff of our services will be involved in either teaching or learning experiences in an ongoing way. This can be seen as the development of a "training milieu" within the entire mental health services. What it really amounts to is institutionalizing the many scattered in-service training experiences which have always been present and relating this more specifically to the program's continuing needs for new skills and expansion of professional role identities.

In another vein, our demonstration officer, whose work has focused upon the programming and training needs of mental health professionals from throughout the nation, has designed an "Institute for Training in Community Mental Health Systems Operation." This format, produced under an NIMH-supported project, will utilize a series of seven documentary films and a detailed institute manual, which have been produced during the past two years. It will also use such techniques as management games, various types of observations, and so on.

We have also taken initial steps to tie in all the above training experiences to the rest of our own professional community and to several neighboring training institutions. In these, we see excellent resources for exposure to basic and clinical research and behavior sciences, to psychoanalytic therapies, and to more advanced and specialized didactic courses in community psychiatry.

With the elaboration of these various training experiences, we can anticipate that many newly graduated or inexperienced mental health professionals in the various disciplines would find it highly desirable to come to work in such a system, at staff salaries, with the expectation that, over a period of two or three years, they could become quite skilled in the community mental health field and then perhaps move on to positions of leadership in their disciplines in our own or other programs. In addition, we would hope that many professionals in private practice within our own community would eventually become involved to some extent, perhaps in an ongoing way, in these learning experiences.

Eventually, we hope to have an integrated network of various kinds of training activities at various levels, extending throughout our central and regionalized services and into our professional community. This network will evolve in a dynamic way in response to the developing needs of our services and the professional community. For want of a better term, we have chosen to call this venture a "System for Continuing Education in Community Mental Health."

In concluding, it would seem fitting to consider some of the broader implications of our experience. The single most important condition for a satisfactory resolution of the integration of training into a service system has been the strong administrative sanction and support we have received. From this we conclude that the administration must be certain at the outset that it wants a training program—for training, that is, and not simply as an additional source of manpower. It must be ready to pay the price of a significant commitment of staff time and energy in undertaking any serious training effort. It has been our experience, however, that eventually we reap a significant return of service of a high quality from the trainees whose needs have been thus respected. Far more important, however, is the overall stimulating effect of training programs on the services themselves.

We feel it is important for newly developing mental health programs to recognize the great potential and necessity for serious training efforts. These should preferably be included in the early phases of program planning so that the training function may grow and develop along with the rest of the mental health program. The relationship of training activities to the services should be such that there is a resonating interaction, each contributing to the other's growth and development.

With regard to those existing community mental health programs who would consider initiating a training program, it would be folly to underestimate the amount of work necessary and the difficulties to be encountered. Critical issues are the process of change within the system, the need to develop a mutually acceptable commitment to realistic training requirements on the part of all the service staff, and a consequent adjustment in their priorities. However, if someone is willing to make the effort and if administrative support is clearly present, it is undoubtedly worth all the trouble. As indicated earlier, such ventures are absolutely necessary if the community mental health movement is to survive and grow.

A very obvious implication of our experience is the great need for active support for the growth of high quality training programs within the larger and more sophisticated community mental health centers as they develop. These programs should associate themselves with university or other academic centers, but this should be a reciprocal relationship—that is, not just to infuse an academic atmosphere into the service-oriented community programs, but also to offer to the academic programs an opportunity to discover the excitement and gratification of a more intensive involvement with the community—to share in the tasks of finding new applications for traditional clinical skills and of seeking new approaches to newly discovered needs.

Finally, it would seem in order here to comment on the general question of the feasibility of such a deep and pervasive involvement in training activities by essentially service-oriented, tax-supported community mental health programs.

We used to think that community mental health primarily involved providing service, and that training was a separate function, often impinging upon staff time and conflicting with service demands. What we are beginning to discover, however, is that community mental health is in itself a largely educative function. Certainly, in our indirect service activities, most of our work involves educating the community—both lay and professional—about mental illness and mental health. Through entertaining professional visitors from other programs in this country and abroad, we have attempted to make an educative contribution to the mental health field. Even in our direct services, we have worked to enlarge the understanding and skills of volunteers and other non-mental health professionals with whom we have worked collaboratively. And some even choose to see our work with patients as largely an educative process.

It is not surprising, therefore, that the interests and aptitudes that draw people to this field should also lead them to be enthusiastic participants in the development of training activities. Hence, the development of training programs can only enhance the enthusiasm and gratification of the staff in their work, as well as enlarge their competence and make a significant contribution to the overall development of the community mental health field.

PART **V**

*In* planning and designing a new regional community mental health center to serve about one-fourth (approximately 150,000) of the county's citizens, San Mateo's Mental Health Services Division was influenced by many of its own experiences, in addition to programming methods and empirical models developed elsewhere. Prior to the appearance of this new center in 1965, the service region was virtually without any locally-based mental health services—private, public, or voluntary. The single notable exception to this was a rudimentary county outpatient facility operated by two part-time professionals out of an office in the business district of the city of Pacifica.

The nonconforming service patterns and operational rationale for the north county region were intended to respond to local demands

# STRATEGY OF
# REGIONALIZATION

*and needs with greater sensitivity than had other programming previously carried out in the county. A major thrust for this regional center was to insert a public health orientation that would assure ongoing attention to changing community needs, collaboration with the community in evolving promptly available and accessible services, and evaluation to assess results.*

*Required, above all, was an experimental attitude, since conventional deployment of limited staff would fail to meet anticipated needs. There was also a keen awareness that there was little experience, in San Mateo or elsewhere, to guide us in balancing our responsibilities and those of the community in the programming process. By accepting a popular but seldom-tested hypothesis that communities must be collaborators with professionals in service design and operational decisions, this new center was faced with a multitude of puz-*

*zling questions. Many of these reduce to a fundamental problem: professionals, who may willingly agree about the fallacy of unilaterally imposing their own viewpoints and prejudices upon a community, face a serious risk that the community may be ill-prepared to collaborate wisely; community perceptions and attitudes may well reflect a lack of familiarity with even conventional service patterns, let alone those included in a prevention-oriented service configuration.*

*How do professionals achieve reasonable collaborative contracts with their communities? To what extent can an alarming community demand (for example, for an unrealistic volume of patient treatment services) be met by "educating the community"? On the other hand, to what extent are other demands (for example, that mental health professionals participate in broad social movements) reasonable, albeit anxiety-producing, requests which ought to be met by flexible professionals willing to adapt to their communities? In short, what are the limits and ground rules that help us decide when to be flexible and when to draw the line in departing from traditional service models?*

*It is not the intent here to supply final answers to such questions. Indeed, these central issues are being explored by those involved in community mental health wherever it is found. Instead, a detailed exposition of San Mateo's first regionalization endeavor may help to clarify and redefine some of these questions for those who are, like all of us, still dedicated to the quest for more efficacious methods of prevention, treatment, evaluation, and training.*

*The chapters to follow describe the steps taken in developing the North County Mental Health Center (Chapter 17). They turn, then, to the operational aspects of the new program, suggesting how the accessibility of the shopping-center-based program and its ambitious outreach have produced certain challenges not often shared by conventionally-designed mental health services (Chapter 18). And, finally, there is an attempt to pinpoint factors that have influenced staff responses since the initiation of the new center; these enthusiasms, resistances, and dilemmas, in many respects, recapitulate on a microcosmic scale the contemporary drama of professional readjustment and reorientation (Chapter 19).*

CHAPTER 17

# Programming in
# a New Region

### *Howard Gurevitz, Don Heath*

ᶠᵃᶠᵃᶠᵃᶠᵃᶠᵃᶠᵃᶠᵃᶠᵃᶠᵃᶠᵃᶠᵃᶠᵃᶠᵃᶠᵃᶠᵃᶠᵃᶠᵃ

$W$ith the formulation of the concept of the community mental health center, mental health workers have sought to modify and redefine their services, consonant with guidelines from the models of medicine, the behavioral sciences, and the field of public health with its tripartite approach to prevention. In addition, a growing awareness of the interactive relationship of the individual and the community (Klein and Lindemann, 1961; Duhl, 1963)—as embodied in the thinking of social psychiatry and those pioneering what are termed social systems approaches—has profoundly shaped the thinking and planning about the nature and function of mental health services. Many of the basic issues were either foreshadowed or summarized in the Joint Commission Report (1961).

391

From a century of public health practice have come some of the dominant community mental health themes. These include the tripartite approach to prevention (Caplan, 1964; Hume, 1964), a focus upon the total population (Lemkau, 1955; USPHS, 1964), and the consequent emphasis upon epidemiology (Srole *et al.*, 1962; Leighton, 1959), as well as upon certain modalities of prevention, including mental health consultation, education, and community organization.

The experiences of Kiesler (1964; 1965) and his colleagues in the Range program in Minnesota helped to reinforce a strongly developed local theme of indirect service delivery to strategic gatekeeper agencies and individuals. For a description of the rich climate which stimulated the development of San Mateo's emphatic indirect service orientation, see Chapter 12. Also influential in the development of the North County Regional Mental Health Center were the theory and techniques of crisis intervention (see Chapter 9) and the recognition that partial hospitalization can serve as an effective alternative to twenty-four-hour hospitalization for a significant number of patients (see Chapter 5).

San Mateo also followed the work of Peck and his staff at the Lincoln Hospital in the South Bronx; their development of neighborhood service centers and their pioneering work in establishing a complex new careerist approach to meeting the manifold social and environmental needs of a severely disadvantaged neighborhood was evolving simultaneously with our north county center. The strong inducements inserted into the various Office of Economic Opportunity programs to collaborate with those for whom new services were to be delivered were evident influences in our thinking, though for the most part these, like the Albert Einstein project at Lincoln Hospital, were materializing at about the time our own plans were being shaped in north county. Among the most significant documents to which we have subsequently turned for stimulation have been those which have helped to introduce and develop the new careers concepts (Riessman, 1964; Pearl and Riessman, 1965).

Finally, it should be mentioned that the north county multipurpose team developed concurrently with the geographical teams operating at Fort Logan Mental Health Center, Denver. Fort Logan visitors, plus visits made to that program by our administration and staff people over a period of several years, provided us with the major sources of information about that highly interesting program. We were convinced that such teams could successfully accommodate themselves to a responsibility for delivering indirect services, as well as clinical treatment.

Among the requisites of the new center we were to design were the following: (1) prompt availability of and easy access to services; (2) effective continuity of service within identified primary mental health systems—hospitals, clinics, and private psychiatrists—and from these systems to other systems whose mental health function is subsumed under their basic responsibilities—schools, clergy, probation, and nonpsychiatric medicine, among others; (3) centralization of responsibility and communications for the mental health care of individuals and their families; that is, the linking of services to produce a *center;* (4) development of a wider range of knowledge about the individual and his relationship to the community; (5) stimulation of increased capacity to utilize other services within the community to deal with mental health issues; (6) enhancement of the community potential to increase its own resources for working with the emotional and mental health problems of its inhabitants; (7) development of a service pattern which takes account of and compensates for the critical and increasing shortages of specialized personnel to develop and deliver mental health services; and (8) insertion of a continuous data collection system of proven merit to support a wide range of ongoing program evaluation and research.

Much of what happens in community mental health is, in our experience, opportunistic and expedient. In common with many others who have concerned themselves with community mental health programming issues, we had for some years recognized the value of service decentralization into regions (Brown and Cain, 1964; USPHS, 1964). This seemed the essential answer to the problems presented by demographic and socioeconomic variations between neighborhoods and communities within the county. An important stimulus to this thinking was the participation of our administration and certain staff in a case-study of a community mental health center, subsequently published in book form by the United States Public Health Service (1965).

Regionalization actually received its major impetus following a 1963 amendment to the Short-Doyle (California Local Mental

Health Services) Act. This new legislation authorized the state to increase its subvention of local programs from 50 to 75 per cent reimbursement. Since this money was not available for capital improvements, which could have been used to strengthen the centralized services, it was decided to institute the first of four proposed regions.

A number of considerations were involved in the choice to develop the north county region first. It was, from the standpoint of geographical distance from the central county base of existing public
mental health services, the most remote heavily populated sector of the
county. Coupled with this remoteness was the virtual absence of public
transportation between north county and central county—indeed, for
those in many north county neighborhoods existing bus routes required
them to travel to downtown San Francisco and, after a delay in changing to another bus, ride for an hour to the city of San Mateo in central county.

The distance from Redwood City, the county seat—even far-
ther away, in the southern quadrant of the county—tended also to
persuade these communities that they were out of the sphere of influence in determining total county policies. North county newspapers
and community leaders had long insisted upon the establishment of
major county government branch offices in their area. Among the
services they actively sought and accurately accused of being inaccessi-
ble to them were mental health services. This evident readiness, even
eagerness, for our proposed new program was an important plus, as
far as the Mental Health Services Division was concerned. It seemed
equally evident that the county Board of Supervisors also welcomed
the plan, since it helped to portray to these critics that concrete efforts
were being made in Redwood City to supply adequate tax-supported
services in north county.

### Assessing the Region

Since we were interested in dividing the 457 square-mile county
with its population of 550,000 into four regions, several parameters
were reviewed to identify reasonable boundaries for our catchment
area. This basic planning, in itself, was a demonstration of what community mental health seems to involve, when it is truly taken to be a
valid response to unique local conditions. This early phase of the planning process made us very much aware of the problems and factors

inherent in learning to understand and to relate to the community.

We viewed this preliminary fact-finding as an opportunity to begin to develop a partnership with the community. Our goal was to choose an area large enough to support a mental health center and one which, at the same time, would present a certain general cohesiveness. The center would be most effective, we believed, if it limited its service region to an area that shared some basic characteristics and, thereby, took on a certain distinct identity, despite various internal differences. The criteria and issues we examined can be clustered within four general categories.

*Demographic Factors.* As a division of the county Department of Public Health and Welfare, the mental health program had ready access to a wealth of data. With assistance from the biostatistical section, we made an intensive review of relevant information collected in the 1960 Census, as well as more current health and welfare statistics. Using these data, we attempted to produce a profile of the north county population and to assess socioeconomic and cultural homogeneity.

We early noted certain characteristics held in common by those who lived in the six municipalities clustered just south of and contiguous to the city of San Francisco. This population was younger than that of most of the county. These communities shared a rapid population growth and an extremely high birth rate. Income was slightly less than the county average, and coupled with this was a tendency toward more families in which both parents were employed in order to maintain a level of income. Because of the proximity to San Francisco, the bulk of the labor force was employed there rather than in San Mateo County. To a significant extent, the region seemed to be attitudinally linked to San Francisco, to which it turned for many services. It was remarkably ambivalent about its jurisdictionally-enforced relationship to San Mateo County.

There were fewer people over sixty-five years of age in the area; the Negro population was much less than the already low county rate (2.8 per cent in 1960); however, persons of Oriental descent and those having Spanish surnames constituted a larger fraction of the north county population than they did of the county as a whole.

This population resided in the twenty-two most northerly census tracts in the county. Included in these census tracts were the cities and towns of Daly City, Pacifica, South San Francisco, Colma, Brisbane, and Broadmoor. Approximately 150,000 people, just over one-quarter of the currently estimated county population, lived in this area.

The process of gathering and evaluating this information produced for all of us a strikingly different image of this region than we had previously entertained. Moreover, it seemed to suggest some important clues for potential mental health priorities. We began to see this as a group of mostly new neighborhoods in which people lived in relatively close confinement, primarily in tract houses, under a considerable pressure to move up and out. Growth and expansion were rapid. Planning was hurried and pressured. Transiency, instability of the population, a high percentage of problems of young adults and young children were some of the characteristics that tended to bind together the population and the individual communities in this proposed service region.

Added complications were occasioned by San Francisco urban renewal programs, which had peremptorily dislodged lower income populations in the inner city and accelerated a tendency for them to relocate astride the southern city limits. This produced a noticeable influx of minority groups into deteriorating sections of the north county. There was, as a consequence, a heightening of the sense of rapid change with which local resources appeared ill-equipped to cope.

Furthermore, the preponderance of young people in north county presented difficulties for the institutions (schools, police, probation) which were hard put to react other than negatively and punitively to the flagrant idiom of the contemporary adolescent scene (drugs, protest, lack of commitment to the establishment).

*Epidemiological Factors.* A review of case loads of agencies that had met needs in the past was our major means of obtaining information about the mental health problems of the region. These agencies, for the most part located in the central county, were units of the existing public mental health program. We found, for example, that the north county representation within the case loads of both the child guidance and adult clinics constituted roughly one-quarter of the total cases served. This was proportional to the north county's share of the total county population. However, the state hospital reported a more than proportional number of north county residents. This led us to speculate that several factors might be among the significant variables

that a new center should consider. For one thing, north county is far-
ther away from the San Mateo regionalized state hospital service—
located at San Jose, to the south—than the rest of the county. Perhaps
this greater distance, as well as certain socioeconomic factors, would
make it more difficult for people in this area to be released back to the
community in the most prompt and timely manner. More than that,
however, it appeared likely, also, that lack of local resources might
well have forced people to delay seeking care until they were sicker.

Many unknowns confronted us. Our data failed to supply more
than an inkling about a base rate of mental illness incidence, although
the negative correlation between state hospital and county outpatient
services utilization helped to prepare us for the influx of previously
undiagnosed patients who flocked to our door soon after our more
accessible facility was opened. One of the most important trends we
could not measure was the reliance upon non-county-based facilities in
San Francisco. Knowing that the labor force was preponderantly employed there, we suspected a considerable portion of the region's health
needs were being met there, as well. This fact tended to be borne out
by statistics showing that most births for north county occurred in out-
of-county hospitals.

A different, less precise, but probably more significant source
of epidemiological data was produced in the course of our visits to
local resources and services. School personnel, local police departments,
clergymen, welfare workers, and public health nurses working within
this region all conveyed their impressions about the prevalence, incidence, and types of mental and emotional problems they encountered
in their work with people. This was seldom communicated to us with
statistical precision, but it helped us to see the needs through the eyes
of key caregivers. Even more important from our point of view were
the insights these discussions generated as to the variations between
these resources in their perceptions as to what constituted mental
health problems, which of these problems the existing agencies believed themselves able to handle, and which they wished to refer to
mental health services.

*Local Resources and Services.* A major block of time was devoted to contacts with every caregiving agent and agency that we could
think of. In addition to those mentioned above, these agencies included
city government personnel, recreation departments, voluntary agencies,

probation workers, chambers of commerce, service clubs, parent-teach-
ers associations, and any other formal, informal, or unofficial helping
source that we learned about. Beyond their epidemiological value,
these contacts were an invaluable introduction to the community,
opening the channels to an early alliance between ourselves and these
future partners. It was an opportunity to orient and educate our staff,
as well as to understand how we might relate at a later date. Early
concepts of our own program goals and policies were interpreted, and
our mutual ideas about preventive programs were explored. This was
of special importance, since the delivery of north county mental health
services was to be organized in patterns that would be considerably
different than the pre-existing county services.

From these visits, which proved the most enlightening in sensitizing us to the nature of the community and its problems, we obtained
a rather accurate picture of the distribution of existing services and
resources in the region, the extent to which there were overlap, redupli-
cation, logical definition, and separation of services.

In the most rapidly growing and compacted city, the elementary school district had developed an extremely progressive and flexible philosophy—viewing itself as the agency responsible for giving
children a sense of belonging, in which individualistic behavior was
accepted and encouraged. It was the conviction of this district that
parents had abdicated that task in the hectic climate of striving for
economic and social status. Conflicting with this attitude, however,
was the narrower, more traditional view of the high school district.
This lack of congruence between the educational philosophies of the
two districts resulted in understandable difficulty for children passing
from one system to another; from our point of view, it seemed a reflection of some of this community's confusion and lack of consensus
about its goals and responsibilities.

Very divergent views and practices were encountered among
the region's clergy. Each city had a loose alliance of them in a ministerial association. Despite a large Roman Catholic church membership
in the north county, few Catholic priests were actively working with
other clergy. One association was vigorously involved in protesting
housing discrimination. The others seemed much more insular in their
views about their roles.

Local police proved the most informative and involved agency in one community. This law enforcement agency had developed an extremely effective and friendly relationship with the people it served. Being innovative and flexible, it found many opportunities for new roles or grounds for collaboration. Police functions and responsibilities, as viewed by other local law enforcement agencies, proved much more traditional and limited in scope.

Ultimately these meetings with formal, as well as informal, groups proved to highlight the differences between cities, and, of major significance, the differences between the "official" view of the community and that of the residents. Clearly, local resources and institutions through which people could relate to each other or seek help did not seem adequate. Recreation areas were few. Community centers were lacking. More often than not physician and hospital services were supplied by doctors and facilities based outside the region (a private general hospital, the first to be located in north county, was then being constructed in the area but was not destined to open until some months after the North County Mental Health Center started). A sense of community involvement and relevance was noticeably absent. Many people, being new to the community and, indeed, new to the Bay Area, were separated from their extended families and the familiar institutions they had relied upon for support in the past.

*Cultural Factors and History.* A most elusive aspect of this fact-finding concerned our attempt to understand how people perceived themselves in their communities. Some sense of this became apparent during the early planning stages. But it is evident that we missed certain cues which, as it transpired, might have served as accurate auguries of future difficulties.

One city was bisected by a major thoroughfare between its old and new sections. This dichotomy symbolized and reinforced the division between the old, established resident and the newcomer. Power alliances, tradition, sentiment, and control issues dominated as central themes in discussions with people at all levels of community life. This city, the largest of the three major municipalities in north county, had virtually no industry and, therefore, homeowners bore the highest tax burden. The amount of sentiment these issues aroused was considerable. Our own choice of a physical site for our facility involved us (without our knowledge at the time) in the competitive strivings between this community's old and new neighborhoods, as well as between this city and another, older municipality. Like it or not, we later discovered we had inadvertently, though inevitably, identified ourselves with the goals and problems of the community and neighborhood in which we settled.

A second community tended to view itself as having no voice in the determination of its own destiny, believing itself disenfranchised from the rest of the county by virtue of its lower socioeconomic status. This self-image was given as a reason for the considerable apathy and sense of futility on the part of residents about their ability to provide or augment necessary services. Being heavily industrialized (that is, by San Mateo County standards), this city was most responsive to changes in economic and labor factors—strikes, increased costs of living, unemployment, and the like. Since this was the oldest, and second largest, city in the region, there was a great deal of competitive striving for political and economic dominance with the next largest city.

Another city viewed itself as being cut off from services and alienated from the entire county; to some extent, indeed, it was unable to see itself, nor was it seen by other cities, as an integral part of the north county region we had selected as our catchment area. This isolated community relied upon others for services, had the lowest tax base, was growing rapidly, and was the youngest community in the area. It had an unenviable reputation for having a considerable amount of social and emotional disruption, perhaps as much because its youthful families seemed less restrained than families in the more settled communities in overt acting-out in response to social, economic, domestic, and emotional stresses. In an almost adolescent fashion, interest and activity levels were high with a great deal of exhibition of energy. However, planning and coordination were disorganized.

Reviewing the geographic and historical factors in the development of the community was another source of important information about attitudes, services, and expectations. The cities had been in existence long enough to have developed very separate and distinct identities, in spite of the many shared factors that united them. Although the various cities were at different levels of development and maturity, there was an overwhelming similarity in the regional striving to cope with problems of rapid growth. Competitive issues, the search for new monies, the sharing of services, taxation problems, and collaborative ventures devoted to development of mutual regional resources, such as roads and hospitals, were all reviewed in the course of our introduction to the region.

A major unifying factor was the isolation and compactness of the region, as typified by the truly wretched transportation problems encountered by those having the need to travel to other sections of the county. This sense of being fractured and cut off from the mainstream of county life was given vocal expression in a variety of ways. The difficulty these communities experienced in obtaining their share of county tax-supported services led to a stereotype that the county neither cared to, nor would, provide the same quality or quantity of services for the region that it did for other areas. Viewing this negative stereotype as a cohesive force enabled us to define with a high degree of accuracy some boundaries of our catchment area. This sense of discontent, isolation, and alienation—and the demarcation between communities that possessed it and those that did not—was quite dramatic and proved a surprisingly appropriate means of drawing the lines of our service region.

## Programming for Community Characteristics

A paramount concern, in programming for this catchment area, was to produce a center design calculated to reinforce the community mental health orientation. Service patterns, we recognized, would have to include ingredients that would encourage staff to identify with the community. To the extent possible, the design should also convey inducements to the community to join with the staff in collaborative and partnership efforts of many kinds.

It was this conviction that motivated us in adapting to our situation the geographic team idea. The three regional teams we developed were to serve the major cities in north county. Each team consisted initially of psychiatrist, psychologist, and social worker—a choice that seems, in retrospect, somewhat less than creative. This composition was dictated, first of all, by expediency—there was some urgency, and these were the most immediately available trained personnel. Nevertheless, this decision clearly reflects our professional stereotyping, as well as the timidity of our imagination. The opportunity to use other types of personnel—public health nurses, activity therapists, anthropologists, and new careerists from our disadvantaged neighborhoods—

was postponed. There was, however, a somewhat vague intent (one that, in any case, has not been fully realized to date) that the teams would slowly develop a wide network of caregiving partnerships as they carried on indirect service work in their communities. It was hoped these partnerships might actually take on the characteristics of an "extended team." In effect, each regional team would then consist of our mental health professionals plus representatives of the many so-called gatekeeper and human service agencies with which collaborative work-sharing had been achieved. In practice, teams have experienecd mixed degrees of success in achieving partnerships that might fulfill the extended team definition. Public health nurses, for example, have been highly receptive, so that they are included in team meetings on a regular basis. Certain of our north county welfare colleagues have been equally willing and able to join with the teams in this way as needs arise. In general, however, the teams have found most agencies reluctant to make the transition from collaboration on single cases or problems to a kind of open-end collaboration on a long-term basis. It appears this may be due, in part, to the fact that our teams have not been highly skilled in carrying on the community or indirect phases of their work or that other priorities and time needs interfere; however, it is a realistic experience, also encountered elsewhere, that the development of close partnership alliances that run across agency lines is, under the best of circumstances, a goal that may take years to achieve.

Our mandate to the teams was clearcut and ambitious: each team was to have full responsibility for the community mental health work required in its service area. Basic planning for programs calculated to meet the indigenous problems of their communities was, for example, an integral part of this. We knew that in visiting in the community and learning to understand it, the teams would become intimately involved and identified with the issues the community presented.

Intrinsic to this mandate was the concept of the mental health generalist, a worker who would function clinically—providing treatment to both adults and children, as well as filling the manifold roles subsumed by the term *indirect services*—as a mental health consultant, educator, community organizer, and mental health resource person.

Underlying the development of this team rationale was our desire to upgrade continuity of care. From its inception in 1958, the San

Mateo Mental Health Services Division had given high priority to preventive services aimed at working with a wide range of non-mental health professionals (see Chapter 12). Our experiences in both the juvenile and adult probation systems had confirmed the value of mingling direct and indirect service work (see Chapters 10, 14). The mental health units in these settings had evolved multifaceted relationships in which direct services were supplied but indirect service was given major emphasis.

When clinical and preventive work are administratively separated, particularly in a situation that involves coverage of a very wide geographic area, a tendency exists for the indirect and direct services to lose a sense of immediacy and relevance to each other's practices. Aftercare opportunities and optimum utilization of community resources tend to be sacrificed; treatment plans and admission criteria, which may be significantly influenced by the clinic's ability to utilize the adjunctive services of other strategically placed caregivers, can be far more sensitively keyed to community aptitudes and resources when direct and indirect services are intimately linked in the same staff or the same individual.

Ranged against these advantages are some admittedly important considerations. The consultant, for instance, sacrifices a certain degree of objectivity and experiences a greater burden of vulnerability to demands for direct treatment when it is to him that the consultee hopes to refer a difficult case. Moreover, the indirect services call for highly specialized skills not easily acquired. It may well be argued, therefore, that those who possess such skills be utilized as full-time experts in the much-needed preventive aspects of community mental health work. These are the kinds of considerations that must be weighed by administrators in making a fundamental choice between optimum continuity of care and optimum deployment of the prevention-oriented specialist. In north county, our decision—which was at the time far less well illuminated by the logic of these pros and cons—was forthrightly in the interests of continuity, a characteristic that had been notably unsatisfactory in central county.

Inpatient psychiatric services were and continue to be unavailable in the center's catchment area. This element, as well as twenty-four-hour emergency services, are the two essentials missing from the north county program. Both continue to be centralized at the county hospital, with which fairly close liaison is possible to expedite patient referral, admission, and discharge bilaterally.

However, we were soon able to phase into operation a day hospital that was specifically designed to serve as a closer-to-home alternative for persons who would otherwise have to be admitted to a full-time hospital. In our initial enthusiasm for the policy of staff integration, we envisioned this partial hospitalization element as being staffed by team members already carrying outpatient and community service responsibilities.

If it is to serve as a viable alternative to hospitalization for acutely and chronically disturbed patients, however, such a facility must be prepared to supply a very active, intensive, goal-oriented program making full use of therapeutic community concepts. Although team involvement is still essential, we have from the beginning provided a separate staff whose responsibility it is to maintain the therapeutic milieu and carry out the day-to-day therapy activities.

With time and experience, we have gradually worked toward a model of collaboration very similar to that of private practice. Each patient admitted to the day hospital has a responsible therapist on the team serving the area where the patient lives. This therapist is responsible for admitting and discharging the patient and is expected to have at least weekly contacts with him. Contacts with families and arrangements with other community agencies for ancillary and follow-up services are also the responsibility of the team therapist, ensuring development of meaningful continuity of care.

The day hospital also proved a convenient portal through which patients returning from the inpatient services at County General Hospital or Agnews State Hospital could be received. Availability of day hospital follow-up is one of the major factors permitting the county inpatient unit to maintain its brief average length of stay and reinforcing its consequent ability to meet the heavy demands for local admissions (see Chapter 4). A very large percentage of north county patients, discharged from this centralized facility, require a day hospital program as their next phase of treatment. Because of the pace of the central county inpatient program and the fact that treatment and discharge planning are done by a staff of resident psychiatrists that is subject to rotation every four or six months, effective communication about policies and procedures needs close attention. Nevertheless, we are able to "weekend" patients on that service, as well as to have patients admitted overnight—expedients which often prove absolutely necessary when an acutely disturbed day hospital patient shows signs of serious decompensation toward the end of the day or week or when a new patient, suffering a transient crisis reaction, is to begin outpatient treatment a day or so later.

Our linkage with the San Mateo County wards at Agnews State Hospital was improvised by the day hospital, because it was there that we had begun to develop a range of social and activity therapies, specifically designed to meet the aftercare needs of chronically disabled, long-term patients. These individuals are routinely admitted to the day hospital when it is seen that an active and intensive intervention is needed to help them deal with a new, acute episode in their illness. They are not, however, maintained in the day hospital on an extended care basis; instead, we have attempted to produce less intensive but continuous aftercare services that permit us to maintain contact with them and to assist them in making the most effective possible adjustment to the demands of community life.

These social and activity groups, often operated as ex-patient clubs and staffed sometimes exclusively by volunteers, have been of great value in meeting the needs of many of the long-term patients that have been discharged in recent years from the state hospital.

To minimize difficulty in the transitional phase between state and local care, the day hospital social worker has been delegated state hospital liaison responsibilities. This weekly contact, which included participation with state hospital staff in therapeutic as well as discharge planning activities, has led to subregionalization at Agnews (see Chapter 2), so that all north county patients occupy a single ward.

This personal contact with the entire contingent of north county patients has served to facilitate an almost fail-safe method of state-local transition. Nearly 95 per cent of all north county patients discharged from Agnews come to the center for some form of transitional and dispositional service, which, in many cases, may lead to outpatient follow-up, day hospital admission, or participation in a social therapy group. In addition, this example of community interest in the state hospital patient has proved an impetus to motivate state hospital personnel to think, plan, and actually work in community-oriented programs.

### Pre-Admission Screening Intake

Owing to the absence of an emergency service, the center has found it more difficult to initiate effective precare routines. Referral sources and families have been encouraged to call or come to the center during its regular work day (8:00 A.M. to 8:00 P.M. weekdays), as needed for emergency intake. Weekend and evening screening and inpatient admissions are, of course, handled by the central county emergency service, without our prior knowledge.

Teams have accepted responsibility for the pre-commitment home-visit services (see Chapter 4) in their communities. These activities, however, have been reserved to a limited number of patients who were resistive to hospitalization and for whom petitions for court commitment to the state hospital were being sought by relatives. Pre-commitment home visits have to be done by psychiatrists, since medical decisions are often needed (such as prescriptions for medications or use of the seventy-two-hour "hold" that must be signed by a deputy health officer). Initially, most psychiatrists were reluctant to undertake this task, which often is crisis-oriented. With time, however, this timidity disappeared, and the task was accepted as a job expectation. Referrals for this are lower in north county than in other regions, possibly because alternative evaluations at a local center are more available or that the distance from County General Hospital prohibits early home intervention. Home visiting for purposes other than pre-commitment screening has become a standard practice involving all disciplines on the staff.

Intake was assigned to teams in rotation on an O.D. basis. Wherever possible, it was the policy for the team member handling the initial evaluation to follow up on the case without collaboration. This plan was designed to minimize transfer of patients, to avoid needless multiplication of professionals in the screening process, and to cut down on the volume of communication required to clarify and focus treatment and diagnostic goals. The intake work, like all other team functions, was shared by each of the disciplines. It involved follow-up contacts with families of applicants (rather than "farming out" the necessary collateral work to another professional). From the intake interview, regardless of what phase of treatment a patient might find himself in, the team member assuming original responsibility was considered the responsible therapist, an administrative mechanism predicated on preserving continuity of care to a greater degree than had been possible in the past.

The direct service intake was emphasized to the teams as a convenient and continuous indicator of the kind, incidence, and prevalence of mental health problems in their team regions, as well as the most sensitive measure of the adequacy of their communities in serving mental health issues.

Initially, the referral process was seen as a key link between the individual and the community. Accordingly, our policy was to minimize self-referral—a procedure that has never been fully understood by some of our colleagues elsewhere in the mental health division. The self-referral restriction was by no means an ironclad stricture; its intent was to reinforce heavy emphasis upon contacts with other helping sources in the community. When families applied without prior referral, it was the policy to learn whether anyone else in the community was familiar with the problem, and, if so, to seek family approval to contact that prior source of help. In the rare instances in which the family had not previously turned to other caregivers, team personnel were expected to help the family identify others who might logically become involved in some adjunctive and supportive fashion. No family was turned away for lack of a referral source.

The contact between the center's staff and the referral source was expected to help us trace the patient's needs back to a system that was potentially in the position to continue offering services. In addition, this was an opportunity to develop a fuller knowledge of the community, a more accurate picture of the circumstances surrounding the patient's mental health problem, and a tentative judgment whether there might be a potential for a working relationship with the particular caregiver involved. This procedure has been less successful than we had hoped at the outset. The problems have almost entirely related to lack of team confidence in offering and supplying a wide and varied range of indirect services to referral sources, many of whom were somewhat less than eager to become engaged in such partnership ventures.

Unlike conventional clinics, the teams have been explicitly prohibited from establishing a waiting list, which is, of course, the tacit expedient by which outpatient services—including those in our central county complex—limit the availability of their services. Generally speaking, the intake techniques followed in the north county center helped staff to respond to the need for prompt, appropriate disposition. This pressure led to more selective screening of patients and earlier decisions about what was possible as opposed to what might have been ideal.

The concept of utilizing referral as an entrée to a consultative relationship with a non-mental health system remains valid, in our view. It does, at least, constitute a more definitive and positive expedient than the sterile one of sweeping mental health casualties into the limbo of the waiting list. More will be said later about the general issues of staff attitudes toward the altered focus of their comprehensive mental health assignments; at this point, however, it should be observed that a routine policy of offering and delivering indirect services to those who have previously decided to ship the case over to the mental health center presents difficulties that can be a substantial challenge for a seasoned indirect service worker, one which a less well-trained consultant is hardly likely to be able to master without considerable support and sensitive supervision. In any case, some of the most remarkable individual accomplishments of the center have, in fact, stemmed from a team's recognition that its treatment resources could not possibly encompass the volume of referrals from an individual source (for example, programs of demonstration counseling groups led jointly, in one high school facing an epidemic of teenage acting out, by a team member and a school counselor).

## Using Nonprofessionals

One dominant theme in the predominantly middle-class value system of our north county catchment area has been a sense of alienation expressed, at one level, by institutional patterns that tend to foster isolation rather than sharing. In our early exploratory work, we were struck by the extent to which the community expressed the desire to "send problems away," an attitude implied by the expressed hope for development of agencies, in or out of the community, that would take care of the kinds of concerns that trouble most human beings. The concept of neighborhood centers and the development of a strong network of indigenous institutions that deal with both normal and deviant behavior at all levels was not well developed.

One goal that we had in community organization has been the implementation of planning for effective services that would have a self-help focus. In facing this, it has seemed feasible and advantageous to think of using nonprofessionals, volunteers or paid, within the framework of other agencies and resources, such as churches, recreation departments, and schools. Thus we have begun to establish a series of gradated groups—discussion, planning, and social activity groups, for instance—within churches and other community resources. These groups, sometimes co-led by our staff along with volunteers, or led entirely by volunteers with consultation from our staff, have dealt with a variety of populations that would not usually be accessible to or involved in mental health activities.

In addition, some community groups utilize the facilities of the center for non-mental health activities. For example, a group of mothers living in a tightly compacted apartment complex began to meet, utilizing a social worker as a resource, in order to discuss the problems and feelings about coping in this kind of community. The population density contrasted with the emotional isolation was one of the most remarkable disparities this group experienced, and the lack of sharing —indeed, the feeling of not knowing where to turn in order to share and obtain some kind of assistance—was striking. This group has continued and expanded; it has become a most useful kind of self-help group, which now actually serves the center by helping to identify and make available resources for new families and young mothers living in the area.

Considerable interest in ex-patient activity groups has been displayed, making it possible for us to move some of these out of the center and into the community. Some of the churches have shown particular interest in sponsoring such groups, quickly developing programs either co-led by our staff and volunteers from their organizations or led by volunteers with consultation from the staff.

Volunteer services were supported in the center by provision of a separate office to house the daily volunteer chairman. Months prior to the opening of the facilities, volunteers had been recruited, screened, and oriented to the new program. This was done in collaboration with

the Mental Health Association of San Mateo County, which had previously organized an extensive program of volunteer services to the
central county facilities and the regionalized wards at the state hospital. Our opening day ceremonies—a civic luncheon and open house
—were planned, publicized, and executed largely under the supervision of our volunteers. These workers have developed ties with local
garden clubs (to beautify the lightwells on our second-floor facility).
They have arranged with local art clubs and painters to circulate their
works in the center (sales of paintings from our walls result in a small
income that helps support volunteer projects); and an annual volun-
teer-sponsored art auction and wine-tasting is held in the center to encourage heightened community visibility, as well as to raise additional
funds for volunteer services.

The day hospital has served as a core experience for the training of volunteers, since it offers a more structured setting for both
training and supervision. The variety of volunteer activities includes
provision of specific types of crafts and skills, transportation, assistance
in research (gathering and collating data), co-leading groups, providing public information and public relations services, leading commu-
nity-centered social activity groups, home visiting, assisting in development of liaison with other community agencies or agencies outside the
community (for example, state hospital), and educational efforts in
the community.

### Training

In the beginning, training was characterized by a heavy emphasis upon in-service needs, supplying help to our own staff in areas
where they lacked special skills or would be called upon to provide
certain types of services with which they were not conversant. These
included work with children, consultation, community organization,
mental health education, working with volunteers, family therapy,
group therapy, and crisis intervention.

Because we had considerable interest in enlisting the services of
others in the community, as well as in experimenting to determine how
other disciplines and professionals could be used, we welcomed field
placements from a variety of sources. To date, these have included
undergraduate nurses (assigned to the day hospital and to the teams),
graduate public health nurses (deployed into outpatient and preven-

tive service work), post-master's degree social workers and public health nurses receiving specialized training in community mental health, vocational rehabilitation students, recreation students, health education students, social work students completing work toward the M.S.W., psychologists in master's degree programs in both clinical and education fields, pastoral counselors at the doctoral level, and psychiatrists.

Our contacts with these trainees has been stimulating to the staff, instructive in supplying clues for program development, and, above all, a vital additional link with key training centers in the Bay Area. In a sense, the center has been willing to be highly experimental in responding to requests for such field placements, for it has been our conviction that we could seldom hazard a clear conclusion as to the nature of the training experience we might offer to those who have not usually been received for training in mental health programs until after we had engaged in a mutual process of discovery.

This point of view has led to some innovative programs that would not have been feasible otherwise. For instance, the availability of a well-qualified trainee in public health nursing (acquiring a doctorate in community mental health nursing) enabled us to formulate and establish a program with police in early intervention in family disturbance cases. A health education trainee did an outstanding job in community organization in helping us establish liaison and joint planning with the minority group in the community that was trying to achieve recognition and develop services within one of the cities. Another trainee in mental health social work was instrumental in doing an initial survey about attitudes toward drug use that led to continuing dialogues and activities about this problem with the high school districts. A survey of physician attitudes and interests that has been most useful in suggesting how we might adapt our service to meet the needs of nonpsychiatric physicians was developed by another health education student. Under supervision, some trainees have undertaken various kinds of community and consultative tasks that have significantly extended center services to teachers of the mentally retarded, Red Cross workers, police, and local recreation departments.

### Choosing a Location

Looking for appropriate space in a practical location immediately involved us in the competitive vying among the cities—each aspiring to augment local services. The site decision is, in every respect, highly revealing of our attitudes and those of the service area. In part, it was dictated by the various realistic factors—considerations of the costs involved in leasing the amount of space necessary, availability of accessible locations, and the fact that various local interests were in a position to influence the final judgment which was, of course, made by the county governing body and not by the mental health division or the Department of Public Health and Welfare (although it must be emphasized that all of those parties concurred in the final decision).

We selected an unfinished 8,500-square-foot second floor located in a large shopping center in the newly developed area of the largest city in our catchment area. Clearly recognizing that transportation, even within the north county region we had selected, was very inconvenient owing to a sparsity of connecting highways, the presence of geographic barriers (hills, coastal ridges, and the like), and the virtual absence of public transit, we assumed the accessibility studies that had culminated in the private enterprise decision concerning the location of the large regional shopping center would similarly predispose us to choose the same location. As it happened, the shopping center owners were eager to receive us and submitted a most attractive bid on the lease arrangement.

Originally, we had planned to phase in services, but the opportunity to obtain the necessary space in a single location made it easier for us to develop our family-centered outpatient, day hospital, and preventive services simultaneously; this lent itself neatly to our ideas of a coordinated and integrated multipurpose center and staff. The fact that the physical space was unfinished was equally advantageous, enabling us to work with architects and contractors in designing spaces to suit our anticipated needs. Consequently, we were able to earmark office space for the volunteer chairman and for certain community agencies, which (as was often the case in our region) might serve case loads in north county out of facilities located in other areas. In addition, we planned our staff room as a multipurpose unit that could accommodate small community meetings during periods of the day and week when it was not in use by our own staff and patients.

Inevitably, of course, our communities interpreted location in one place or another from the perspective of their set and preexisting attitudes. Our site decision—putting us into the densely populated, predominantly middle-class, newer section of one city—tended to alienate minority groups in other areas and to identify us with the rapidly developing and "successful" power group rather than with the older, more established and currently deteriorating former "center" of the city.

This was one of our early definitive decisions. It provided a valuable lesson, for it made us more sensitive to the consequences of our choices by demonstrating that many imponderables may lurk beneath what seem to be quite sound and reasonable decisions.

CHAPTER **18**

# The Community and Clinical Practice

*Howard Gurevitz, Don Heath*

ⅅⅆⅅ✳ⅅⅆⅅ✳ⅅⅆⅅ✳ⅅⅆⅅ✳ⅅⅆⅅ✳ⅅⅆⅅ✳ⅅⅆⅅ✳ⅅⅆⅅ✳ⅅⅆⅅ✳ⅅⅆⅅ

Community mental health programs confront a baffling problem when they present themselves to the population to be served. They are concerned, at once, about unmet treatment needs and about the all-important preventive work that must also be done if a reasonable balance is to be struck between available resources and community needs. With a flurry of publicity and fanfare, the North County Mental Health Center opened its second-floor suite, overlooking the Westlake shopping center in Daly City, on January 14, 1965. From that day forward, the new community mental health center struggled to find ways to assert, at one and the same time, that it was available to help meet total community mental health

414

needs but that it was not able to provide therapy for all who might be referred.

This is not a new dilemma. It faces every mental health service, not excluding private practice. For the most part, however, it may be uneasily ignored—hidden in the implicit message of the waiting list and spiraling state hospital admissions, which covertly bespeak the inability to take into local treatment all those who present themselves. The community mental health center, however, has a clear mandate to serve a total catchment area; having limited resources at its disposal, it must consider expedients other than those of direct treatment. In the broadest sense, it must enlist other resources in a community-wide self-help enterprise calculated to upgrade the community's ability to cope with mental and emotional problems. Some may argue that utilization of non-mental health agents and agencies constitutes a second-class approach using fifth-rate methods. It does, in any case, honestly respond to the underlying professional manpower scarcity that must be balanced against the magnitude of community needs. Moreover, even the least charitable critic will perhaps agree that any real heightening of the community's coping ability constitutes a distinct improvement over the time-honored pattern of shipping the difficult psychiatric problems to remote institutions where they can be comfortably ignored.

Second-class or not (and we emphatically deny that it is), the approach seems to be the best devised to date. It faces, directly and unambiguously, the reality that there is not enough group and individual therapy available from the limited mental health manpower to justify an open invitation to all who wish treatment and to all who wish to refer. The North County Mental Health Center was the first unit in our mental health division to state this simple, ever-present fact of life in clear, explicit language—and to face the consequences.

However, it should be stated here that we do not view increasing the manpower reservoir or expanding therapeutic modalities as second-class treatment. Implicit in our approach has been the belief that these approaches to mental health issues have as much validity and impact as any of the traditional methods which have gained acceptance over the years. Our stance has not been one of developing "junior psychiatrists" out of "subprofessionals," but of developing roles for new professionals offering services heretofore not available to troubled people.

There is, however, an added ingredient in the apostasy practiced by community mental health. In the course of their work, the north county staff have found themselves dealing with sociopolitical issues somewhat remote from the immediate sphere of patient treatment. These have included civil rights, poverty, school bonds, school busing, garbage dumping, city planning, and many other such concerns. It is as decisions are entered on the ledgers of such key community controversies as these that the very environment is shaped.

Mental health professionals, it is sometimes argued, have no special disciplinary credentials that would legitimize their contributions to such issues. We have come to see this argument as reflecting a narrow, insular view of professional responsibility and as an attempt to remain professionally comfortable. Concern over expertise and proper role development is important, but it is not a basis for remaining uninvolved. Community mental health, which may be only marginally prepared for these tasks, not only wants to become involved but, in fact, *is* squarely involved, whether one likes it or not.

It may pique the fancies of some to discover a certain quixotic element in this strange (for mental health), bustling involvement with social forces and large human movements. But it does, at least, imply encouraging progress toward increased maturity. It reflects a keener awareness of mental health personnel that they need not be omniscient, despite the false expectations that may be focused upon them. They, like other specialists, need not contribute the whole answer, or even, in some cases, any part of an answer to the great issues of our time. Being available and involved, they may do no more than help to bring together those whose talents and credentials can be expected to produce answers. The mental health professional in the north county has been able to function as an expediter, a change agent, an enabler, a facilitator—essentially, he has been a middle-man—to promote more effective communication from one group to another.

Our work of enlisting community resources and our participation in shaping the environment of our communities have been the two articles of the north county policy that have most often defined us as "different," marking us as practitioners who have cut themselves loose from the restraints of a buoyant, secure, albeit slightly imperfect, tradition. Other specifics were often seized upon as ostensive flaws in our armor: the "generalist" idea was criticized by those who still found it imperative that a professional have something of his own that no one else could really do; the absence of the conventional child guidance format was even more often deplored. But these penetrating and not irrelevant criticisms of our program were, in fact, the verbalized discomfort felt by our colleagues as they witnessed our difficult struggle to couple a population-wide outreach with a limited and realistic service pattern.

Complex and potent issues are exposed when mental health services develop in close juxtaposition to the community. Essentially, in establishing local services, one is faced with the reality that in order to change or make an impact upon the community and its existing or needed resources, the very nature of clinical practice may be altered.

It has become a cliché in community mental health to recite the principle that "we start where the patient is." This same principle, extrapolated in terminology to describe our approach to indirect, preventive services, is supposed to connote an egalitarianism, an openness, and a willingness to work in new relationships. Applied to groups and particularly to communities with complex identities and multiple needs, however, it becomes very difficult to assess where the community really is and what it wants. Often, in desperation, having failed to get the community to express its needs in discrete or lucid terms, mental health professionals have tended to fall back upon doing what they thought the community needed. Not surprisingly, this frequently proved to be what mental health workers were most comfortable in offering to begin with.

Provision of direct treatment and evaluation services is widely expected by the lay community as the chief stock in trade of mental health services. In our catchment area, we found the citizens with whom we came into contact agreed, or at least did not disagree, when our preventive goals were described; full understanding and grasp of these issues, we sensed, were often lacking. When mental health services were advocated by community spokesmen as essential to the well-being of the north county region, we could be relatively sure the enthusiasm was based upon the conviction that the new program would become actively involved in and mainly responsible for the direct treatment of patients.

It has been a constant source of discouragement for many of our staff to meet with repeated traditional direct service demands that were couched in contexts which clearly implied we were not being helpful if such services were not forthcoming. A major goal of our center was community involvement at many levels. The identity we wished to establish was that of an agency supplying an essential level of treatment-oriented patient services together with an increasing measure of preventive services designed to integrate mental health concepts into the broad institutional tapestry of the community. The insistent demands for direct treatment were sometimes heard by our staff as messages of rejection of our efforts and thus of our skill and identity. Despite such disappointing interpretations, however, we came to realize that efforts to listen to and adapt ourselves to the expression of these needs was extremely important. Attentive discussion of these demands with those expressing them offered an effective medium or communicational forum in which to initiate and pursue our goal of educating the community concerning the potential value of working together.

We learned how to pay attention both to what the community said it wanted and the form in which it saw these needs being met, as well as to its unspoken needs. By seizing repeated opportunities to carry out a long-range (indeed, interminable) demonstration to community caregivers that our model and goals were different and involved an ongoing collaboration with them, it became possible to begin to modify this distortion.

Our accessible location was interpreted by the community to mean that we were prepared to accept patients and families on a drop-in basis. Nor was this wholly erroneous. Because ours was the only psychiatric service available, public or private, we had no intention of retreating behind bureaucratic routines as a means of barring those who clearly needed urgent help. But our limitations were clear. Accessibility often implied not treatment but immediate screening, planning, and disposition elsewhere (perhaps to the central county inpatient unit or the state hospital; perhaps to another community caregiver).

To begin with, we suggested to the teams that available time be divided equally between direct and indirect service—a goal that was not achieved. Team members, fatigued and anxious because of multiple responsibilities and keenly aware of the dearth of alternative services in the region, retreated into the therapist role. This effectively minimized the time available for paying attention to the community.

In order to impose realistic limits upon services to applicants, the emphasis was upon short-term treatment goals, and we encouraged crisis-oriented approaches. The referral source was, to the extent possible, included in the decision-making process. Rapid evaluation, early decision-making about the nature of the problem, and appropriate disposition were the key considerations. In the course of this process, we carefully clarified with the referral source that we saw this as a mutual responsibility, an extremely important concept, since it helped to dissipate the perception that our request for collaboration was a thinly disguised rejection of the case.

Not all of the intricacies of this approach were readily understood by the staff of the new center. Because we had explicitly assumed fuller responsibility for community mental health needs and because there were no other mental health services in the region, the staff found it difficult to balance center priorities. Frequently, it was hard to sort out requests for services that were appropriate from those that were not. In addition, our personnel often felt personally responsible and rather guilty at having to explain to patients that "optimal" treatment was not available. Strong administrative backing was necessary for any limitation of service. There was fear that our total and global responsibility for "comprehensiveness" made it impossible for an individual staff member to set limits individually, since this might be perceived as an admission of inadequacy.

Because of such problems, there was a gradual relaxation of intake ground rules. As a practical matter, staff themselves frequently felt direct treatment was the only effective skill they had to offer. These personnel themselves felt that attempts to use the referral process as a basis for collaboration or consultation were, in fact, rejections. Until they had sufficient training and positive experience as consultants, they simply did not feel comfortable or adequate in relating to referrals in this manner.

We also urged the teams to divide the areas of responsibility in their community work. Each team member would serve as coordinator of the indirect services delivered to a particular system: the social worker, for instance, coordinating work with the elementary school; the psychiatrist overseeing the work with public health nursing; and the psychologist serving as coordinator of the work with clergy. The coordinator would be expected to develop a relationship with the social system; it would be his function to identify spheres of mutual interest and potential collaboration. The hope was that this would stimulate development of consultative relationships and lead toward a mutually supportive stance between our system and that of the other caregiver.

To some extent, of course, introduction of any new service means more work for existing agencies. They have to learn how the service is organized, who is staffing it, what the policies are, and how the new services can be utilized most quickly. Agencies which were not themselves regionalized and which provided county-wide service faced some special problems in revising their procedures to fit themselves into the new service pattern we were introducing in the region. This kind of complementary adaptation by other agencies and institutions has been an interesting and gratifying phenomenon. For instance, two of the private voluntary social service agencies have either regionalized in accordance with our pattern or else have reinstated regional practices that had been abandoned.

Our own service region assignments, based upon specific clusters of census tracts, were, so far as possible, coordinated with the census tract assignments that had been given to the north county public health nursing and welfare family and children's units. These programs, administratively based within our own department (but located in an adjacent city), and such services as schools and police were already organized in service delivery patterns that approximated ours.

### Indirect Services

Working in multifaceted relationships, such as the center was seeking to create, provided an opportunity for mutual problem-solving not available when one's role is limited to a more narrow focus. Innovation, collaboration, mutual program planning, and a more effective sharing of problems often were by-products. The information one gained as a consultant about the social system in which one was working was often invaluable in making decisions about the therapy or disposition for an individual when one was, at another point, operating in a direct service capacity. Although multiple roles (consultant, educator, therapist) create problems in interpreting and separating functions, it was assumed that the advantages to be gained in adapting the mental health system outweighed the disadvantages.

There has been a stereotyping of the mental health professions as being distant and removed from "where the action is." The continuity of care, greater accessibility, and immediacy of our services thus served as an important selling point, demonstrating our involvement. Willingness to collaborate, whether in the form of consultation, direct evaluation, home visiting, or joint planning, has been an essential means of correcting the distortion of mental health workers as aloof and removed from the mainstream of problem-solving.

To be sure, there are many things we need to learn in settings new to us in order to adapt our services in a useful way to the community. A clinical issue requiring close attention and study has to do with formulation of new concepts governing our responsibility to work in new ways when we face unmotivated individuals who are clearly in crisis. The same is true of critical community mental health problems which seem to be denied by the community. In such instances, ethical conduct may require us to invent and perfect new methods that are directed toward the need by means of intermediaries who are more strategically positioned and have the required sanction to intervene.

In collaboration with police, a program of early intervention in instances of family disturbances investigated by police was initiated. A postgraduate public health nurse trainee was assigned to make home visits to families referred by police. Using an entry technique we have found effective in our adult courts and correction unit, she began by obtaining police permission to accompany officers during routine evening patrols. This gave her an opportunity to see the problem of family disturbances from the viewpoint of the peace officer (it is, incidentally, widely recognized as a phase of police work which is highly dangerous, with a higher mortality rate for investigating officers than any other category of police activity). The nurse soon achieved excellent rapport with the police departments. She produced a referral procedure, as well as written materials which police investigators could leave with families whose domestic quarrels had resulted in police intervention. Daily reports listing each call were sent to the center by each police department. The nurse then followed up with calls and visits to the homes listed, and short-term, goal-limited couples groups were organized in the community rather than at the center for those families which indicated willingness to discuss their problems.

Inevitably, this led to consultation and training of police handling these cases. It also resulted in better service to the families which otherwise might not have been referred or which might have been reluctant to follow through on a referral. Fewer repeated incidents of trouble in such families were reported, and we had an opportunity to involve other community caregivers in the design of joint services for this high risk group.

In addition to home visiting, we have experimentally initiated many programs within schools and developed new community services within churches. We think there is much merit in the idea of part-time satellite centers for screening, referral, and on-the-spot consultation to the community in key neighborhoods (the relatively isolated, disadvantaged neighborhoods, in particular) that may be of high need and difficult to reach.

This openness to the possibility of relevant collaboration—which results from the clear recognition of the center's limitations as well as its realistic potentials—has resulted in a number of unusual encounters that have been both highly spontaneous and extremely useful. The assassination of Martin Luther King, for instance, led to the establishment of a rather informal luncheon meeting with community people from various formal and informal circles of concern to discuss problems facing the community as the consequence of civil disorder, civil rights agitation, and the ever-present threat of violence. Out of this has come a greater sense of security and willingness on the part of the staff to involve themselves actively in community affairs when violence threatened. They often take the initiative in making overtures to other agencies to determine, when crises occur, whether there may be some basis upon which we can help or collaborate. In this way, we have been able to approach the police and schools on our own initiative—a strategy which has helped to create a foundation of trust based upon mutually perceived and legitimized sharing of community problems.

Psychiatry has been much criticized, both internally and externally, for its preoccupation with the individual confined to office practice (Felix, 1964). Our experiences have led us to believe that we no longer have the privilege of being able to disentangle ourselves from complex, affectively charged issues that impinge upon large groups. If, for instance, we expect to work with those who do not perceive mental health services as being helpful or who do not seek our services, then we must be prepared to work in a different fashion. If we can justify not approaching these groups on the basis of their lack of readiness, poor motivation, or inappropriate expansion of our roles, then we need not be troubled. If, however, these groups happen to be minority groups, as they often are, then we are also in the position of ignoring the problems of the poor, the disadvantaged, and the disenfranchised.

Since the north county center chose to see these as mental health issues or as derivatives of mental health issues, it also concomitantly accepted the fact that it would be identified with these issues in the eyes of other groups. In the process, of course, we have had to think carefully about the bases of our contributions. It has been necessary to conceptualize our actions and our participation on clinically sound grounds.

A particular example of this was our early identification with a community action group in a deprived area of north county. The group sought better representation for itself within the community. Our work with the group, assisting in the development of an indigenous leader, gave them the time and the training necessary to carry out an effective plan. The result was the initiation, under indigenous leadership, of an information and referral center, funded by the Office of Economic Opportunity, with the north county center as the delegate agency in the community. Our sponsorship of this community action project put us in the role of supporting the neighborhood efforts to establish a dialogue with the many officials and departments of the city from which inhabitants in the target area felt alienated. If one is sensitive about loyalties or identity between "the establishment" and "the dissidents," this kind of role can be very uncomfortable. Moreover, of course, if it cannot be clearly shown that there are mental health implications that can be reasonably defined and understood by all parties involved, such work becomes impossible.

As services become more intimate and accessible, in a small community or within a defined catchment area, confidentiality and its derivative issues become important factors influencing program operation and service delivery. Although it is often mentioned by professionals, the problem of patient anonymity—avoiding the stigma attached to those who seek psychiatric help—has not proved to be a major difficulty in our center.

It has been quite impossible to insure against others finding out that an individual is in treatment or has sought services. However, there is little evidence that either the number or the type of individuals who come to us has been limited by this consideration. For only a few patients has it seemed that issues of confidentiality significantly entered into the decision to seek or to continue therapy. When it has come up, it has proved, more often than not, one more manifestation of the basic psychopathology. In such instances, the discussion of the issue has served as a vehicle to work through the question of basic trust.

In our experience nothing is more often held forth as a basis for declining to create reasonable community-focused mental health services than the question of confidentiality. There is, of course, no simple prescription that can be offered to cover all instances that will arise in community work. The dedicated community mental health worker will no doubt find, as we have in our center, that each new situation may require a different assessment and conclusion concerning the professional basis of one's conduct. Just the problems of working and living in the community where one frequently sees patients or where patients are aware that others know about their treatment and need for services will be handled in a manner directly reflecting the professional's own comfort and security in dealing with the type of intimacy that develops in a small community.

It is, however, when we begin to work with other professionals in joint preventive endeavors that we are confronted by some of the most troublesome aspects of this general problem. It was difficult for us, at first, to accept the implications of our conviction that mental health principles and services should be widely sown throughout the people-serving agencies of our communities. If such principles and services are, in fact, to be integrated within the network of existing services, we are really declaring that other caregivers have significant mental health concerns and responsibilities as an essential part of their jobs. This immediately requires our sanction to allow these nonpsychiatric professionals to have some type of access, on a selective basis, to case information.

To suppose this selective sharing of information is capable of being achieved easily—for instance, by means of some administrative policy decision—is both naive and potentially dangerous. Often what is involved is a very large task of education at various levels of community life. Only as significant work relationships are achieved, and as the various parties to such relationships gain solid experience in working together successfully, can the barriers to sharing of confidential information be revised. Furthermore, this is a two-way street. Schools, especially, as well as police, the courts, and various other strategically situated caregivers are equally protective of certain kinds of sensitive information.

Our mutual access to information from each other, coupled with the ease of entry into various levels of shared activities, greatly facilitates our work in the north county. One of the most effective roles we can play is that of pointing out and reinforcing the need to integrate mental health principles within the broad social and institutional fabric of the community. This can hardly be done convincingly if we are found to be holding, at the same time, that our "secrets" are both too profound and too important to be shared. We have come to be quite comfortable in the north county in sharing many kinds of information that we could not have considered sharing when we opened our center in 1965.

Indirect service work also presents demands for differential judgments about information handling. Usually the problems encountered in handling case information have to do with sharing for collaborative purposes. In performing indirect service work, the problems often relate to questions of utilizing privileged information in program planning, research, training, and epidemiology.

In delivering indirect services, one gets definite impressions about how community caregivers operate. Judgments about their styles, effectiveness, and idiosyncrasies—both personal and professional—are formed. We soon become privy to the way agencies are structured (their implicit, as well as explicit structure). Often we learn of internal agency or personal conflicts and tensions.

Since the preventive services are currently developing as new and largely unsystematized practices, there is a need for detailed and accurate record-keeping and study. As Haylett points out (see Chapter 13), this involves setting down the consultative process in a candid and explicit manner. On the one hand, we are trying to establish what has been referred to as an egalitarian relationship in consultation and to promote basic trust and respect between professionals (Caplan, 1964). On the other hand, we are also studying the community and the groups within it. These are goals that present conflicting concerns; such problems should be frankly discussed in the development of any community mental health program.

The fact that our north county personnel often had multiple roles, providing indirect services and receiving direct service referrals from the same agency, added to the depth and breadth of the picture we got as to agency and community functioning. Although this intimate and comprehensive view constituted a valuable source of epidemiology, workers had to exercise caution. Sometimes, it appeared injudicious to communicate certain kinds of information to one's colleagues within the center. However, there are methods of unblocking such barriers to information flow. The consultant, in his contacts with the consultee, can encourage and support the idea that sensitive information be communicated by the consultee himself to appropriate receivers; realistic difficulties standing in the way of this, as well as resistances based on other factors, are among the kinds of work problems consultants often help to resolve.

In record keeping, in cross contacts with a variety of caregivers, in staff meetings, and in casual conversation, staff had to school themselves to be aware of the trust and responsibility vested in them, so that inadvertent lapses would be avoided. Violations of trust at this level are sometimes even more devastating than those which might occur in direct patient care, since they may well prove more difficult to repair and may vitiate the establishment or promotion of effective relationships with agencies serving large groups of people.

### Regional Versus Central Services

Not all services lend themselves well to the regionalization strategy. Some may best be centralized for both practical and therapeutic reasons. Others might be made available centrally, as well as regionally. Decisions concerning these questions must, of course, be decided with reference to the reality considerations presented by each community mental health program.

It was our concept that our regional pattern would be adequate, if not ideal, with the following: outpatient services for children and adults, rehabilitation services—including day hospital, transitional placement in the community, and aftercare—pre-commitment home visiting, and the community-oriented services—consultation, education, and community organization. Had the option been available, we would have added two other elements, twenty-four-hour emergency (which we would articulate into a brief treatment, walk-in clinic) and inpatient services. The need for these is underscored by problems of continuity of care and basic communication that are unnecessarily complicated when these key elements are missing.

Services that can be established centrally, to be called into play by regional centers, include, in our county, mental retardation diagnostic services (which would, of course, supply neurological work-ups when brain damage and perceptual difficulties are suspected). These services have proved necessary in such a small number of instances in our region as to militate against the cost of regional duplication. Vocational rehabilitation programs, including testing, the vocational workshop, and counseling services, are equally impractical to regionalize. If, as in our county, such services are available centrally, and if counseling time is assigned in sufficient quantity to screen potential candidates in each region, we have found little to justify provision of such high-cost services in the several regions.

Certain services require central coordination but must be represented at decentralized levels. These include research and program evaluation and basic residency training, both of which must be in a position to view possibilities and needs throughout the entire structure of a multi-regional system.

Several service elements appear to require both centralized and decentralized levels of care. Some increments may be supplied as central resources to be called into play by the regions, whereas others must be available on a decentralized basis. These include children's services, programs to serve alcoholics, and drug abuse programs, as well as the whole complex of indirect services.

Our regional teams supply outpatient services to children, as well as to adults. Nevertheless, these generalists found many occasions when it was essential to turn to specialists in the field of child guidance. Thus, a full-time child psychiatrist was added to the center staff. Further, our central child guidance clinic, staffed by personnel primarily trained for working in this demanding field, has been a source

of enrichment and service augmentation. Such a staff can be very useful in supervising, training, and consulting with regional staff in the
process of program development. As described in Chapter 10, the central child guidance service is also needed to develop and supervise
such county-wide services as the juvenile probation mental health unit
and the summer activity program. We have not yet found it possible
to develop within our county the range of inpatient and day care programs required for fully comprehensive community services for children. It seems abundantly clear, however, that regional duplication of
such costly facilities and programs will long be impractical.

As we have explored and developed our regionalized pattern,
it has become apparent there should be close collaboration in program
planning by the region and the central children's services. Essentially
the same thing can be said for the indirect services. Here, too, regional
teams have been given substantial service delivery responsibilities.
However, we followed a pattern of gradual transition in delegating to
the teams the indirect service relationships that previously had been
established in north county by the centralized consultation service.

This phasing-in process proved wise. Most of the staff in our region were not wholly conversant with the service techniques involved;
nor were they entirely comfortable in assuming the mantle of consultant or educator. We found they functioned most effectively after a
period of in-service training and supervised experience was provided
under the tutelage of the seasoned central county staff. It should be
obvious to anyone skilled in the indirect service sphere that to step
into established indirect service relationships with other community
caregivers calls for different and somewhat more demanding skills
than are required in accepting transfer of an individual patient from
another therapist.

In addition to the training and support the regional staff have
obtained from their central county consultation colleagues, there is
another important benefit to be realized from maintaining the centralized indirect service unit. Some community services simply do not
fit logically into one region or another. These are agencies which may
have regional components but which also have strong central coordinating and administrative units. We have found the specialized consultation service in central county is in the best position to initiate development of indirect services or to continue to work with such services.

Administrative coordination and liaison between the central services and the regionalized center have not been fully satisfactory. As further regional centers are developed, we can foresee the need for more efficient mechanisms that will be more sensitive measures of quality control and more timely in supplying routine information flow. Program planning and development is likely to be delegated to a central staff, at least for purposes of coordination and setting of priorities. This will, of course, infringe upon the autonomy of the regional centers. It will be necessary, therefore, that some checks and balances be built in to assure that regionalized programs continue to have the scope necessary to respond to the particular needs and opportunities that present themselves in each catchment area.

CHAPTER **19**

# Prevention and Professional Response

*Howard Gurevitz, Don Heath*

Introduction of a regionalized center to respond to the preventive and treatment needs of communities comprising San Mateo County's northern population quadrant provided an excellent opportunity not previously available to us. On a scale small enough to assure a vigorous outreach and easy accessibility, we could put into practice many of the emerging principles of preventive psychiatry that had been tested in the mid-county program and in other localities. Each innovation in the design of the North County Mental Health Center was consciously intended to achieve standards of clinical practice which had been incorporated into our thinking by 1965.

Some of the most important design conclusions were calculated to remedy certain evident shortcomings in continuity of care and service integration that we had come to recognize in our rather traditionally organized central county pattern. Others were taken from the wide variety of projects, services, and investigations that had been carried out within the division from the time of its formation in 1958 up to the period of the evolution of the new center. Thus, the north county program constitutes a kind of recapitulation of much of what we had considered the best of our mid-county experience. Coming almost a decade after the division itself was created, the new center also had the benefit of a rich body of community experience that had swiftly produced the transformation sometimes referred to as the third revolution in psychiatry (Bellak, 1964).

From chapter to chapter throughout this book, the reader will have discerned the crucial ingredients in the experiences of the comprehensive program that shaped our professional planning for this first regionalized venture in service delivery. The fertile public health philosophy and the administrative climate favoring innovation and autonomy were most influential and were repeated in our regional pattern. Our links with a regionalized state hospital service were further strengthened with an improved version of liaison that became feasible for a new center having a more limited catchment area and more intimate and immediate contact with its population.

Despite our lack of inpatient and emergency services, the highly sophisticated development of these services in the county hospital had shown us the validity of the principle of early definitive diagnosis and treatment as a means of reducing lengthy care and preventing unnecessary hospitalization. They also schooled us in a more realistic and effective utilization of milieu techniques; and home visiting, which we had seen pioneered locally by this inpatient service, was instituted as a major function of our multipurpose teams. A day hospital—and, in particular, the research that validated this as a significant alternative to full-time hospitalization—was also programmed into the new center in a format that duplicated the mid-county emphasis upon intensive, goal-oriented interventions calculated to serve the acutely as well as the chronically ill person on a time-limited basis. Our vigorous utilization of activity and socializing groups was a direct outgrowth of the ex-patient club that had been long operated by staff attached to the mid-county day center.

Because we were frankly dissatisfied with the limitations (portrayed monthly by continuous program evaluation) that seemed intrinsic to the organizational pattern of our two mid-county outpatient clinics, we consciously imposed upon ourselves in north county a family-centered format that asked our team members to see both children and adults. In addition, we ruled out the luxury of the waiting list, substituting the principles of crisis intervention, service limitation, and heavy utilization of alternative resources—those already available, as well as those that might be generated through skillful community organization work.

Nor was this organizational decision wholly based upon negative considerations. At least equally responsible were the positive lessons we had learned in our units dealing with juvenile and adult courts and corrections, public welfare, and public health nursing agencies. We had seen in each of these, one after another, that non-mental health professionals can, in fact, assume, under optimum circumstances, major and highly skilled therapeutic responsibilities for those who constitute their caseloads. These experiences in collaboration, consultation, mental health education and community organization proved to have been powerful demonstrations. Having observed this at first hand, some of us could no longer deny the overwhelming confirmation of this cardinal principle of preventive psychiatry.

What is of foremost importance from the standpoint of our discussion in this chapter is the experience we have collected in staff responses to the kinds of change imposed upon them by a comprehensive program carefully designed, for the first time in our county, to incorporate some of the most basic and vital principles of preventive psychiatry.

Two other chapters of this book (see Chapters 1, 15) explicitly refer to the "changing of the old order," a fundamental and fateful transformation in professional orientation clearly subsumed and conveyed by community mental health. Professionals, deeply concerned about the values that dominate their most intimate professional identities, display behavior that may be taken as sheer, stubborn resistance by those who indignantly demand overnight change. The same behavior can be excused as a last, desperate gesture by embattled champions of a valued and scientifically validated tradition of psychiatric therapy. Each of these divergent attitudes, although not without merit, is likely to do a disservice to our overriding contemporary social need for improved utilization of our limited numbers of professional manpower.

## Recruitment

We have learned that personnel trained in even the finest residency programs, departments of psychology, schools of social work, and schools of nursing are not prepared, without further training, to work in the patterns which we built into the north county center. Nevertheless, we have found this training can be provided on the job (though not without a significant sacrifice in service). This lesson warrants grave consideration from those who seriously intend to stimulate development of prevention-oriented programs, as well as by administrators planning such programs.

The staff of the north county center, although generally younger and less experienced professionally than their mid-county colleagues, have been quite gifted, more so, perhaps, than the average mental health worker. Without exception, their basic professional training has been excellent. They would undoubtedly agree, however, that what was asked of them by the north county program proved a most burdensome challenge. Most eagerly sought and studiously pursued the in-service training offered to them.

It should be emphasized this is not merely a scarcity of qualified manpower. We are convinced that a truly preventive program, one which articulates sensitively with its community, requires essential retraining and continuing education of all manpower, regardless of prior experience. Professionals need on-the-job training to supply the additional education necessary, if they are to gear their responses to the unique interlocked pattern of opportunities and needs presented by each catchment area to be served. Or, to put it differently, there is, in fact, no trained manpower available. There is a limited reservoir of more or less well-prepared candidates for training.

Incidentally, we found that professionals, regardless of styles, personality, and training can adapt and broaden their skills, if the organization demands, sanctions, and supports this. Each program will find it imperative, we believe, to develop multifaceted training oppor-

tunities which will, in time, produce community mental health workers that possess the skills required by each center. Ultimately, but still
beyond the foreseeable future, some of these training deficiences may
be alleviated by incorporation into existing training centers of more
serviceable and functional (that is, systems-oriented) community mental health curricula. Until that day comes, however, it is folly for a
new community mental health center to suppose it can attract staff
who will be prepared upon employment to assume the responsibilities
and undertake the tasks mandated by community mental health and
community psychiatry.

Younger people, somewhat less experienced in their basic professional identities, were attracted to the north county program. Often
they came in response to the opportunities the new center offered to
gain experience and training in several different spheres of community mental health work. Many functions and program attributes not
widely available to younger professionals were included in the center's
service pattern.

Major recruitment problems were concerned with judging the
ability of an individual to adapt to this multidimensional program and
to assess the candidate's potential for growth in several different areas.
Since these included consultation and community work, spheres that
are in preliminary stages of development, staff selection criteria were
somewhat uncertain.

Few professionals who possess knowledge and sensitivity in psychotherapy are also well-trained in preventive techniques. Staff, in our
judgment, must be basically well-trained in their disciplines, having
experience and maturity as diagnosticians and psychotherapists, in order to provide a basis for their work in consultation and community
work. Continuing psychotherapeutic activity is essential to refining and
reinforcing skills in the preventive services and underlies one major
justification for the generalist.

Our goals specifically included the exploration and development of new skills and new roles for professionals. This desirable openness to change met with some unfavorable consequences. "Newness"
became an attraction, a challenge, and a virtue in itself. The heavy
emphasis upon the "generalist" approach, which included greater responsibility, promoted independence and flexibility. But this, too, ex-
acted a certain price. Personnel who had difficulty with problems of

authority, autonomy, and status, often underwent a very rocky adjustment period.

Asked to achieve a very aggressive outreach into the community, personnel (and the program as a whole) were often overextended. Ensuing stresses sometimes led to feelings of frustration and guilt about not being able to do "all things for all people," which was how some staff identified program intent. Although challenged by the opportunity to grow and develop new roles, staff might overextend themselves. Commonly the reaction to this anxiety was to become "overwhelmed" with direct patient contacts through diagnostic and treatment work. Younger staff were understandably uncomfortable in the role of consultant and, being uncertain as to how systems changed, would betray unrealistic self-expectations concerning their own abilities to be helpful in promoting such change.

Simultaneously, the need to assess the community and its protean aspects and problems proved very baffling to many personnel who had responsibility for planning, developing program priorities, and setting goals. People experienced a great deal of difficulty in making decisions about where they would invest time. They felt themselves to be exceedingly visible and vulnerable, a conviction reinforced by the center's location in the heart of a shopping center. At times there was a longing for the anonymity and protection of a medical facility setting. This kind of anxiety was sometimes disclosed in the terminology chosen by staff to describe our program to visitors. Some readily chose to call it a "center"; others referred to it as a "clinic." The former was the preferred term, since it connoted an open, receptive attitude rather than a closed or restricted position.

### Administrative Structuring

Support, supervision, consultation, and training were to be accomplished through senior staff experienced in these functions. This backing was to be made available to team members in order to help them expedite and process their work. It was anticipated from the beginning that team personnel would require training in such phases of basic work as child therapy, family therapy, mental health consultation, mental health education, and community organization. What we did not anticipate was the amount of support, supervision, and training that would be required.

As time went on, it became apparent this training had to be much more skillfully focused and supervised and built right into the daily and weekly team activities. As more structured support was provided, staff members became more comfortable in making responses based upon their own individuality. These began to reflect the variable interests and needs of each person, rather than solely certain external mandates (either real or suspected) imposed by the center or the community. Simultaneously, the teams succeeded in maintaining the pattern of sharing among members, so that we found teams exhibiting greater interest and willingness to respond more flexibly to community needs.

Although the teams consisted of three disciplines, each team member was assigned equal responsibility. Each person was expected to participate in consultation, community organization, education, diagnosis, and psychotherapy. This structure was intended to nurture role diffusion, upgrade continuity of care, and minimize the time spent conferencing about cases. Hampering optimum realization of this goal were certain administrative and organization problems. For instance, barriers tended to be erected by differences in salary scales and legal requirements that must be followed in writing prescriptions, or in establishing a diagnosis. Teams had difficulties balancing such conflicting trends without administrative intervention. Some attempts to supply this needed administrative guidance are now being tried in the center, but the question, still not resolved, is how this can be provided without limiting creativity, interest, initiative, and innovation that an indigenous mental health team provides.

Supervision often has been too scanty. Because of the needs impinging upon professionals from all directions, it seemed, at times, to run the risk of being overlooked. Orientation of new staff proved unsatisfactory, and after repeated mistakes in our supervisory patterns were observed, we began to put a new emphasis upon this kind of guidance. We now take pains to give supervision not only when staff feel they need it but have also retained the option to give supervision whenever our administrative staff feels it is required. This is, of course, taken for granted in many places. Nevertheless, it does not always happen, in fact, and care must be taken to make sure that it does.

At first, we found it difficult to find competent people to fill our supervisorial echelon. Gradually, however, as our center established a reputation, we were able to obtain supervisors who could inspire the confidence of the staff and who could develop packages or sequences of programs that readily adapted themselves to both supervision and training.

Within the center, the administrative staff consisted of the regional program chief, a clinical director (who supplied coordination between teams and the day hospital and provided supervision of all clinical services), the mental health consultant, the mental health educator, the social work supervisor, and the psychiatrist in charge of the day hospital. The weekly meeting of this group was an occasion for discussion of problems in developing new patterns of service and how best to cope with the difficulties staff were experiencing in absorbing new skills and the demands made upon their time and energy.

All personnel of the center attended a weekly, two-hour general staff meeting. In the beginning, it was suggested this be kept open and unstructured to permit people to discuss in an uncritical fashion their concerns about what they were being asked to do and how they were doing it. A considerable amount of feeling was elicited, as staff aired issues seriously affecting their motivation and work. Among these were problems of differential pay rates in a setting in which basic equality of responsibility was delegated. Some care had to be exercised to avoid confusing this work-focused meeting with "sensitivity training."

Our teams, at least in the beginning, scheduled two meetings per week for themselves. One conference was devoted to reviewing and processing all cases received during the week. The second was generally set aside to consider community work; guests or resource people from the community were frequently invited, and both the mental health consultant and the health educator routinely attended.

The day hospital, because of its more tightly structured and highly developed program, organized its own series of staff meetings, chiefly devoted to discussion of day-to-day operation and case management. Team members were invited to attend on a selected basis, at first, later being required to attend one such meeting weekly, if they had patients in day treatment. Other meetings, such as day hospital intakes, were attended by staff from the teams as well as from the day program and often by persons from the community, including the patient and his family. These were usually focused upon admission questions or upon issues relating to significant change in status for a patient (that is, periodic evaluation of treatment goals). These discussions helped to interpret to patients and families what might be expected of day treatment; they also provided an opportunity to produce consensus between the day program and the responsible team as to the various roles and responsibilities that would be mutually expected.

As referrals and case loads rapidly increased, anticipated problems of selection of patients, avoidance of waiting lists, and service limitations presented themselves. Three basic outpatient patterns emerged: brief, crisis-oriented therapy, group therapy, and social activity therapy. Frequently, family members were seen, either during the actual intake interview with the designated patient, or at another time to complete the evaluation. A family conference became a fairly common intake procedure.

Crisis therapy was directed to individuals, couples, and families for time-limited and goal-limited ventures designed to bring about resolution of conflicts arising out of recent upsetting precipitants. This proved most satisfactory in correlating with our pattern of accessibility and staffing. Because of our ease of access to other caregiving services, we were often able to discover collaborators or adjunctive services when they were appropriate.

Patients whose needs for therapy extended beyond the brief treatment episode were evaluated and placed in one of a variety of groups. These included couples, single parents, alcoholics, family, and parents groups. Occasionally, because of individual attitudes or problems, a few individual interviews were needed beyond intake to assist patients in getting started in group therapy, but, for the most part, we have found people are quite willing to accept group treatment.

Social activity therapy was both a preventive and an adjunctive service primarily for patients who needed experience in socialization or who had difficulty in accepting or profiting from the more traditional types of psychotherapy. To a large extent, these groups served high risk groups, such as patients returning from the state hospital. Frequently such patients also received help from our public welfare workers, public health nurses, and other local agencies. Consequently, we placed some emphasis upon introducing social activity group techniques to other caregiving systems, including recreation departments and churches. Volunteers, as well as personnel working in other systems (such as public welfare), often assumed total responsibility for these group techniques.

Treatment orientations among the staff varied widely. Some came to the center with analytically oriented approaches. At the other end of the spectrum were those who wished to try confrontation and encounter groups, as well as sensory awareness techniques. Drug therapy, of course, was a major modality available to patients as needed.

Introduction of the crisis approach in the center triggered a problem that frequently came up as we attempted to initiate change. We found many professionals assumed their basic education had prepared them to perform crisis interventions, and, in the beginning, we did not question this assuredness. What we found, of course, was that most staff tended to suppose that crisis treatment was simply shorter-term therapy. There was a glaring lack of skill in the specific techniques that have been elaborated as the consequence of considerable empirical experience. The same problem was encountered in group therapy, family therapy, and mental health consultation. We soon realized that basic professional training imparts a good grounding in individual psychotherapy and, to a lesser extent, in group and family therapy.

Staff members often were reluctant to reveal the areas of deficiencies in their skills. Often there was a sense of frustration and personal defeat involved. Perhaps our tendency to emphasize the goal of independent and autonomous responsibility by the teams whatever their capacities made it difficult to indicate inadequacies. Eventually, however, we learned of these feelings and recognized the importance of being open among ourselves about the need for intensive support and training in order to help staff achieve the skills that were lacking.

Of all the specialized techniques programmed into the center, the indirect services were the ones for which basic training proved most inadequate. Having served previously as chief of the mid-county indirect service unit, the regional program chief had no illusions about the possibility of finding a number of skilled consultants, educators, and community organizers to man the new program. He was, however, not fully prepared for the magnitude of the training and supervision that proved necessary to help the staff establish identities as consultants and to impart the necessary skills.

Mental health professionals often draw from their experiences in psychotherapy the various expectations they apply to indirect service work. Unless they can be helped to revise such estimates as the time required for results to be seen, it is inevitable that much frustration is in store for them.

A substantial amount of retraining and reorientation was required to help this staff grasp the difficult and tedious processes through which change takes place at the system level. When acting as consultants or community organizers, staff felt lost and discouraged by their inability to determine their impact upon the structures or the operating procedures of a system with which they were working.

Even more perplexing for some was the concept that many community agency demands made upon us for direct services represented unrealistic or inappropriate dependency needs on the part of the agency. Thus, repeated demands that the center display its usefulness in the single idiom that the community could understand—direct service—sometimes evoked a hostile response from staff. When an analogous experience is encountered in therapy—the patient testing the situation or the roles—the therapist is quite comfortable in clarifying or interpreting these concerns. However, we found many of our personnel were surprised and reacted negatively when this same circumstance came up in consultation.

By and large, the major problems arose in the entry phases—the initial contacts with agencies. Commonly, there was a reluctance to demonstrate expertness or to indicate a desire to learn from the consultee the essential nature and structure of his task—information that underlies any successful consultation. Coupled with this was the fact that personnel had to be acquainted with the very substantial and important contributions that potentially could be obtained by working with others in this way. For instance, if a staff person did not truly believe the police or the clergy had a legitimate and significant mental health role, it was highly unlikely he could operate as an effective consultant. It was virtually impossible to tell in advance whether a new staff member felt this way. Opportunities first had to be provided to engage a professional in actual field experience—something that generally had not been provided in his basic educational preparation.

This was the most serious training gap we encountered. It was met by increasing the planned in-service training and supervision that we obtained from the mid-county indirect service staff. Still later, however, this training need was met more comprehensively when the central county unit established an intensive year-long seminar in indirect service delivery. This seminar (see Chapter 16) was a major staff enrichment activity designed to meet needs for didactic schooling, as well as supervised field experience.

Roles and responsibilities for subprofessionals and volunteers were developed in the north county center. This deployment of nonprofessional personnel was not achieved, however, without some painstaking work of clarifying tasks and roles and building a climate of professional acceptance. Our trained mental health workers were reluctant initially to delegate certain significant case management activities to these "outsiders." Concern was voiced about matters of confidentiality, control, communication, levels of training, and experience.

Sometimes the staff reactions would manifest themselves in patterns of vague difficulties surrounding the development of a given activity or the training designed to prepare nonprofessionals for an assignment. Occasionally there was apathy or inadequate supervision, and this led to early demise of a volunteer activity.

We devised some methods of altering professional attitudes. These included provision of a series of structured placements within activities of the center as a means of orientation, training, and "job promotion" for volunteers. With continued demonstration of volunteer effectiveness, the staff took more interest, began to realize the usefulness of nonprofessionals, and became open to their being involved in many of the "professional" activities.

By 1968, after three years of experience, the entire staff of the center carried out an extensive review of preventive and treatment services. This analysis led to decisions to modify the supervision and delivery of preventive services, to clarify role function among staff members, to permit greater specialization, where indicated, and to provide better coordination of both types of services. The mental health consultant, a social worker who was already functioning as a trainer and coordinator, has been assigned to supervise all preventive services. Each community system to which indirect services are offered now has a coordinator on the staff (often a team member); this coordinator is responsible to the mental health consultant (see Chapter 12). Work in each system is done by staff from across the center. In this way, virtually all team personnel remain involved in both treatment and preventive services, but a more direct and comprehensive supervisory line is established. This helps to give greater continuity to indirect services and assures the team greater access to administrative support and supervision.

We have retained the geographic team concept, and the day hospital continues to receive patients from all three teams. Referring team members no longer remain in a "liaison" capacity, however. They have begun to participate actively in the day hospital treatment of their patients.

The social work supervisor has been named director of training at the center, in addition to other duties, with responsibility for planning and coordinating the programs for the twenty to thirty students and trainees who come on field placement each year. The senior psychologist at the center has been given responsibility for program evaluation and research. The mental health educator now supervises community organization and mental health education, working with all preventive systems units, as well as with the teams. Finally, we have recruited a child psychiatrist, who is developing improved preventive and treatment services for children, and supplying major new in-service training resources for team members who require additional training to serve the needs of children in their team areas.

Significant change in any system is always anxiety-provoking. In mounting the north county program, we were planning not merely regionalization of services but were, in fact, implementing a detailed program of prevention in community mental health. We were cutting a new template for service delivery in the county. New positions had to be created for the division. There were questions about how the regional program chief and the clinical director were to fit into the hierarchy of division administration.

The pattern of a single regional administration was taken by some as a tacit criticism of our familiar organizational structure in mid-county. The global approach to community with emphasis upon prevention stirred up a great deal of feeling among staff who had operated primarily on a patient-therapist model. Use of the three mental health disciplines in teams calculated to diffuse the distinctions between them raised questions of competence, supervision, and quality of care, in the minds of some. The concept of the generalist provoked great concern. Formulation of a family-centered outpatient service was viewed as regressive from the child guidance viewpoint.

As the planning and programming took place, anxieties rose to a high pitch within the division. Bitter exchanges were not uncommon, since this new design was frequently taken as a threat. The new center was the first of four regionalized services that were to be created. Many assumed (though this was repeatedly denied) our design was to be a prototype that would be imposed, willy-nilly, upon the other three regions when they were established. Comfortable and entrenched in one way of working, staff in mid-county could not easily imagine themselves adapting to this unconventional new pattern.

We had an opportunity to recruit for an entirely new staff. This option was taken, since we believed some of the difficulties of initiating this program would be reduced by bringing in personnel who would not already have allegiances in the mid-county that might further complicate their ability to remain objective and optimistic in the face of the serious implementation problems that would confront them in the early stages. This did prove to make it easier to develop a cohesive staff with relatively high morale. However, it created a new set of problems by highlighting the differences between old and new staff —thus, old and new programs. New staff without the same perception of history, tradition, and practice often tended to feel cut off and isolated from the older staff working centrally.

As our service pattern developed, we found ourselves interpreting to our catchment area ideas about community mental health services, priorities that emphasized preventive approaches, and a wide range of choices that governed our decisions about treatment that were somewhat irreconcilable with the messages that had long been communicated (by deed, perhaps, even more than by word) by the central county services down through the years. This virtually inevitable lack of congruence between ourselves and our central county colleagues was also expressed in other ways. The fact that the north county center was more accessible to its service region, offering a relative ease of entry, was contrasted with the waiting list barriers that had always hampered quick access to the centralized services. On the other hand, our center de-emphasized prolonged therapy in favor of short-term treatment—heavily reinforced by adjunctive resources that we enlisted to

## FIGURE 1—ORGANIZATION CHART

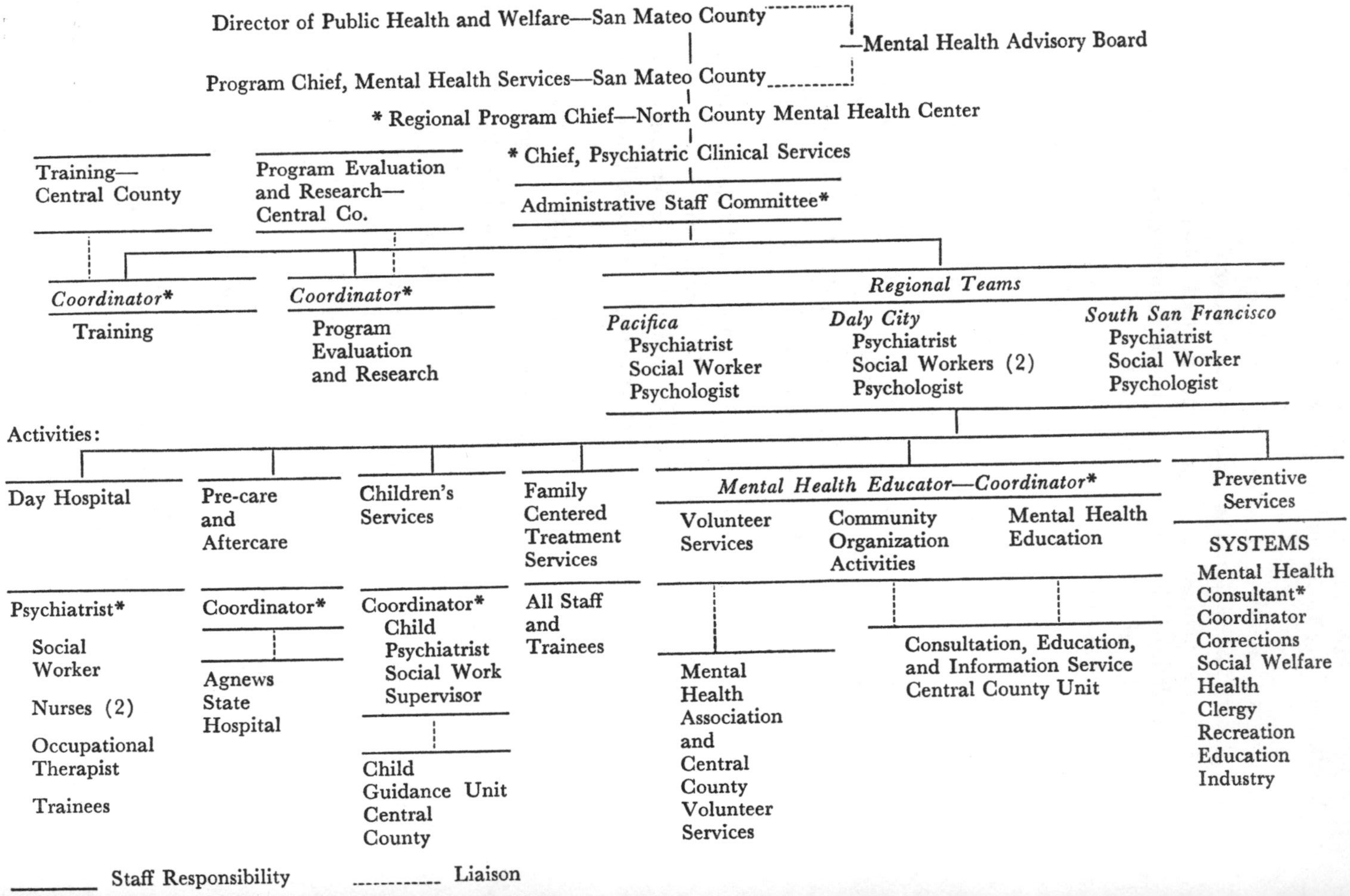

Director of Public Health and Welfare—San Mateo County ----- Mental Health Advisory Board

Program Chief, Mental Health Services—San Mateo County

* Regional Program Chief—North County Mental Health Center

* Chief, Psychiatric Clinical Services

Administrative Staff Committee*

Training—Central County
Coordinator*
Training

Program Evaluation and Research—Central Co.
Coordinator*
Program Evaluation and Research

*Regional Teams*

Pacifica
Psychiatrist
Social Worker
Psychologist

Daly City
Psychiatrist
Social Workers (2)
Psychologist

South San Francisco
Psychiatrist
Social Worker
Psychologist

*Mental Health Educator—Coordinator**

Volunteer Services

Community Organization Activities

Mental Health Education

Preventive Services

Consultation, Education, and Information Service Central County Unit

Mental Health Association and Central County Volunteer Services

SYSTEMS
Mental Health Consultant*
Coordinator
Corrections
Social Welfare
Health
Clergy
Recreation
Education
Industry

Activities:

Day Hospital
Psychiatrist*
Social Worker
Nurses (2)
Occupational Therapist
Trainees

Pre-care and Aftercare
Coordinator*
Agnews State Hospital

Children's Services
Coordinator*
Child Psychiatrist
Social Work Supervisor
Child Guidance Unit Central County

Family Centered Treatment Services
All Staff and Trainees

——— Staff Responsibility        --------- Liaison

collaborate with us. This, too, produced predictable conflict. Some saw this as a progressive and positive step; others condemned it. Among resource agencies, some were pleased to collaborate; others were dissatisfied and compared us unfavorably with the central county services.

The lag time necessary to develop children's services—that is, the time required to supply training to team members—was a source of major dissatisfaction. Indeed, those who identified themselves with what they chose to define as the "traditional" child guidance format, found the whole idea of the "generalist" most unpalatable.

This recitation of the factors that produced tension between north county and the established centralized program is intended to supply in some detail the ingredients that appear to be involved at the national level in producing stress between community mental health and other psychiatric orientations. The issues may vary, depending upon the context of a given discussion or situation. But implicit within them are the underlying principles that produced a local manifestation of this quite historic debate in San Mateo County.

If community mental health is to have a distinctive form rather than to become the captive of more traditional orientations, it must face squarely the implications of its defining characteristics. They include the commitment to serve a total population; a willingness to utilize manpower—professional as well as nonprofessional—in new and perhaps unconventional ways; the tolerance to limit service to realistic potentials, coupled with the all-important emphasis upon indirect service as a means of tapping into adjunctive resources (those that exist, as well as those that can be created) to supplement limited care; far more attention to the tasks that produce bridges between resources; and heavy stress upon methods that can be reasonably expected to help reduce the prevalence of illness and raise immunity levels throughout the community.

Facing these demands does require workers to present themselves and their services in new words and new deeds. It demands a willingness to face the tension that results from the searching questions —many of which are asked by people of high principle and undoubted sincerity in both the professional and the lay community. It is a tall order. If, as one suspects, it is to be placed, as it was in our north county center, upon the shoulders of relatively young men and women, who have not enjoyed a period of professional seasoning and maturity, it may well prove too great a trial.

At this early period in its history, community mental health urgently needs the vigorous leadership of reputable and respected professionals in all disciplines, as well as a creative and balanced presentation of its goals and implications to the informed and articulate community at large. Without this kind of thoughtful and encouraging support, an already overextended band of young professionals may well find it expedient to retreat into the comfortable and familiar grind of diagnosis and remedy. This, in turn, will surely result in the creation of new warehouses for the untended thousands who cannot be accommodated within the limited number of fifty-minute-hours that will be available.

San Mateo's north county center, having weathered this trial for three years, appears to have developed the professional sinews necessary for its survival. Although it has not added immensely to the sum total of information needed to tell us whether a program of preventive psychiatry is entirely valid, it has demonstrated that such a program, in fact, can be sustained in the face of the grave (as well as the litigious and the querulous) questions that are raised wherever community mental health is discussed. It stands as a kind of inadvertent symbol to the aspirations of community mental health: although it has not proved the basic assumptions, it has diligently pioneered a position from which some of them, perhaps, can be investigated.

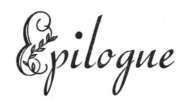

# From Experience
# to Principles

*Portia Bell Hume*

The San Mateo County mental health services are the embodiment of a public mental health program with the potentiality of serving, both directly and indirectly, the whole population of a particular community. It is a program which seeks to integrate psychiatric with nonpsychiatric services to people, and to maximize both comprehensiveness and the continuity of these components by means of interagency and interprofessional sanctions and relationships that are both ethically considered and technically refined. Guided by public health concepts, such a program epitomizes the principles of preventive psychiatry with respect to both clinical and nonclinical psychiatric practices. But the feature that gives added depth to the San Mateo program is its recognition of the men-

447

tal health functions performed by the nonpsychiatric agencies and professions in behalf of individuals who either are at risk of, or have already experienced, mental breakdown: (1) the psychosocially deprived, (2) persons experiencing a life crisis, (3) cases requiring referral for psychiatric evaluation, and (4) the mentally disabled who need either habilitation or rehabilitation. It is for all of these reasons that the San Mateo County mental health services may be said to exemplify several sound principles of public mental health, which are expressed through program policy in terms of goals and functions; through the processes of administration, research, and preventive intervention; through organizational, epidemiological, and psychodynamic methods; and through characteristic patterns of services, staffing, and leadership.

Many, if not most, of the community mental health programs which have been springing up at an accelerated rate during the past twenty years are opportunistic endeavors which share a weakness in favor of the quick answer or the easy, specific remedy which does not require time-consuming studies, planning, or the discipline of thought. Such well-intended efforts appear to be based upon the limitations inherent in the two main kinds of community mental health services with which psychiatric practitioners outside of large public mental hospitals have had the most experience, namely, outpatient psychiatric clinics and psychiatric services in general hospitals. In such settings, the private practice model of clinical psychiatry taught in most medical schools has flourished. Consequently it has sometimes been mistakenly assumed that a community mental health program could qualify for a construction or staffing grant merely by tacking onto the inpatient service a twenty-four-hour telephone answering service for emergencies, the admission of daytime patients, and a clinical consultation service. Or, when the program takes off from an outpatient clinic, the recipe may consist of a written contract to share patients and their records with a nearby hospital for partial to full-time hospitalization of psychiatric patients, including emergency services, and assignment of a modicum of the clinic's staff time for mental health education and consultation to those community agencies and professionals that constitute any clinic's chief sources of referrals. It must be said in favor of such action for mental health that, at the very least, it is based upon professional experience and expresses a human impulse to do what comes most naturally; thus the effect upon the patients involved may, under favorable circumstances, represent a very high quality of clinical care, indeed.

The trouble with the private practice model of community psychiatry is the dilemma encountered when the community mental health center or program is supposed to cover all the potential patients in its catchment area. On the one hand, there is a limit to both the manpower and the funds required by such a goal; on the other hand, there are persons who steadfastly refuse to become patients. Thus another model of community mental health services, sometimes described as a revolutionary change from traditional clinical psychiatry, has emerged in reaction to the dilemma mentioned above. This newer model, associated with social psychiatry in Great Britain, relies heavily upon therapeutic communities and various other forms of group activity for severely mentally ill patients, and also, in this country, for nonpatients who are grouped or categorized as troublesome. The latter individuals are generally identified in terms of deviant social behavior. The absence of clinical, diagnostic services in these cases may be rationalized in a number of ways: (1) the program is more immediately responsive to people's "mental health needs"; (2) it spares its recipients' feelings about authoritarian doctors; (3) it saves staff time and money by dispensing with "labels"; or (4) after all, the dual objectives of social psychiatry are to alter the environment which is held responsible for mental illness and social deviancy, and to correct the social behavior of the deviant, so as to bring the two into greater harmony as quickly as possible.

The trouble with the American version of the social psychiatry model is that it is simplistic on a number of counts. It discounts epidemiological studies which reveal the complexity of biological, psychological, and psychosocial factors present in those afflicted with mental or emotional disorders, or in those at risk of mental breakdown. It fails to distinguish between epidemiology and psychiatric sociology. It suffers from such corrective zeal that the end justifies almost any means of social reconditioning. It concerns itself mainly with the present, blurring the past or the future of either the social disturbance or the socially disturbed. The idea of prevention, even with respect to possible, iatrogenic components in the remedies employed, is relatively foreign to this model of community mental health services. In its favor, however, is its undoubted usefulness in dealing retrospectively with the social concomitants and sequels of the gravest mental disorders.

The public health model, of which the San Mateo County mental health services are an example, incorporates some features of both the medical and the sociological models. As a public mental health program with some claim to comprehensiveness, however, it integrates direct, clinical services to patients with indirect services whose scope extends beyond the purely remedial, restorative, or corrective features of private clinical practice or of social psychiatry. Nevertheless, historically speaking, the San Mateo County program was grounded upon, and overshadowed by, the private practice model of clinical psychiatry during the first ten years of the program. The major innovation, which ushered in the second decade of the program's development, was the establishment of a therapeutic community for psychiatric inpatients on a county hospital ward. Thus the social psychiatry model in its most clinically oriented and defensible form was introduced in a clinical setting and significantly modified the pre-existing traditional forms of treating the community's severest cases of mental illness or abuse of mind-altering substances like alcohol. This bringing together in 1958 of the two best-known models for delivering psychiatric services in a public program made it possible for San Mateo County to develop a continuum of clinical psychiatric services that is representative of the major kinds of direct, clinical interventions, from the point of view of what a patient needs at different times in the course of a mental disorder. Such a spectrum of diagnostic and remedial services together with general medical and other nonpsychiatric forms of care is, furthermore, considerably enhanced when viewed the other way around; that is, when the primary responsibility for mentally and emotionally disabled persons has been taken by a nonpsychiatric (medical or nonmedical) professional, the collaboration of the clinical facilities and personnel of the San Mateo program is available as a supportive, psychiatric service that does not require the transfer of primary responsibility for the patient. The number of psychiatric patients who can thus be served is obviously greater when there is a mutual sharing of them by true collaborators than when exclusive possession of the patient is demanded by either the psychiatric or nonpsychiatric resource which has the patient.

Another parameter of comprehensiveness is demonstrable

through the attempted coverage of all age-groups in the population of San Mateo County, not only through direct, clinical services to children and youth or to adults, but also through indirect, consultative services to personnel in the traditional health, education, and welfare agencies, or to special organizations and professions serving specific age-groups, from the unborn to the very aged. Furthermore, in the San Mateo program, there are formal contracts including financial arrangements with, for example, a private, pediatrically directed agency serving emotionally and mentally afflicted children, or with a different kind of voluntary agency offering day care to mentally and emotionally disturbed youth.

The principle of comprehensiveness is often violated by community mental health programs which ignore a third parameter, namely, the inclusion of all kinds of psychiatric patients, particularly those who are the least attractive and the hardest to treat. These are the patients who wait the longest for any kind of psychiatric attention, and who end up being the most expensive (in both manpower and dollars) to help; in short, they are alcoholics, psychotics, and the severely retarded about whom the general public and its elected officials are particularly concerned. The Prologue and Chapter 1 of this book make it clear that, during the first decade of the San Mateo program, it managed to a considerable degree to ignore the county's most mentally afflicted citizens. During the second decade, however, the program gave increasing clinical attention to such patients and, most significantly, promoted both collaborative treatment and the earliest possible casefinding by means of consultation.

The twenty-year history of the San Mateo County mental health services reveals that both the program and its director played a role in bringing about, as well as responding to, an event which reinforced the turning point in the program coincident with the establishment of the therapeutic community. The California Community Mental Health Services Act, more familiarly known as the Short-Doyle Act, was passed in 1957. It provided for state financial aid, in the form of a 50 per cent reimbursement* after January 1, 1958, for all the major kinds of local mental health services that might be operated by cities or counties. At that time, a number of counties in California were already providing one or more types of mental health services

---

* As of 1965, 75 per cent and increased to 90 per cent in 1969.

and thus, rather than being in the position of initiating a program from scratch, as was the case in other localities, they could either expand or augment their existing services with the aid of the state reimbursement, that is, redouble their efforts without encumbering additional property taxes. San Mateo County was among the few California counties with significant mental health services before 1958, not only in regard to the amount of service per capita of general population, but also with respect to the variety of services provided. As described in the Prologue to this book, the first of San Mateo County's mental health services had been developed slowly, over a period of ten years prior to 1958, as additions to the established program of a county hospital already integrated with public health and welfare services. Thus the effect of the Short-Doyle Act upon San Mateo County was to accelerate the maturation, during the ten years 1958 to 1968, of a program destined by its enlightened and experienced leadership to reflect a public health approach which had been latent throughout the program's first decade of growing up.

It is clear that the current status of the San Mateo County program, delineated in the previous chapters, illustrates an important administrative principle of community psychiatry, to wit: for community mental health programs to have some claim to being comprehensive and to achieve either their short-term or their long-range objectives, they need time to grow and develop, and the chance to engage in time-consuming processes, rather than responding hastily and prematurely to the urge to establish services on the basis of rapidly erected structural elements prescribed by legislative fiats or induced by financial windfalls. When placed in historical perspective, such events as federal or state mental health acts offer once-in-a-lifetime opportunities that may either initiate a new program or invigorate an existing one; but in certain circumstances, such events may be taken as invitations to both professionals and lay leaders with the best of intentions to pursue a headlong course of heedless and instant action.

In sophisticated, viable, mental health programs, such as San Mateo's, every day is a day for reevaluation and readaptation to changing conditions and demands; on the other hand, in more rigidly structured and prefabricated programs, change in any element is viewed with disproportionate alarm because of the enhanced risk of collapse. Quality control, desirable as it may be, is hardly a substitute for program evaluation, and so the day of reckoning is postponed or ignored as long as possible. In an atomic age characterized by rapid change on every front, the viability of a mental health program is proportionate to its flexibility, both structural and functional. Flexibility is a bonus that accrues to a program out of its day-to-day functioning, above and beyond the structural provisions for it in any blueprint or organization chart. Functional flexibility, meaning adaptability, needs of course to be limited and disciplined in ways that avoid bringing down the whole structure. But enduring stability in most instances can be more readily achieved by renovating or remodeling the structural elements of a program in response to changing functions, than by relying too exclusively upon the strength and solidity of the structure to perpetuate purposes which all too soon become outmoded.

A review of the ingredients which currently make up the San Mateo County program shows that it meets the specifications of a comprehensive community mental health center as defined in the federal guidelines for implementation of the National Mental Health Act of 1963. However, the San Mateo County program is far more than a consortium of services for a population of half a million, in the sense that the whole program is more than the sum of its parts. Thus, when the program is regarded less superficially and is scrutinized for the components that are visible evidence of its development, a number of features which do not appear in any list of mere ingredients are discoverable. These are the dynamic elements of the San Mateo County program shown in the accompanying table, in terms which attempt to account for how the program got to be the way it is, since it is certainly not a carbon copy of any prescribed model.

The life style of the San Mateo County mental health services has its origin in a rational and practical general policy consistently expressive of the public mental health functions of the program. The ways in which the program has changed and grown reflect the fundamental, dynamic interrelationships between the seven long-range objectives (functionally defined in Table 3 as purposes) which give the program its direction. In between policy and the never complete achievement of purposes lie the processes which give order to the undertaking (despite blunders and roadblocks), and which determine the feasibility of short-term objectives or target-areas in a given year. When related purposes, processes, methods, and program components

# Table 3

## Dynamic Elements in the San Mateo Program

| PURPOSES OR FUNCTIONS | MAIN PROCESSES | CHIEF METHODS | PROGRAM COMPONENTS | GUIDING PRINCIPLES |
|---|---|---|---|---|
| I. *Reduction of mental disorders* | 1. Fact-finding and forecasting<br>2. Development and communication of policy | 1. Analysis of trends (demographic and epidemiological)<br>2. Persuasion<br>3. Diplomacy | 1. Authorization of the program (legal sanctions)<br>2. Leadership and public relations (Prologue and Chapter 1) | A. *Orderly planning for prevention on a comprehensive scale* |
| II. *Implementation and program development* | 1. Legislation<br>2. Financing<br>3. Organization<br>4. Staff development | 1. Management<br>2. Fiscal and professional accounting<br>3. Monitoring of records<br>4. Contracting for services | 1. Recruitment of staff<br>2. Structuring of chain of command<br>3. Supervision<br>4. In-service training Chapters 1, 13, and 16) | B. *Delegation of authority commensurate with assigned responsibility* |
| III. *Accommodation of the program to the community* | 1. Surveying of mental health needs, resources, and gaps in between<br>2. Interpretation of findings<br>3. Determination of priorities | 1. Community organization and education in response to concerns expressed by the community | 1. Augmentation<br>2. Innovation<br>3. Reorganization (Chapters 2, 17, 18, and 19) | C. *Timely, relevant, flexible and coordinated adaptation* |

| Goal | | | | Prevention |
|---|---|---|---|---|
| IV. *Reduction in the incidence of mental disorders* | 1. Development of consultant-consultee relationships: the consultation process | 1. Identification and facilitation of the mental health functions of nonpsychiatric agencies and professions (consultees) | 1. Mental health education and consultation: indirect services<br>2. Clinical consultation: direct service (Chapters 12 and 13) | D. *Primary prevention* (of breakdown due to deficits in necessary supplies or to life crises) |
| V. *Reduction in the duration of a mental disorder in an individual* | 1. Diagnostic evaluation<br>2. Prognostication<br>3. Preventive-therapeutic interventions | 1. Prompt assessment and remedial measures<br>2. Cooperative diagnosis and treatment | 1. Clinical psychiatric services<br>2. Collaboration with other psychiatric resources (Chapters 3, 4, 5, 6, 7, 9, and 10) | E. *Secondary prevention* (of secondary symptoms or handicaps) |
| VI. *Reduction in disability due to a mental disorder* | 1. Assessment and<br>2. Alleviation of the sequels of intractable or recurrent illnesses | 1. Physical, psychosocial and vocational rehabilitation<br>2. Habilitation | 1. Clinical services<br>2. Nonmedical services<br>3. Collaboration with other such resources (Chapters 8, 11, and 14) | F. *Tertiary prevention* (of neglected or extreme disability) |
| VII. *Evaluation of the effectiveness of the program* | 1. Applied research | 1. Descriptive studies<br>2. Biostatistical studies<br>3. Epidemiological research<br>4. Program evaluation | 1. Record keeping and validation<br>2. Experimentation<br>3. Comparative studies (Chapter 15) | G. *Program change based on investigation of evidence* |

are put together, it is possible to identify, to derive, or to abstract the guiding principles inherent in each means-end continuum, of which seven are represented in the table.

The first and overriding purpose of public mental health is the reduction to a minimum of all forms of mental breakdown in the entire population of an area, which in this instance is San Mateo County, California, but which theoretically may range from the over-populated neighborhood of a metropolis to an entire region with a low density of inhabitants. Of the remaining six purposes shown in the first vertical column of the table, three (IV, V, and VI) focus upon the different levels of prevention, all of which must to some extent be undertaken by any public mental health program to accomplish an appreciable lowering of the incidence or prevalence rates indicating the extent of some forms of mental breakdown in the particular population at risk. The remaining three purposes (II, III, and VII) focus upon the developmental, adaptive, and reality-testing functions that are involved in the delivery of comprehensive mental health services in a designated community. In other words, the mental health purposes of a program like San Mateo's take into account both the entire population (host) and the particular community (environment) in which mental breakdown occurs.

The table may also be read vertically for an overview of the main processes, chief methods, program components, and guiding principles. In the fourth vertical column, there are references to the chapters in this book, in which the descriptions of the various aspects of the program appear. The table, however, should be read from left to right for the purpose of seeking the principle which is exemplified by the processes and methods employed to field a special service or to take a particular action with a specific direction and purpose (long-range objective) in mind. The program elements of each horizontal series are not only functionally connected as means to ends, but also are dynamically related with respect to both direction and time—without, however, implying a necessarily simple and straightforward type of linear progression. Indeed, the path of progress in mental health programs is rarely as visible or evenly paced as it could be with the sort of forecasting and planning demonstrated by the San Mateo program.

# Bibliography

BARTON, W. E. "An Editorial: The Reluctance to Lead," *Hospital and Community Psychiatry,* 1967, *18,* 7.

BEARD, J. H., SCHMIDT, J. R., SMITH, M. M., and DINCIN, J. "Three Aspects of Psychiatric Rehabilitation at Fountain House," *Mental Hygiene,* 1964, *48,* 11–20.

BEARD, J. H., SMITH, M. M., and SOROKIN, F. "An Apartment Program for Post-Hospitalized Psychiatric Patients." In Grob, S. (Ed.), *The Community Social Club and the Returning Mental Patient.* Proceedings of a Conference in Framingham, Mass., 1963.

BELLAK, L. *Handbook of Community Psychiatry and Community Mental Health.* New York: Grune and Stratton, 1964.

BENNEY, C., and WALTZER, S. "Treatment of the Ambulatory Schizophrenic in a Rehabilitation Center," *Mental Hygiene,* 1958, *42,* 332–339.

BERLIN, I. N. "Mental Health Consultation in Schools as a Means of Communicating Mental Health Principles," *Journal of the American Academy of Child Psychiatry,* 1962, *1,* 671–679.

457

BERNARD, V. W. "Education for Community Psychiatry in a University Medical Center; with Emphasis on the Rationale and Objectives of Training." In Bellak, L. (Ed.), *Handbook of Community Psychiatry and Community Mental Health*. New York: Grune and Stratton, 1964, 82–122.

BIBRING, E. "The Mechanism of Depression." In Greenacre, P. (Ed.), *Affective Disorders*. New York: International Universities Press, 1953, 13–48.

BINNER, P. R. "The Team and the Concept of Democracy," *Journal of the Fort Logan Mental Health Center*, 1967, *4*, 115–124.

BLACK, B. J. *Industrial Therapy for the Mentally Ill in Western Europe: Report of NIMH Project NH-1405*. New York: Altro Service Bureau, 1965.

BLANE, H. T., MULLER, J. J., and CHAFETZ, M. E. "Acute Psychiatric Services in the General Hospital. II. Current Status of Emergency Psychiatric Services," *American Journal of Psychiatry*, 1967 (October supplement), *124*, 37–45.

BLUM, R. H., and DOWNING, J. J. "Staff Response to Innovation in a Mental Health Service," *American Journal of Public Health*, 1964, *54*, 1230–1240.

BLUM, R. H., and EZEKIEL, J. *Clinical Records for Mental Health Services*. Springfield, Ill.: Thomas, 1962.

BLUM, H. L., and LEONARD, A. R. *Public Administration: A Public Health Viewpoint*. New York: Macmillan, 1963.

BROWN, B. S. "Psychiatric Practice and Public Policy," *American Journal of Psychiatry*, 1968, *125*, 141–146.

BROWN, B. S., and CAIN, H. P. "The Many Meanings of 'Comprehensive': Underlying Issues in Implementing the Community Mental Health Center Program," *American Journal of Orthopsychiatry*, 1964, *34*, 834–839.

BRYANT, C. M. "Training in Mental Health: A Community Model." Paper presented at the annual meeting of the American Orthopsychiatric Association, San Francisco, April, 1966.

BURLING, T. "The Vocational Rehabilitation of the Mentally Handicapped," *American Journal of Orthopsychiatry*, 1950, *20*, 202–207.

CALIFORNIA DEPARTMENT OF MENTAL HYGIENE. *Long Range Plan for Mental Health Services in California*. Sacramento: California Department of Mental Hygiene, 1962.

CAPLAN, G. *An Approach to Community Mental Health*. New York: Grune and Stratton, 1961.

CAPLAN, G. *Principles of Preventive Psychiatry*. New York: Basic Books, 1964.

CAPLAN, G. "Community Psychiatry—Introduction and Overview." In

Goldston, S. E. (Ed.), *Concepts of Community Psychiatry: A Framework for Training.* Public Health Service Publication, 1965, *1319,* 3–18.

CAPLAN, G. "Perspectives on Primary Prevention, a Review." *Archives of General Psychiatry,* 1967, *17,* 331–346.

CARLSON, D. A., COLEMAN, J. V., ERRERA, P., and HARRISON, R. W. "Problems in Treating the Lower Class Psychotic," *Archives of General Psychiatry,* 1965, *13,* 269–274.

CARMICHAEL, D. M. "Day Hospital Program with Emphasis on Translatable Skills." In Epps, R. L., and Hanes, L. D. (Eds.), *Day Care of Psychiatric Patients.* Springfield, Ill.: Thomas, 1964, 66–78.

CHAFETZ, M. E., BLANE, H. T., and MULLER, J. J. "Acute Psychiatric Services in the General Hospital. I. Implications for Psychiatry in Emergency Admissions," *American Journal of Psychiatry,* 1966, *123,* 664–670.

CHILDERS, B. "A Ward Program Based on Graduated Activities and Group Effort," *Hospital and Community Psychiatry,* 1967, *18,* 289–295.

CHIN, A. H. *A Study of the Characteristics of Recidivists on the Inpatients Psychiatric Service.* Unpublished study (mimeographed), 1965.

CHODOFF, P., FRIEDMAN, S. B., and HAMBURG, D. A. "Stress, Defenses and Coping Behavior: Observations in Parents of Children with Malignant Disease," *American Journal of Psychiatry,* 1964, *120,* 743–749.

CLARK, D. H. "The Therapeutic Community Concept, Practice and Future," *British Journal of Psychiatry,* 1965, *13,* 947–954.

COLLARD, E. J. "Public Health Nurse in Aftercare Program for the Mentally Ill: The Present Status," *American Journal of Public Health,* 1966, *56,* 210–217.

CUMMING, J., and CUMMING, E. *Ego and Milieu.* New York: Atherton Press, 1962.

DANIELS, D. N., and RUBIN, R. S. "The Community Meeting," *Archives of General Psychiatry,* 1968, *18,* 60–75.

DONNELLY, E. M., AUSTIN, F. C., KETTLE, R. H., STEWARD, J. R., and VERDE, C. W. "A Cooperative Program Between State Hospital and Public Health Nursing Agency for Psychiatric Aftercare," *American Journal of Public Health,* 1962, *52,* 1084–1094.

DUHL, L. *The Urban Condition.* New York: Basic Books, 1963, 3–10 and 59–73.

DUVAL, P. R. "The Problem of Smallness in a Rehabilitation Agency," *Journal of Rehabilitation,* 1968, *34,* 16–40.

EDELSON, M. "The Sociotherapeutic Function in a Psychiatric Hospital," *Journal of the Fort Logan Mental Health Center,* 1967, *4,* 1–45.

EISENBERG, L. "An Evaluation of Psychiatric Consultation Service for a Public Agency," *American Journal of Public Health*, 1958, *48*, 742–749.

ERICKSON, M. *Consultation Practice in Community Mental Health Services*. Unpublished D.S.W. dissertation, University of Southern California, 1966.

ERIKSON, E. H. *Childhood and Society*. New York: Norton, 1950.

ERIKSON, E. "Identity and the Life Cycle," *Psychological Issues*, 1959, *1*.

ETHRIDGE, D. A. "Pre-Vocational Assessment of Rehabilitation Potential of Psychiatric Patients," *American Journal of Occupational Therapy*, 1968, *22*, 161–167.

FAIRWEATHER, G. W. *Social Psychology in Treating Mental Illness*. New York: Wiley, 1964.

FAIRWEATHER, G. W., SANDERS, D. H., MAYNARD, H., and CRESSLER, D. L. *Community Life for the Mentally Ill: An Alternative to Institutional Care*. Chicago, Ill.: Aldine, 1969.

FAIRWEATHER, G. W., SIMON, R., GEBHARD, M. E., WEINGARTEN, E., HOLLAND, J. L., and SANDERS, R. "Relative Effectiveness of Psychotherapeutic Programs: A Multi-Criteria Comparison of Four Programs for Three Different Patient Groups," *Psychological Monograph*, 1960, *74*, No. 492.

FELIX, R. H. "The Image of the Psychiatrist: Past, Present and Future," Address to American Psychiatric Association, Los Angeles, May 6, 1964.

FINK, L., ASBURY, D. M., and DOWNING, J. J. *The San Mateo County Pre-Admission Home Visiting Program*. Unpublished preliminary study (mimeographed), 1963.

FISH, B. "Drug Therapy in Child Psychiatry: Psychological Aspects," *Comprehensive Psychiatry*, 1960, *1*, 212–227.

FISH, B. "Drug Use in Psychiatric Disorders of Children," *American Journal of Psychiatry*, 1968 (February Supplement), *124*, 31–36.

FLEISHMAN, M. "Will the Real Third Revolution Please Stand UP?," *American Journal of Psychiatry*, 1968, *124*, 1260–1262.

FREEMAN, H. E., and SIMMONS, O. G. *The Mental Patient Comes Home*. New York: Wiley, 1963.

FREUD, A. *Introduction to Psychoanalysis for Teachers*. London: Allen and Unwin, 1931.

FREUD, S. "Analysis of a Phobia in a Five Year Old Boy." In *The Complete Psychological Works of Sigmund Freud*, 1909, Vol. 10. London: The Hogarth Press, 1955, 3–149.

FRIEDMAN, T. T., BECKER, A., and WEINER, L. "The Psychiatric Home Treatment Service: Preliminary Report of Five Years of Clinical Experience," *American Journal of Psychiatry*, 1964, *120*, 782–788.

FRIEDMAN, T. T., and WEINER, L. "Psychiatric Home Treatment Services,

Public Health Aspects." In *Current Psychiatric Therapies, Vol. 5.* New York: Grune and Stratton, 1965.

GARCIA, L. "The Clarinda Plan: An Ecological Approach to Hospital Organization," *Mental Hospitals,* 1960, *11,* 30–31.

GASKILL, H. S., and NORTON, J. E. "Observations on Psychiatric Residency Training," *Archives of General Psychiatry,* 1968, *18,* 7–15.

GILBERT, R. "Functions of the Consultant," *Teachers College Record,* 1960, *61.*

GLADIS M., and HALE, P. "Schizophrenia, Motility and Counseling," *Personnel and Guidance Journal,* 1965, *41,* 808–810.

GLASSCOTE, R., SANDERS, D., FORSTENZER, H. M., and FOLEY, A. R. *The Community Mental Health Center: An Analysis of Existing Models.* Washington, D.C.: Joint Information Service of the American Psychiatric Association and the National Association for Mental Health, 1964.

GOERTZEL, V. "Evaluation of Halfway House Programs," *Quarterly of Camarillo,* 1965, *1,* No. 3.

GOLDFARB, A. "Application of Scientific Procedures in an Essentially Service Oriented Setting." Paper presented at a conference on Research in Community Mental Health, Asbury Park, New Jersey, September 22, 1965.

GOLDFARB, A. "Current Mental Health Program Evaluation in San Mateo County," *Community Mental Health Journal,* 1967, *3,* 284–289.

GOLDFARB, A., MOSES, L. E., and DOWNING, J. J. "Reliability of Psychiatrists' Ratings in Community Case Finding," *American Journal of Public Health,* 1967, *57,* 94–106.

GOLDFARB, A., MOSES, L. E., and DOWNING, J. J. "Reliability of Newly Trained Raters in Community Case Finding," *American Journal of Public Health,* 1967, *57,* 2149–2157.

GOLDSTON, S. E. "Concepts of Community Psychiatry: A Framework for Training," *Public Health Service Publication,* 1965, No. 1319.

GOODMAN, G. "Companionship as Therapy: The Use of Non-Professional Talent." In Hart, J. T., and Tomlenson, T. M. (Eds.), *New Directions in Client Centered Psychotherapy.* New York: Houghton Mifflin, 1969.

GREENBLATT, M., MOORE, R. F., ALBERT, R. S., and SOLOMON, M. H. *The Prevention of Hospitalization.* New York: Grune and Stratton, 1963.

GROUP FOR THE ADVANCEMENT OF PSYCHIATRY. *Mental Retardation, A Family Crisis—The Therapeutic Role of the Physician.* G.A.P. Report No. 56. New York: Group for the Advancement of Psychiatry, 1963.

GROUP FOR THE ADVANCEMENT OF PSYCHIATRY. *Education for Community Psychiatry Committee on Medical Education.* G.A.P. Report

No. 64. New York: Group for the Advancement of Psychiatry, 1967.

GROUP FOR THE ADVANCEMENT OF PSYCHIATRY. *Mild Mental Retardation, A Growing Challenge to the Physician.* G.A.P. Report No. 66. New York: Group for the Advancement of Psychiatry, 1967.

GROUP FOR THE ADVANCEMENT OF PSYCHIATRY. *The Dimensions of Community Psychiatry.* G.A.P. Report No. 69. New York: Group for the Advancement of Psychiatry, 1967.

GRUENBERG, E. M. "The Social Breakdown Syndrome—Some Origins," *American Journal of Psychiatry,* 1967, *123,* 1481–1489.

GULICK, L. "Notes on the Theory of Organization." In Gulick, L., and Urwick, L. (Eds.), *Papers on the Science of Management.* New York: Institute of Public Administration, 1937.

GUMRUKCU, P. Personal Communication, 1966.

GURIN, G., VEROFF, J., and FELD, S. *Americans View Their Mental Health.* Joint Commission on Mental Illness and Health Monograph No. 4. New York: Basic Books, 1960.

HALLECK, S. L., and MILLER, M. H. "The Psychiatric Consultation: Questionable Social Precedents of Some Current Practices." *American Journal of Psychiatry,* 1963, *120,* 164–169.

HALLECK, S. L. "Psychiatry and the Status Quo," *Archives of General Psychiatry,* 1968, *19,* 257–265.

HALLOCK, A., and VAUGHAN, W. T. "Community Organization—A Dynamic Component of Community Mental Health Practice," *American Journal of Orthopsychiatry,* 1956, *26,* 691–708.

HAMMERSLEY, D. W. (Ed.) *Training the Psychiatrist to Meet Changing Needs: Report on the 1962 Conference on Graduate Psychiatric Education.* Washington, D.C.: American Psychiatric Association, 1964.

HAYLETT, C. H., and RAPOPORT, L. "Mental Health Consultation." In Bellak, L. (Ed.), *Handbook of Community Psychiatry and Community Mental Health.* New York: Grune and Stratton, 1964, 319–339.

HEATH, D. *San Mateo Plans for Health Action.* Unpublished report, Redwood City, Calif., 1965.

HEDIGER, M. "Vocational Counseling of the Emotionally Disturbed: An Assessment," *Illinois Journal of Mental Health Rehabilitation Counseling,* 1967, *2,* 1–8.

HENRY, J. "The Formal Structure of a Psychiatric Hospital," *Psychiatry,* 1954, *17,* 139–151.

HEYMANN, G. M., and DOWNING, J. J. "Some Initial Approaches to Continuous Evaluation of a County Mental Health Program—An Interim Report," *American Journal of Public Health,* 1961, *51,* 980–989.

HODGSON, R. C., LEVINSON, D. J., and ZALEZNIK, A. "The Executive Role Constellation: An Analysis of Personality and Role-Relations in Management," Cambridge, Mass.: Division of Research, Harvard Business School, 1965.

HOFLING, C. K., and LEININGER, M. M. *Basic Psychiatric Concepts in Nursing.* Philadelphia, Pa.: Lippincott, 1960, 481–482.

HOGARTY, G. E., DENNIS, H., GUY, W., and GROSS, G. M. "Who Goes There? A Critical Evaluation of Admissions to a Psychiatric Day Hospital," *American Journal of Psychiatry,* 1968, *124,* 934–944.

HOLLINGSHEAD, A., and REDLICH, F. *Social Class and Mental Illness.* New York: Wiley, 1958.

HOWE, L. P. "The Concept of the Community—Some Implications for the Development of Community Psychiatry." In Bellak, L. (Ed.), *Handbook of Community Psychiatry and Community Mental Health.* New York: Grune and Stratton, 1964, 16–46.

HUME, P. B. *The Short-Doyle Act for Community Mental Health Services: An Informational Brochure for the Development of Local Mental Health Programs.* Sacramento: State of California Department of Mental Hygiene, 1957.

HUME, P. B. "Principles and Practice of Community Psychiatry: The Role and Training of the Specialist in Community Psychiatry." In Bellak, L. (Ed.), *Handbook of Community Psychiatry and Community Mental Health.* New York: Grune and Stratton, 1964, 66–81.

HUME, P. B. "General Principles of Community Psychiatry." In Aricti, S. (Ed.), *American Handbook of Psychiatry.* New York: Basic Books, 1966, *3,* 515–541.

HUSETH, B. "What is a Halfway House? Function and Types," *Mental Hygiene,* 1961, *45,* 65–76.

HUSETH, B. "Halfway Houses: A New Rehabilitation Measure," *Mental Hospitals,* 1968, *9,* 5–9.

JACKSON, G. W. "The Kansas Plan." In *Decentralization of Psychiatric Services and Continuity of Care.* New York: Milbank Memorial Fund, 1962, 16–21.

JACOBSON, G. F., WILNER, D. M., MORLEY, W. E., SCHNEIDER, S., STRICKLER, M., and SOMMER, G. J. "The Scope and Practice of an Early-Access Brief Treatment Psychiatric Center," *American Journal of Psychiatry,* 1965, *121,* 1176–1182.

JOINT COMMISSION ON MENTAL ILLNESS AND HEALTH. *Action for Mental Health.* Final Report, 1961. New York: Basic Books, 1961.

JONES, M. *The Therapeutic Community.* New York: Basic Books, 1953.

JONES, M. "Report on Social Psychiatry." In Wilmer, H. A. (Ed.), *Research Report.* Bethesda, Md.: Naval Medical Research Institute, 1958, *16,*

JONES, M. *Social Psychiatry.* Springfield, Ill.: Thomas, 1962.

JONES, M. "The Current Place of Therapeutic Communities in Psychiatric Practice." In Freeman, H., and Farndale, J. (Eds.), *New Aspects of the Mental Health Services.* Oxford, England: Pergamon Press, 1967, 465–480.

KAZANJIAN, V., STEIN, S., and WEINBERG, W. "An Introduction to Mental Health Consultation," *U.S. Public Health Monograph,* 1962, *69.*

KIESLER, F. "Whose is the Clinical Task?" In *Proceedings of AMA Second National Congress on Mental Illness and Health.* Chicago, Ill.: 1964.

KIESLER, F. "Is This Psychiatry?" In Goldston, S. E. (Ed.), *Concepts of Community Psychiatry, A Framework for Training.* Washington, D.C.: U. S. Public Health Service Publication, 1965, *1319.*

KLEIN, D. C., and LINDEMANN, E. "Preventive Intervention in Individual and Family Crisis Situations." In Caplan, G. (Ed.), *Prevention of Mental Disorders in Children.* New York: Basic Books, 1961.

KRAFT, A. M. "The Fort Logan Mental Health Center," *Community Mental Health Journal,* 1965, *1,* 99–102.

KRAFT, A. M. "The Therapeutic Community." In Arieti, S. (Ed.), *American Handbook of Psychiatry.* New York: Basic Books, 1966, *3,* 542–551.

KRAFT, A. M., BINNER, P. R., and DICKEY, B. A. "The Community Mental Health Program and the Longer-Stay Patient," *Archives of General Psychiatry,* 1967, *16,* 64–70.

KRAFT, I. A. "The Use of Psychoactive Drugs in the Outpatient Treatment of Psychiatric Disorders of Children," *American Journal of Psychiatry,* 1968, *124,* 1401–1407.

KRAMER, B. M. *Day Hospital.* New York: Grune and Stratton, 1962, 35–36.

KUBIE, L. S. "Pitfalls of Community Psychiatry," *Archives of General Psychiatry,* 1968, *18,* 257–266.

LAMB, H. R. "Chronic Psychiatric Patients in the Day Hospital," *Archives of General Psychiatry,* 1967, *17,* 615–621.

LAMB, H. R. "Aftercare for Former Day Hospital Patients," *Hospital and Community Psychiatry,* 1967, *18,* 44–46.

LAMB, H. R. "Release of Chronic Psychiatric Patients into the Community," *Archives of General Psychiatry,* 1968, *19,* 38–44.

LANDY, D., and GREENBLATT, M. *Halfway House: A Sociocultural and Clinical Study of Rutland Corner House, A Transitional Aftercare Residence for Female Psychiatric Patients.* Washington, D.C.: United States Department of Health, Education, and Welfare, Vocational Rehabilitation Administration, 1965.

LEIGHTON, A. H. *My Name is Legion.* New York: Basic Books, 1959.

LEMKAU, P. N. *Mental Hygiene in Public Health.* Second edition. New York: McGraw-Hill, 1955.

LERNER, M. L., and FAIRWEATHER, G. W. "The Social Behavior of Chronic Schizophrenics in Supervised and Unsupervised Work Groups," *Journal of Abnormal and Social Psychology,* 1963, *67,* 219–225.

LEVINSON, D. J., and KLERMAN, G. L. "The Clinician-Executive: Some Problematic Issues for the Psychiatrist in Mental Health Organizations," *Psychiatry,* 1967, *30,* 3–15.

LEVY, L. "The State Mental Hospital in Transition: A Review of Principles," *Community Mental Health Journal,* 1965, *1,* 353–356.

LIEF, A. *The Commonsense Psychiatry of Dr. Adolph Meyer.* New York: McGraw-Hill, 1948.

LINDEMANN, E. 'Symptomatology and Management of Acute Grief," *American Journal of Psychiatry,* 1944, *101,* 141–148.

LINDEMANN, E. "Health Needs of Communities." In Knowles, J. (Ed.), *Hospitals, Doctors, and the Public Interest.* Cambridge: Harvard University Press, 1966, 271–292.

LINDEMANN, E. "An Introduction to the Indirect Service Aspects of Community Psychiatry," unpublished lecture delivered to trainees in a San Mateo County course, 1968.

LINDNER, M. P., and LANDY, D. "Post-Discharge Experience and Vocational Rehabilitation Needs of Psychiatric Patients," *Mental Hygiene,* 1958, *42,* 29–44.

LUTOVICH, G. *Home Screening and Treatment of the Hospital Bound Patient with Two-Year Follow-up.* Unpublished paper (mimeographed), 1967.

MARMOR, J. "Psychoanalytic Therapy as an Educational Process." In Masserman, J. (Ed.), *Science and Psychoanalysis.* New York: Grune and Stratton, 1962, 286–299.

MATTE, M. W. "Collaboration Between Doctors and Nurses in a Psychiatric Hospital," *Psychiatric Opinion,* 1967, *4,* 33–36.

MCDONOUGH, L. B., and DOWNING, J. J. "The Day Center as an Alternative to the Psychiatric Ward," *Mental Hygiene,* 1965, *49,* 260–264.

MCINNES, R. S., PALMER, J. T., and DOWNING, J. J. "An Analysis of the Service Relationships Between State Mental Hospitals and One Local Mental Health Program," *American Journal of Public Health,* 1964, *54,* 60–68.

MENOLASCINO, F. J. "Emotional Disturbances in Mentally Retarded Children," *Archives of General Psychiatry,* 1968, *19,* 456–464.

MELTZOFF, J., and BLUMENTHAL, R. L. *The Day Treatment Center.* Springfield, Ill.: Thomas, 1966.

MEYER, R. E., SCHIFF, L. F., and BECKER, A. "The Home Treatment of Psychotic Patients: An Analysis of 154 Cases," *American Journal of Psychiatry*, 1967, *123*, 1430–1438.

MILBANK MEMORIAL FUND, *Elements of a Community Mental Health Program*. New York: Milbank Memorial Fund, 1956.

MILBANK MEMORIAL FUND, *Programs for Community Mental Health*. New York: Milbank Memorial Fund, 1957.

MLODNOSKY, L. B. *Summary of Research on Program Planning and Program Evaluation in the Children's Section, Mental Health Services Division of San Mateo County*. Unpublished study (mimeographed), 1964.

MLODNOSKY, L. B. *Outcome of Diagnostic Evaluations in the Children's Section*. Unpublished study (mimeographed), 1964.

MOUW, M. L., and HAYLETT, C. H. "Mental Health Consultation in a Public Health Nursing Service," *American Journal of Nursing*, 1967, *67*, 1447–1450.

NAKAJIMA, J., and ISHII, T. "A Night Hospital in Tokyo," *Hospital and Community Psychiatry*, 1967, *18*, 20–21.

NATIONAL INSTITUTE OF MENTAL HEALTH, *Consultation and Education—A Service of the Community Mental Health Center*. Public Health Service Publication No. 1478.

NEW HAVEN VISITING NURSE ASSOCIATION, "The Role of Public Health Nursing in the Aftercare of the Psychiatric Patient." A report on the participation of the Visiting Nurse Association of New Haven in the Cooperative Care Project, New Haven, Conn., 1960–1965. New Haven: The Association, 1966.

NEWMAN, M. B. "The Challenge of Community Child Psychiatry," *Community Mental Health Journal*, 1966, *2*, 281–284.

NEWTON, H. J. "The Therapeutic Community in a General Hospital," *California Medicine*, 1963, *98*, 243–248.

ODENHEIMER, J. F. "The Day Hospital as an Alternative to the Psychiatric Ward," *Archives of General Psychiatry*, 1965, *13*, 46–53.

OLSHANSKY, S., and UNTERBERGER, N. "The Meaning of Work and Its Implications for the Ex-Mental Hospital Patient," *Mental Hygiene*, 1963, *47*, 139–149.

PARKER, B. *Psychiatric Consultation for Non-Psychiatric Professional Workers*. Washington, D.C.: Public Health Monograph, 1958, *53*.

PARKER, P. *A Study of Indirect Mental Health Services in California*. Final Report of Project Supported by Public Health Service Research Grant No. M.H. 15034, released in May, 1969.

PASAMANICK, B., SCARPITTI, F. R., and DINITZ, S. *Schizophrenics in the Community*. New York: Appleton-Century-Crofts, 1967.

PAUL, L. "Treatment Techniques in a Walk-In Clinic," *Hospital and Community Psychiatry*, 1966, *17*, 49–51.

PEARL, A., and RIESSMAN, F. *New Careers for the Poor.* New York: The Free Press, 1965.

PEPLAU, H. "The Work of Psychiatric Nurses," *Psychiatric Opinion,* 1967, *4,* 5–11.

PRENTICE, N. M., and SPERRY, B. M. "Therapeutically Oriented Tutoring of Children with Primary Learning Inhibitions," *American Journal of Orthopsychiatry,* 1965, *35,* 521–530.

QUERIDO, A. "Experiment in Public Health," *Bulletin World Federal Mental Health,* 1954, *6,* 203–216.

RAPAPORT, W., and DOWNING, J. J. "State-Local Cooperation for Public Psychiatric Services in San Mateo County, California." In *Decentralization of Psychiatric Services and Continuity of Care.* New York: Milbank Memorial Fund, 1962, 94–107.

RAPOPORT, R. N. *Community as Doctor, New Perspectives on a Therapeutic Community.* Springfield, Ill.: Thomas, 1960.

REIK, L. E. "The Halfway House: The Role of Laymen's Organizations in the Rehabilitation of the Mentally Ill," *Mental Hygiene,* 1953, *37,* 615–618.

RIESSMAN, F. *Mental Health of the Poor: New Treatment Approaches for Low Income People.* New York: The Free Press, 1964.

ROBINS, L. N. *Deviant Children Grown Up.* Baltimore: Williams and Wilkins, 1966.

ROGERS, N. R., and DOWNING, J. J. "Regional Integration of Psychiatric Services," *Mental Hospitals,* 1964, *15,* 185–190.

ROSENBAUM, M., and ZWERLING, I. "Impact of Social Psychiatry," *Archives of General Psychiatry,* 1962, *11,* 31–39.

ROTHWELL, N. D., and DONIGER, J. M. *The Psychiatric Halfway House: A Case Study.* Springfield, Ill.: Thomas, 1966.

SANDERS, R., SMITH, R. S., and WEINMAN, B. S. *Chronic Psychoses and Recovery.* San Francisco: Jossey-Bass, 1967, 25–29 and 42–44.

SCHWARTZ, M. S. "What is a Therapeutic Milieu?" In Greenblatt, M., Levinson, D. J., and Williams, R. H. (Eds.), *The Patient and the Mental Hospital.* Chicago: Free Press of Glencoe, 1957, 130–144.

SHAW, C. R. *The Psychiatric Disorders of Childhood.* New York: Appleton-Century-Crofts, 1966.

SNOW, H. B., and BENNETT, C. L. "The Dutchess County Project After Five Years." In "Evaluating the Effectiveness of Mental Health Services," *Milbank Memorial Fund Quarterly,* 1966 (January, Part 2), *44,* 57–89.

SROLE, L., LANGNER, T. S., MICHAEL, S. T., OPLER, M. K., and RENNIE, T. A. C. *Mental Health in the Metropolis: The Midtown Manhattan Study.* New York: McGraw-Hill, 1962.

STANGER, F. M. *South from San Francisco: San Mateo County, Califor-*

*nia, Its History and Heritage.* Redwood City, Calif.: San Mateo County Historical Association, 1963.

STEIN, L. I. "The Doctor-Nurse Game," *Archives of General Psychiatry,* 1967, *16,* 699–703.

STEWART, A., LAFAVE, H. G., GRUNBERG, F., and HERJANIC, M. "Problems in Phasing Out a Large Public Psychiatric Hospital," *American Journal of Psychiatry,* 1968, *125,* 82–88.

STICKNEY, S. B. "Schools Are Our Community Mental Health Centers," *American Journal of Psychiatry,* 1968, *124,* 1407–1414.

STRAUS, R. "Social Factors in General Hospital Patient Care," *American Journal of Psychiatry,* 1968, *124,* 1663–1668.

SUTHERLAND, J. D. "The Psychotherapeutic Clinic and Community Psychiatry," *Bulletin of the Menninger Clinic,* 1966, *30,* 338–350.

TEMPLETON, R., SPERRY, B. M., and PRENTICE, N. M. "Theoretical and Technical Issues in Therapeutic Tutoring of Children with Psychogenic Learning Problems," *Journal of Child Psychiatry,* 1967, *6,* 464–477.

URWICK, L., and METCALF, H. C. *Dynamic Administration: The Collected Papers of Mary Parker Follett.* New York: Harper, 1940.

URWICK, L. *The Elements of Administration.* New York and London: Harper, 1944.

U. S. PUBLIC HEALTH SERVICE. *Regulations: Community Mental Health Centers Act of 1963, Title II, Public Law 88–164.* Washington, D.C.: Federal Register Office, 1964.

U. S. PUBLIC HEALTH SERVICE. *NIMH Planning, Programming, and Design for the Community Mental Health Center.* Washington, D.C.: U. S. Public Health Service, 1965.

WALKER, R., and MCCOURT, J. "Employment Experience Among 200 Schizophrenic Patients in Hospital and After Discharge," *American Journal of Psychiatry,* 1965, *122,* 316–319.

WALLERSTEIN, R. S. "The Challenge of the Community Mental Health Movement to Psychoanalysis," *American Journal of Psychiatry,* 1968, *124,* 1049–1056.

WECHSLER, H. "Transitional Residences for Former Mental Patients: A Survey of Halfway Houses and Related Rehabilitation Facilities," *Mental Hygiene,* 1961, *45,* 65–76.

WILDER, J. F., LEVIN, G., and ZWERLING, I. "A Two-Year Follow-Up Evaluation of Acute Psychotic Patients Treated in a Day Hospital," *American Journal of Psychiatry,* 1966, *122,* 1095–1101.

WILDER, J. F., KESSELL, M., and CAULFIELD, S. C. "Follow-Up of a 'High Expectations' Halfway House," *American Journal of Psychiatry,* 1968, *124,* 103–109.

WILMER, H. A. *Social Psychiatry in Action.* Springfield, Ill.: Thomas, 1958.

WILMER, H. A. "Toward a Definition of the Therapeutic Community," *American Journal of Psychiatry,* 1958, *114,* 824–834.

WILMER, H. A. "Free Association of People: Observations on the Changing Constellations in Large Group Meetings," *International Journal of Social Psychiatry,* 1966, *12,* 44–51.

YOUNG, C. L. "A Therapeutic Community with an Open Door in a Psychiatric Receiving Service," *Archives of Psychiatry and Neurology,* 1959, *81,* 335–340.

ZALEZNIK, A. "The Structure and Dynamics of Leadership," *Hospital and Community Psychiatry,* 1967, *18,* 33–39.

ZOLIK, E. S., LANTZ, E. M., and SOMMERS, R. "Hospital Return Rates and Pre-Release Referrals," *Archives of General Psychiatry,* 1968, *18,* 712–717.

ZUBIN, J., and FREHAN, F. A. *Social Psychiatry.* New York and London: Grune and Stratton, 1968.

# Name Index

# Subject Index